Forensic Medicine

Forensic Medicine
Ninth Edition

Keith Simpson, CBE
MA (Oxon), LLD (Edin), MD (Lond), MD (Ghent), FRCP, FRC Path,
DMJ
Emeritus Professor of Forensic Medicine to the University of London at
Guy's Hospital; Home Office Pathologist

with Bernard Knight
MD (Wales), MRCP, FRC Path, DMJ
Barrister of Gray's Inn
Professor of Forensic Pathology, University of Wales
College of Medicine, Cardiff;
Home Office Pathologist

Edward Arnold

© Keith Simpson and Bernard Knight 1985

First published 1947
by Edward Arnold (Publishers) Ltd,
41 Bedford Square, London WC1B 3DQ

Edward Arnold (Australia) Pty Ltd,
80 Waverley Road, Caulfield East,
Victoria 3145, Australia

Edward Arnold, 3 East Read Street,
Baltimore, Maryland 21202, U.S.A.

Reprinted with amendments 1950
Reprinted 1951
Second edition 1951
Reprinted 1955
Third edition 1958 (awarded The Swiney Prize of the Royal Society of Arts)
Fourth edition 1961
Fifth edition 1964
Reprinted with amendments 1967
Sixth edition 1969
First published in the ELBS edition 1970
Reprinted with amendments 1972
Seventh edition 1974
Eighth edition 1979
Translated into Spanish 1983
Ninth edition 1985
Reprinted 1986

British Library Cataloguing in Publication Data
  Simpson, Keith, *1907–*
  Forensic medicine. —9th ed.
  1. Medical jurisprudence
  I. Title II. Knight, Bernard, *1931–*
  614'.1 RA1051

  ISBN 0-7131-4452-1

Set in 10/11 Times and printed in Great Britain by Butler & Tanner Ltd.,
Frome and London

Preface to the ninth edition

This small textbook has in its 35 years of life passed through eight editions—with very little increase in size—undergoing improvements in its text and photographic illustrations and keeping abreast of changes both in law and in practice. It is in use throughout the English-speaking world—and has been translated into Spanish for the Latin American people. It has managed to survive searching cross-examination in the law courts of many countries without failing in its duty to provide doctors and lawyers, scientists and police with a simple working handbook for the field.

The time has come for this work to undergo the refreshing effects of a co-author, and those who know of the remarkable contributions of Professor Bernard Knight, of Wales, will welcome the choice of this expert. His professional skill and expertise are matched by his great interest in the use of words ... one of the essential qualities of a good witness.

We have together revised the text to keep it up to date, and have replaced or added some 20 illustrations to improve the clarity of many sections. The text on law has been revised where necessary, as in mental health, and statistics have been brought up to date. New sections have been written on anaesthetic deaths, the General Medical Council, sudden infant death and the battered baby, new drink–driving regulations and on currently 'popular' drugs such as paracetamol and habits such as glue and other solvent-sniffing in teenagers. Technical details remain at a minimum.

We hope that this guide to the study and practise of forensic medicine and toxicology will continue to help in student teaching, aid the tyro in acquiring expertise and provide an understandable reference in the courts, as in the past. The senior author was told at a party by an attractive young doctor that her first question in cross-examination by a barrister, who held in his hand a book she recognised by its dustcover, was 'Doctor, are you familiar with "Keith Simpson"?' The judge remarked 'Perhaps the question might be rephrased.' We both hope that our joint authorship will continue to make this book a familiar friend on the shelf of the student and practitioner, lawyer and detective.

1985   BERNARD KNIGHT
                                                         KEITH SIMPSON

Preface to the first edition

The modern medical student's lot is not entirely a happy one, for he is surfeited with much teaching from specialists who naturally regard their own subject as deserving special attention. The case for forensic medicine is a small one by some standards, but it is an important one as well as fascinating, that deserves the close attention of that live and critical body, the medical student.

This short textbook is designed to provide a brief and essentially practical guide—from an English school—to current teaching in forensic medicine. No pains have been spared to give the subject its vivid colours in life, and the amount of technical data and of laboratory procedure (which is properly relegated to the expert in everyday practice) has been reduced to a minimum. The doctor in practice and the barrister at the criminal bar will, it is hoped, find it a reliable guide to their contacts in practice with the law and medicine respectively.

The illustrations are, with few exceptions which are acknowledged individually, from my own cases, and I am grateful to the Director of Public Prosecutions, the Commissioner of Police of the Metropolis, New Scotland Yard, and to the Chief Constables of various home county joint police forces for permission to use them.

Dr P.B. Skeels, solicitor, HM Coroner for Metropolitan Essex, read the legal sections during his tenure of the Presidency of the Coroners' Society of England and Wales, and I am much indebted to him for his painstaking review and many valuable criticisms. The section on toxicology received similar benefit from the experienced advice of Dr J.H. Ryffel, Analyst to the Home Office, and in matters of practical pharmacy I have profited by conversations with Eric Simpson, MPS, Chief Pharmacist to the St Helier Hospital. The many facets of forensic medicine not only justify this recourse to specialists: they also maintain the subject in an ever fresh state, conversant with advances in scientific and allied medical subjects related to the practice of the law.

My secretary during this period, Miss Molly Lefebure, was responsible for the arduous task of typing the entire manuscript. Her patience contributed greatly to the smooth production of the text.

London, 1946   KEITH SIMPSON

Contents

Introduction

Forensic medicine and toxicology

Forensic, or legal, medicine provides one of the most fascinating of all facets of the practice of medicine. The study of the body, often dead, the quiet scientific assembly of the evidence it bears, and the construction of reasonable inferences based on these observations cannot fail to give interest and satisfaction. All branches of medicine, anatomy, pathology, therapeutics, obstetrics, provide the basic knowledge application of which, shaped to conform with the needs of the law, form the body of the subject. Truth—or the nearest reasonable approach to it that is possible from what is observed—is the sole aim. Vagueness and theory have no place in forensic medicine, and the doctor who properly says he does not know, or feels inadequately qualified to advise, acquires more respect than one who 'ventures an opinion'.

The subject has developed from the enlistment of medical and scientific knowledge in relation to the law. It falls very naturally into two sections:

1. *Forensic medicine*, which deals with the broad field where medical matters come into relation with the law—statements on the live and the dead, the study of sudden or violent or unexplained deaths, scientific criminal investigation, matters involving the coroner, court procedure, medical ethics, and civil and criminal procedure.

2. *Toxicology*, which concerns poisons, the law controlling their sale and their effects on the body. The domestic and therapeutic aspects of this part of the subject are becoming increasingly important and the more sensational criminal features less so. Accidental poisoning alone brings 120 000 cases to hospital in England and Wales each year for diagnosis and treatment.

As it is around a body, often a dead body, that the more common exercises in forensic medicine and toxicology develop, it will not be unreasonable to set out the subject with this as the centrepiece. The scene need not be screened by forms and certificates, or overcast by the heavy atmosphere of court procedure—lightened as it may be by discussion of fees. The primary interests of forensic medicine are to give a sound service to the law, and this should have pride of place in a book that is intended to help the practising doctor, and improve the performance of those taking their first steps in this special branch of medicine.

1

Signs of death

What to do with a dead body

When a doctor is called to a person who is thought to be dead he has three principal duties:

1. To make sure that death has, in fact, taken place.
2. To be on the alert for any medical grounds for suspicion.
3. To issue a certificate, if in a position to do so (see p. 4), or to refer the case to the coroner (or procurator fiscal in Scotland) for inquiry (see p. 216).

Has death taken place?

No doubt will exist as to this in the large majority of cases, for death will usually have taken place some time previously; indeed, the body may be already undergoing plainly visible *post mortem* changes. But suspended animation due to shock, as from electrocution or immersion, may give rise to difficulty, and the doctor may not feel happy about leaving the body for disposal. He should not waste time searching for a suitable feather to hold over the nostril or a mirror to look for condensation: no string tied round the finger or feeling with throbbing hands for a thin or non-existent pulse will provide such solid evidence as auscultation for sounds of the heart. This must be continued patiently for some 4 or 5 minutes, if there is any doubt, for only after such a period of time without a heart beat will it be certain that the circulatory and respiratory centres are no longer capable of revival. There must be no doubt about the matter.

A 78-year-old widow was certified dead by a doctor called to examine her as she lay in bed at home. An empty box of sleeping pills and several letters indicating a suicidal intent were by her bed. Undertakers took her in a coffin (with a loose lid) to the mortuary and the coroner was informed. Nearly 6 hours after, just as an autopsy was about to begin, a police officer saw that she was still breathing. She was rushed to hospital, but died next day.

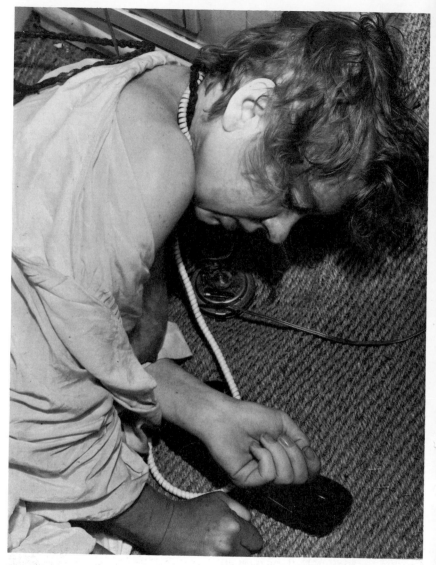

Fig. 1.1 Death requiring careful assessment. Dead girl lying beside bed on floor, with neck entangled in telephone cables; electric lead also nearby and telephone under the left hand. It could be murder by strangling but the cords were loose. Autopsy excluded violence, and analysis revealed high alcohol and barbiturate levels, sufficient to account for confusion, collapse and death.

If there is difficulty because of noise, say, in the street, the doctor is entitled to call an ambulance to have the person removed to a hospital for observation. Attempts at resuscitation should be continued until no possible hope of revival exists: this has proved to be of special value in cases of immersion in water, and in electrocution.

The doctor will often be asked how long ago death occurred. The answer to this is based on the development of *post mortem* changes, and the subject is discussed under that heading in the next chapter. The fall in body temperature should be measured per rectum at the scene, and may be plotted by further readings when the time of death seems likely to have any importance—as in suspected crime. The thermometer must read to 0°C.

Is there any cause for suspicion?

Suspicion may be aroused for a number of reasons. The body may lie in a situation that requires explanation (Fig. 1.1), it may bear injury (Fig. 1.2) or poison may lie nearby (Fig. 1.3). In such cases the doctor should not hesitate when in any doubt to refer the circumstances to the coroner—through his officer or the police, rather than the registrar, so as to avoid delay. It is preferable that no certificate of any kind be issued meanwhile. The doctor is the watchdog of the public, and must keep an ever-open eye for the kinds of deaths that require investigation. Common sense should be the guide to safety in such matters. Where injury is present no possible harm can come of an investigation into its nature and the establishment of its correct relationship with death; its real extent and nature may only become apparent upon autopsy.

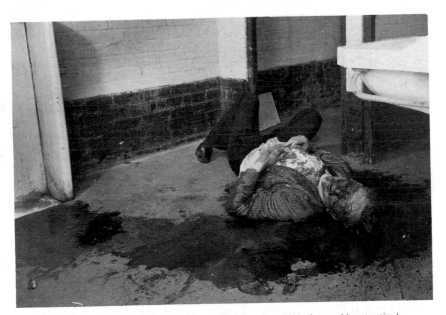

Fig. 1.2 Man found dead in public toilet with blunt head injuries and 'protective' bruising of the hands. The multiplicity of the head wounds excluded the possibility that they were due simply to collapse, and much blood-splashing round the head showed that battering had continued after he had been felled. Photography at the scene before moving the body was important.

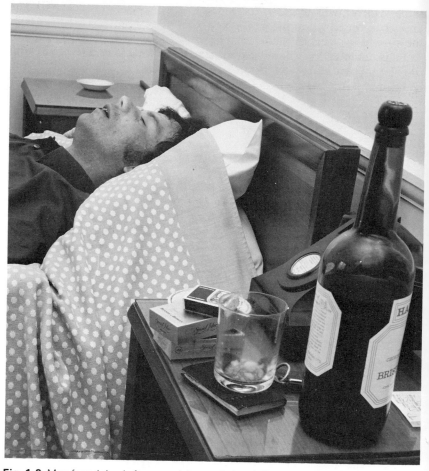

Fig. 1.3 Man found dead after overnight stay in hotel. The part-emptied sherry bottle and remains of tablets in the glass give strong grounds for a supposition of overdosage (and alcohol) at any age, but especially in such a young man.

Where suspicion of foul play is strong it is most important that nothing shall be moved before its exact position has been recorded—by photograph if possible. Should it be necessary to move a body before this—as when still alive—a chalk line may be traced around it as it lies. When any poison—or remains of it—in a cup or bottle is found, the doctor should see that some responsible person—not relatives or friends—take charge of it. It is all too often thrown away. Urine and vomit should also be kept for the time being.

Shall the doctor issue a certificate?

The subject of certification of death is dealt with in Chapter 14; suffice to say here that where a doctor:

1. is duly qualified and registered as a medical practitioner,
2. has been in professional attendance during the deceased's last illness—within a period of 14 days, and
3. is satisfied that the cause of death is a natural one (and knows what it is),

he need have no qualms about the issue of a certificate without further delay.

2

Changes after death. The time of death

Coincident with death, both breathing and circulation cease. Voluntary movement ceases also, but for some time, often several hours, voluntary muscle may flicker when pinched, and spasms of both kinds of muscle may occur.

The skin may redden as lividity develops, and later the generation of gases from decomposition may evacuate faeces, urine, vomit—even the contents of a pregnant uterus. All of these changes may simulate life in a dead body. The principal changes taking place after death are cadaveric spasm, cooling, lividity, rigor mortis, decomposition and mummification.

Cadaveric spasm

This is an uncommon event consisting of a violent spasm of the muscles at the moment of death. The change most frequently involves the hand, which may thus remain gripping a weapon, clothing or grass (Fig. 2.1), etc., affording evidence assisting in the reconstruction of events immediately preceding deaths from violence. Occasionally, in circumstances of extreme nervous tension, the whole body may go rigid at death.

Cooling

This is the only real guide to the lapse of time during the first 18 hours after death, and its *early* measurement is often vital to the establishment of an approximate time of death. Under average conditions the clothed body will cool in air at the rate of about 1.5 degree Celsius an hour for the first 6 hours and average a loss of some 1.0 degree Celsius for the first 12. The body will lose heat more slowly as the temperature comes nearer to that of its surroundings. It should feel cold in about 12 hours and the temperature of the internal organs should be the same as the environment in 18–24 hours. Any thermometer reading to zero will suffice, the most accurate readings coming from the rectum. The vagina should be avoided.

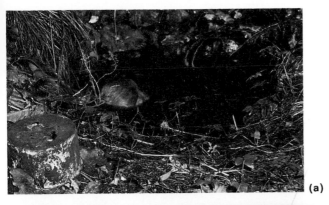

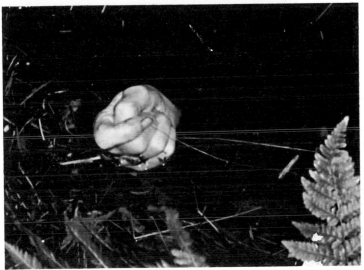

Fig. 2.1 (a) Elderly woman found dead in a well in her own garden. The house had not been ransacked and she bore no injuries. (b) The hand had grasped weeds as she (it was thought) tripped or fell in: such hand gripping (cadaveric spasm) occurs only if life is still present.

Factors which slow the rate of cooling are a warm atmosphere, clothing and bedding, obesity and lack of ventilation.

The temperatures of a coal-gas suicide-pact couple, one of whom wore *nine layers of clothing*, differed by 3 degrees when circumstances showed both deaths must have occurred within minutes of each other some 6 hours previously. Solicitors wished to know who died first.

Cerebral haemorrhage, asphyxia from constriction of the neck, or the arrival of maggots may all raise the temperature of a body. I have seen an initial temperature at death of 42.8°C (109°F) in a case of pontine haemorrhage, a temperature of 37.4°C (99.4°F) some 3 hours after death

Table 2.1 Approximate lapse of time since death by body changes: equitable climates

Period*	Land	Water
Hours	*Cooling*	
0–12	1°C (approx.) per hour.	1.5°C (average) per hour.
12–24	0.5°C (approx.) per hour.	0.75°C (average) per hour.
10–12	Body *feels* cold.	At 5–6 hours, body *feels* cold.
20–24	Body *is* cold.	At 8–10 hours, body *is* cold.
Hours	*Lividity*	
3–5	*Post mortem* lividity developing.	Cutis anserina and whitening of skin. No lividity until at rest.
Hours	*Chemical changes*	
12–72	Vitreous humour K rises steadily.	Slight retardation only.
Hours	*Rigor mortis*	
5–7	Rigor appearing in face, jaw and neck muscles.	Onset delayed by cold and often lasting longer.
7–9	Spread to arms and trunk, and reaching legs.	
12–18	Rigor fully established.	
24–36	Rigor passing away in same order.	Rigor may still be present. Skin markedly wrinkled in hands and feet, sodden. Rigor passing off 2–4 days.
Days	*Putrefaction*	
2	Green staining in flanks.	
2–3	Green and purple staining over abdomen and some distension.	
3–4	Marbling of veins. Further spread of stains into neck and limbs.	Discoloration at root of neck.
5–6	Gaseous swelling and distuption internally. Skin blebs.	Neck and face discoloured and swollen. Body floats 5–8 days (period halved in hot weather).
Weeks		
2	Abdomen distended to tight tension. Swelling of body marked, and blebbing with purple transudate widespread. All organs disrupted by gas.	Decomposition well established in trunk, but little distension. Cutis peeling and hair loosening, easily pulled out. Nails pulled out with difficulty. Face bloated. Eyes and tongue protruding.
3	Vesicles bursting, and tissues sofening and disrupting. Eyes bulging. Organs and cavities bursting. Disfiguration to extreme.	
4	General slimy liquefaction and disruption of all soft tissues.	Body greatly swollen with gases and organs crepitant. Hair easily wiped away. Nails (fingers easily, toes less easily) pulled away. Casts of hands and feet separating.

Months	*Adipocere* (if conditions suitable)	
4–5	Adipocere of face, head and breasts.	Slightly slower adipocere development in proportion to lower temperature.
	Adipocere of arms, legs and internally.	

Note. In hot climates these processes are accelerated. Bodies may warm up in the tropics or in a hot bath. Putrefaction may be well established in air at 24 hours. Bodies in water may float in from 2 or 3 days. In cold months, the processes are decelerated. Putrefaction may not start, and the body may not float, until the temperature rises sufficiently to permit the growth of gas-forming organisms.

in a case of manual strangling, and measured a reading of 25.6°C (78°F) 6 weeks after death in maggot-infested tissues.

Cooling when naked is half again as fast as when clothed, and in water it is twice as fast. These figures are, of course, working approximations. Note the clothing, physique, ventilation and room temperature when making a rectal reading of temperature at the scene, and some allowance can then be made for these corrective factors: it can never be pretended that such estimations point to the exact hour of death, only to a 'peak of probability' (Table 2.1).

Lividity

This change, which consists of a deep staining of the skin and organs of dependent parts of the body, results from the passive distension by blood of the inert vessels of underlying parts. It commences to develop within an hour or so of death, becoming marked in 5 or 6 hours, remaining unless the body is turned to a new position, and eventually becoming dispersed by the evolution of gases of decomposition which dissipate the blood from the vessels. Livid stains cannot develop where pressure of clothing or the weight of the body lying on parts such as the shoulder-blades, spine or buttocks prevent the vessels from filling.

Such stains may afford striking evidence of the position of the body at and after death, as, for instance, in children found dead face down in their cots or in epileptic subjects suffocating on their faces. Relatives who find the body cannot always remember exactly how it lay, and livid stains may provide the evidence required.

Changes of position after death may cause the livid stains to fade from one surface of the body, only to reappear, so long as the blood is fluid, in another, becoming dispersed eventually by decomposition.

One other feature of lividity has special interest. Its hue is similar to that of the blood—which may have been cyanosed, pink (as in CO poisoning) or brown (as in methaemoglobinaemia).

Little difficulty will be experienced in distinguishing these stains from bruises if they are incised, for blood drains freely from the vessels of a livid stain leaving the tissues unstained, whereas in a bruise the blood lies firmly entangled in the tissue spaces. Examination of the cuticle may

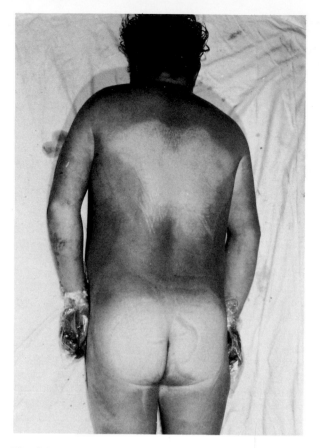

Fig. 2.2 Normal livid stains over the back of a body lying face up after death.

also show some injury—if only a faint graze—over a bruise. Microscopy will dispel any uncertainty.

It must be remembered that hypostatic stains may develop internally, notably in the lungs and the dependent loops of intestine.

> Suspicion that a man who had died suddenly had been poisoned by his wife with arsenic was aroused owing to failure to recognise livid reddening of the intestines as due to simple hypostasis. Suspicion of foul play was raised in another case owing to misinterpreting livid stains in the face of a drowned man as bruising.

Rigor mortis

The best-known though the most uncertain and unreliable of *post mortem* events, this change results from a stiffening of the fibres of all muscles, voluntary and involuntary. It is closely related to the breakdown of ATP after death, for as this proceeds the quantity of adenosine phosphate increases, and both lactates and phosphates accumulate in increasing amounts from its breakdown. Some physical change develops in the muscle as these salts accumulate. The fibres shorten and stiffen, and all groups of muscles become prominent and rigid, fixing the limbs. The quantity of lactates in muscle fixed by rigor is about ten times that in resting muscle in life. Perfusion with saline, or abundant oxygenation together with icing to retard the rate of autolysis, will prevent its development.

Rigor can be detected most easily in the face at some 5-7 hours, during the next 2-3 hours in the shoulders and arms, and finally in the bulky leg muscles. It becomes fully established in about 12 hours, lasts some 12 hours, and takes some 12 hours further to pass off, appearing to leave the body in the same order as it came. Rigor mortis may thus help to establish the time of death over a period of some 36 hours following death. Temperature measurements provide more reliable evidence in the first 18-24 hours of this period (Fig. 2.3).

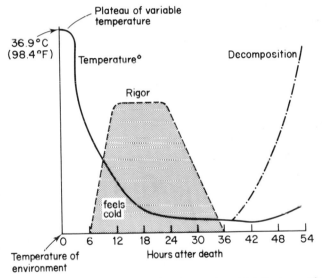

Fig. 2.3 Chart showing the major changes by which the lapse of time after death might be estimated. The first hour often shows little fall in temperature.

It is unfortunate that rigor is uncertain in its timing. It may come early when metabolism is pronounced at death, as in fever and exercise, or in summer, or it may fail to develop properly at any stage. Breaking down the stiffness by stretching a muscle disperses the rigidity for good. It develops earlier in babies and disappears more quickly also. No close estimate of the time of death can, under these circumstances, follow from observation of rigor mortis alone.

A commonly observed skin change—'goosefleshing' (cutis anscrina)—due to contraction of the erector muscles of the hairs is seen in life as well as during rigor.

Heat-stiffening, a coagulation of the muscle proteins by intense heat, may obscure rigor. The effects are further described in Chapter 9.

Freezing may also cause confusion by stiffening the muscles. It will postpone rigor, which will set in as soon as thawing permits.

Decomposition

Some 48 hours after death in mild weather a greenish staining of the skin develops in both flanks of the abdomen. Soon a reddish discoloation of the veins converging on the root of the neck, over the shoulders and running into the groins brings them into prominence, often as a 'marbled' reticule of branching veins (Fig. 2.4). Incision shows them to be

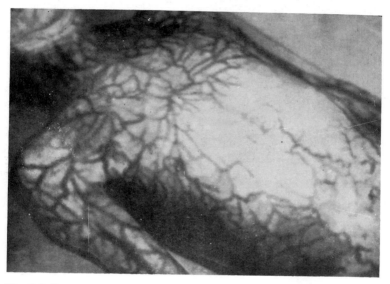

Fig. 2.4 *Post mortem* changes. 'Marbling' of the skin due to the growth of organisms of decomposition from the abdomen into the system of veins entering the root of the neck and the abdomen.

filled with gas bubbles and haemolysing blood. Organisms of the anaerobic gas-forming type have been growing from the intestines into the adjacent flank tissues and through the portal system into the main systemic veins, disrupting the blood and staining the tissues first red, then green, as haemolysis is followed by evolution of H_2S and green S-methaemoglobin formation. Small bubbles disrupt the tissues and bleb the skin. The features puff up and become unrecognisable, for the whole body becomes bloated and the tissues, sodden with fluid, eventually liquefy and disintegrate. Although most of this process is due to anaerobic intestinal organisms, it is accelerated by airborne bacteria and would be hindered by immersion in water or burial. Maggots, flies and beetles may hasten disintegration of the exposed soft tissues (Fig. 2.5)

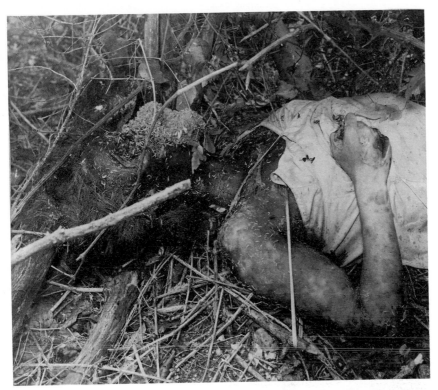

Fig. 2.5 Conditions of putrefaction with swelling by gases in the arm, together with maggot infestation of the face; developed in the summer within 5–7 days.

The usual order of decomposition is:

1. Intestines, stomach, liver blood, heart blood and circulation, heart muscle.
2. Air passages, lungs, liver.
3. Brain and cord.
4. Kidneys and bladder. Testis.
5. Voluntary muscles.
6. Uterus. Prostate.

The importance of autopsy even in states of advanced decomposition is plain, for organs such as the kidney or uterus may still remain to afford vital information.

A warm atmosphere, unless it is so hot as to kill decomposing bacteria, will hasten putrefaction. Exclusion of blood by tight clothing, and of air by burial or immersion, will retard the process.

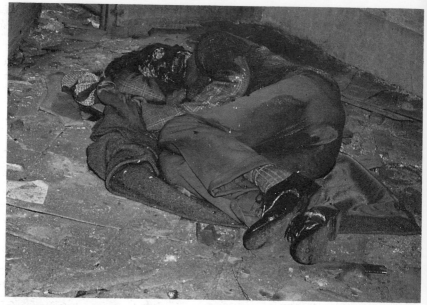

Fig. 2.6 Body of man found dead in deserted city warehouse. The clothing was identified as that of a man (Pettit) wanted for murder, but advanced decomposition made facial identification impossible. A dental card and chart in his pocket proved identity.

Mummification

Dry heat, especially when aided by currents of air, as in the desert or inside a chimney, will prevent bacterial decomposition, and thus prevent putrefaction. Newborn infants, being sterile and the less likely to decompose, more commonly mummify (Fig. 2.7). A progressive drying of the tissue ensues, resulting in leathery hardening and shrivelling, drawing the skin tight over the bony skeleton. Moulds, moths and beetles may hasten the powdery disintegration of tissues which follows. An infant (see Fig. 11.4) placed soon after birth in a cardboard box on a radiator, and the body of a man who lay dead for 4 months in a dry atmosphere above a coffee-shop, became mummified and desiccated.

Changes due to immersion in water

The development of *post mortem* changes is so affected by immersion that a special account of the course of events is desirable.

On immersion in cold water the commonplace cutis anserina or 'goose-flesh' appearance develops owing to cold contraction of the arectores pilorum muscles. The change is not, of course, confined to immersion: a cold wind on the foreshore—before going into water—may cause it to develop, and so may unrelated conditions such as fear with its 'skin-creeping'.

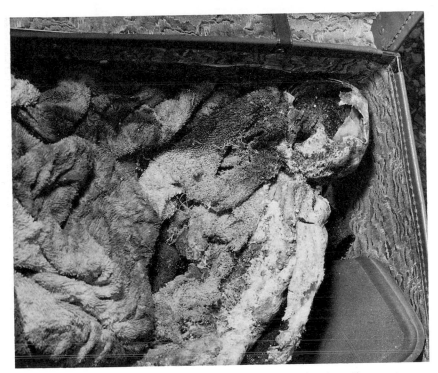

Fig. 2.7 Mummified and disintegrating body of a newborn infant found in an attaché case in the loft of a house unoccupied for 3 years.

Because the head sinks low in water, blood gravitates towards the head and neck, and when decomposition appears it will be likely to do so first in the neck and face. Because heat is lost twice as fast in water as in air, the process of decomposition is retarded. The colour change normally seen in the flank at the second or third day may not appear at the neck until the fifth or sixth, and the generation of gases may not be sufficient to cause the body to float until, in average cool weather, the sixth to tenth day. Warmth or sewage will, of course, greatly accelerate the process of decomposition, whilst a body lying in cool clean river-water may remain in surprisingly good condition for rather longer than the average times stated above. The circumstances must be known before an estimate of the lapse of time is ventured.

Meanwhile the skin is becoming sodden. After 10–12 hours the skin of the hands and feet becomes wrinkled, and if serious decomposition is retarded the affected skin may peel like gloves or socks in 10 days. The hair is, by this time, also becoming loose, and by 3–4 weeks the finger- and toe-nails may be detached without difficulty. In the summer, these periods may be halved.

Finally, as decomposition and sodden disintegration of the tissues proceed, the flesh breaks down into slime and the skeletal frame collapses. (See also the section on drowning in Chapter 7.)

Adipocere, a remarkable stiffening and swelling of the body fats, usually requires some months for development, though exceptional circumstances, such as sun-heat, rain and the warmth of maggot infestation, may greatly accelerate the process. It has been seen in as little as $3\frac{1}{2}$ weeks. Such rapid development is rare in moderate climates, and several months' burial in moist soil, or immersion, is usual. The only essential is moisture.

The change involves the body fats only, consisting of a hydrogenation of the more oily unsaturated oleic acid into higher fatty acids, oleic acid becoming hard opaque stearic acid.

Affected fat becomes swollen, whitened and greatly stiffened, often remaining adherent to the bones or muscle tissues after the skin has become softened and rotted away (Fig. 2.8).

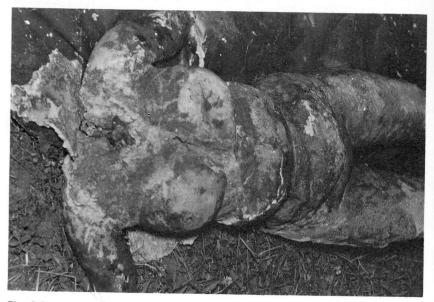

Fig. 2.8 Adipocere in the skin fat of the body of a woman recovered from a Canadian lake 7 years after death. The heavy head had become detached, but the body is held together by stiff adipocere.

'Bluebottle' flies (Calliphora) lay their eggs on moist parts such as the eyes and mouth, or on wounds, soon after death. Minute 'first instar' maggots hatch on the next day, a 'second instar' develops from these by the third day and fat active maggots by the fifth or sixth day, feeding for another 5 or 6 days, then curling up inside a brown pupa case. Samples of these should be preserved.

Injuries to the body after death

The body can be injured in a number of ways after death. The dead skin is commonly injured in handling by undertakers or by chafing in removal to the mortuary: attempts at resuscitation may also mark the skin and fracture ribs. The application of hot-water bottles or electric cradle heat may cause some blistering. Bones may become fractured by handling or flaked by great heat in burning. Soft tissues may become torn or eaten away by cats (Fig. 2.9), rats or fish and passing craft may dismember a body floating in water.

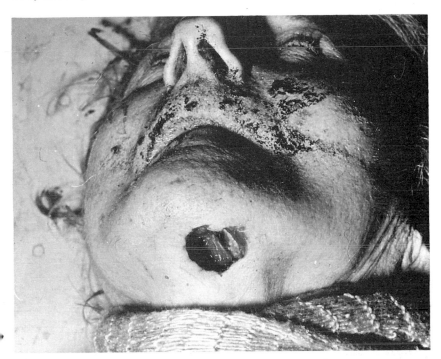

Fig. 2.9 Injuries to the dead body by cat bites. Tooth-marks can be seen on the edges of the hole under the chin. There is no bleeding or tissue reaction.

All such injuries have one thing in common: they lack a vital reaction. Abrasions to the cutis are sharply defined, becoming brown as the raw grazed skin tissue dries, and hardens like parchment. No local flushing is present, for the vessels, being dead, are incapable of such vital change.

Post mortem blistering can result from exposure to heat, for dead tissue fluids may be swollen by heat or even boiled, raising cuticular weals. Blood may boil and congeal after death.

As regards bruising after death, there can be no doubt that it is possible. Heavy blunt injury can tear dead vessels and open up tissue spaces into which blood may seep passively. Such extravasations of blood will not extend far, and the difficulty of distinguishing them from *ante mortem* bruises can be resolved by a little common sense: *there is never any cellular reaction.*

It is fair to add, nevertheless, that when injuries occur closely at or about the time of death it may be impossible to say whether they occurred just before, at or about the time of death. An opinion that they took place 'at about the time of death' is the most that can safely be offered. The blood remains fluid for some time—indeed may never clot at all, and may percolate into spaces opened up by injury at, or after, death.

3

Identification of live and dead human remains

The identification of living persons is increasingly a task for joint medical and police procedure. Immigrants applying for grants, pensions, etc., sometimes without proper documentation, require ageing, and missing or 'wanted' persons' data are useful only when accurate. A lay description of sex, age, height and weight, colouring of hair and eyes, details of teeth, and of special characteristics such as birthmarks or deformities, wounds and scars, tattoos, even some plain natural disease or sign of it may be supplemented by 'Identikit' pictures. A criminal record file may contain further exact details of standard anthropometrical measurements, photographs, and—most damning tally of all—ten finger-prints. The general description contains sufficient information to enable the police to enlist the help of a wide net of their own forces, and of the public, in the tracing of persons 'wanted' or 'missing', but no such general description can ever provide the wealth of detail laid on paper by a single finger-print; nor has it such unalterable individuality. The doctor should know the bare outline of this comparatively modern facet of criminology—dactylography—but has no need to concern himself with its details.

Finger-prints

These are impressions of the balls of the fingers and thumbs either detected at a scene of crime or recorded by moistening the skin with printer's ink and pressing or rolling on prepared paper so that a permanent record results. In Scotland finger-prints may be taken as soon as a person is under arrest, but in England they may not be taken before conviction unless with permission or on authority from a magistrate to whom a police inspector may apply.

A primary classification is based on the arrangement of the lines of the skin pattern into one of four general types (Fig. 3.1). The principal lines fall into arch, loop, whorl or composite form; loops may open towards either radial or ulnar side, permitting a further broad subdivision. Enumeration of lines between, say, core and delta of whorl and

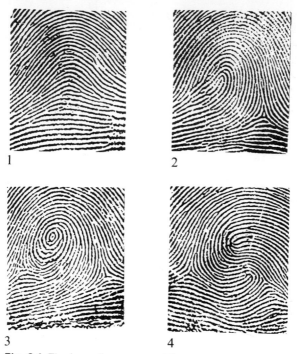

1   2

3   4

Fig. 3.1 The four primary types of finger-print. 1. Arch. 2. Loop. 3. Whorl. 4. Composite: forking, ovals and ridge-ends provide many subsidiary points for identification, and finer ridge characters are present in profusion.

composite forms, and of the precise situation of branching and fusion provides divisional detail. Final individuality lies with the exact position and shape, on these lines, of ridge pockets or indentations caused by the pore sites. Comparison of some 16 or 20 points in a small area, magnified to show the detail of these 'ridge patterns', is best made from photographs (Fig. 3.2).

The doctor called to a scene of crime should never handle any weapon, glass, furniture, telephone or door-knob upon which these tell-tale impressions may have been left. Clothing and the skin of the victim are not of any value for prints, and the doctor may proceed to establish the fact of death without fear of interfering with criminal investigation so long as he disturbs the body and its clothing as little as possible for this vital purpose. A record of temperature may be delayed whilst the clothing is left for photography, but an early reading can be vital and, whenever possible, should be made at the scene—where the body has started to cool. Several readings are desirable, at half-hour intervals. The vagina should always be left well alone, as should the rectum, if there is suspicion of a sex offence.

The individuality of the finger-print never changes though scars may disturb it. Attempts to deface this tell-tale label of identity by deep cuts only add more defacing details to the print.

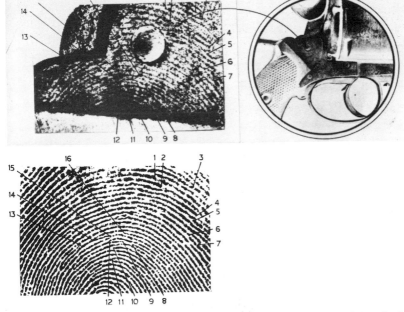

Fig. 3.2 Identity by finger-print on weapons. Identification of print of left thumb of woman found shot dead. Position on pistol to be expected if victim herself held weapon left-handed. Points of comparison numbered in print from left thumb (below). Suspicion dispelled.

Galton estimated that the chance of two prints from different fingers being identical was less than one in sixty-four thousand millions—then some twelve times the world population. It is perhaps more significant that never yet, in the world's crime records, have identical prints come to light unless from the same finger. Even a portion of the palm which bulged between a glove worn by a safebreaker has left sufficient detail for proof of identity by the finger-print expert, and a bare footprint has pointed conclusively at a suspect.

Identification of the dead

The whole body in a varying state of dress, or mere fragmentary remains of human tissues, commonly provide material for studies in identification, and the pathologist should exercise himself in the subject even when the actual necessity of proof does not arise. Sooner or later the test of proving identity from some naked victim or a hank of hair, an odd bone and a few teeth will arise, and the fruits of previous experience will then taste sweet.

The body of a girl was found buried in a shallow grave near Godalming by a party of marines exercising on the heath (Fig. 3.3). *The clothing proved sufficient to identify the victim.* But ample material for the establishment of

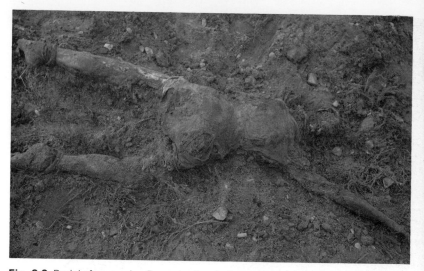

Fig. 3.3 Burial after murder. Example of case demanding careful collection of material (clothing, fragmentary bone, and other tissues, loose teeth and hair) for establishment of identity and reconstruction of circumstances (see Fig. 3.10).

the sex, stature, age, colouring, hair and dental data lay open for study, and much useful experience was gained in confirming the known data of identity by which the individuality of the victim of what proved to be a murder could be clinched.

Finger-pads, although disturbed by *post mortem* change, may still be of the greatest importance in identification. A method of stripping apparently useless skin for reversal-photography has been described by American criminologists, and the doctor should leave the finger-pads untouched as far as possible.

In the case of a woman murdered, stripped of clothing, and wheeled in four sacks on a bicycle through Luton to be tumbled into a stream, identification proved a problem of great difficulty. It was eventually clinched by dental records and the finding of a finger-print on a pickle jar lying on a shelf in the house of the presumed victim, which was shown to be identical with the finger-print details of the dead woman made as a routine at autopsy 3 months previously.

The principal details of identity which require to be established are: (1) that the remains are human; (2) race; (3) sex; (4) stature; (5) age; (6) colour of skin, eyes, hair; (7) dental data; (8) occupational stigmata, scars, tattoos; (9) disease .

Proof that remains are human

When considerable amounts of tissue or whole bones are available, little doubt exists about their being human or otherwise; common sense and a knowledge of elementary human anatomy suffices.

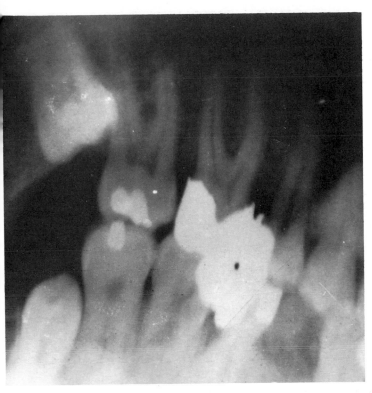

Fig. 3.4 Identification in one of the charred victims of the Barnes Bridge railway disaster—15 dead. X-rays of the suspected victim lying in dental records corresponded in detail.

A length of windpipe from the larynx to the lungs, with attached pericardial sac, but no tongue or heart, was found on the roadside in a tin box in a Surrey country district. The police-surgeon viewed it with suspicion, and it was referred for a skilled examination as possibly 'remains' of the victim of a crime. The trachea was 25 cm long, about twice the length of the human windpipe! The absence of tongue and heart might have suggested it was butcher's refuse. It could not be human.

Smaller fragments of organs or of the skeleton may require the attentions of a skilled anatomist who can identify portions of human bones with accuracy.

Fragments of tissue which lack sufficient data to permit anatomical recognition may be identified as human or not by means of the precipitin test and the antiglobulin inhibition test.

The precipitin test   The test fluid is the serum of a rabbit which has been injected with defibrinated human blood and has developed precipitins to human protein. The laboratory tests for a reaction of prepared extract with test serum in suitable dilutions is now made by the use of electrophoretic methods, and must be left to those with experience of the technique. The minutest stain of blood or a mere tag of tissue may be so tested, for a good test serum is very highly sensitive.

During the search for remains of the victim in the 'acid-bath' case (R. *v.* Haigh) three gallstones were recovered from a mass of some 215 kg of acrid fatty residue. They were intact and one provided sufficient cellular debris in its core to give a positive human precipitin test indicating their human origin.

The antiglobulin inhibition test, which depends on the power of human globulin to protect sensitised human cells from agglutination, is an even more highly sensitive test, but demands a higher technical skill, and should be left to the expert.

Race

The world races are 'mixing' geographically more than ever before, and skin colour, hair texture, skeletal features, facial contours, dental conservation methods—and the genetic blood typing factors—are becoming everyday problems wherever the need for identification arises.

Sex

The nature of the clothing, the tendency for the uterus to resist decomposition to the last among the soft organs and, in the last resort, the sex differences in the skeleton provide evidence which eliminates difficulty in the establishment of sex.

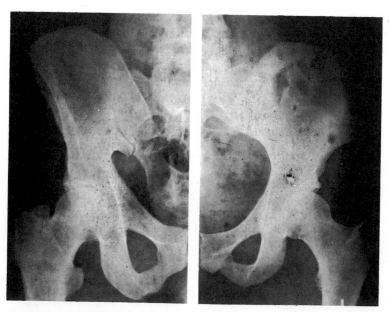

Fig. 3.5 X-ray photographs of male (left) and female (right) half-pelvis, showing striking features of contrast.

Of the bones, those of the pelvis designed with regard to sexual requirements are the most informative (Fig. 3.5), and a sacrum or even a femur will provide ample proof of sex. The lighter form and comparatively lighter muscle markings of the other bones, as in the skull, may make the sex tolerably certain. 'Mathematical' methods of sexing the heads of the humerus and femur have also been devised.

The sternal body is more than twice the length of the manubrium in the male and less than twice in the female.

Hair distribution, especially in the pubic region, and the probability

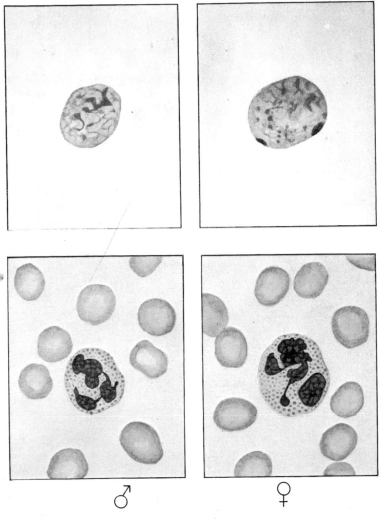

Fig. 3.6 Sex cell characters. Above (right), female cell showing 'Barr bodies' inside the nuclear membrane. Below, male (left) and female (right) form of 'Davidson nuclear drumsticks'.

of long hair on the female head may help to corroborate other evidence. So also may breast tissue and even lineae gravidarum, but none of these data has the finality of a uterus or a testis, prostate or penis.

Cell sexing   A method of sexing cells which relies upon their nuclear chromatin form has now become standard. In cells that are not dividing, the female shows one or more tiny nodes of chromatin attached to the inner surface of the nuclear membrane; males do not have this 'Barr' body. White blood cells show, as their feminine trait, a thin-stalked drumstick projection of the polymorph nucleus—a 'Davidson' body. In cells that are dividing, an expert chromosome count can also identify the sex (XY or XX) chromatin bodies. The Y chromosome (in the male) is fluorescent to quinacrine.

Stature

Where the body can be reassembled or sufficient skeletal remains are available (and allowance is made for scalp and heel-pad thickness) the height may be measured if only roughly.

A rough estimate of height may also be gained from the outstretched arms, finger-tip to finger-tip (or its half in a dismembered body); the

Table 3.1 Stature from bone. Dupertuis and Hadden's general formulae for reconstruction of stature from lengths of dry long bones without cartilage (constant terms in metric and adapted to imperial system)

Sex	Formula	Stature–bone length coefficient(s)	Constant term to be added *after* calculations in previous column (cm)	(in)
Male	(a)	2.238 (femur)	69.089	27.200
	(b)	2.392 (tibia)	81.688	32.161
	(c)	2.970 (humerus)	73.570	28.965
	(d)	3.650 (radius)	80.405	31.655
	(e)	1.255 (femur + tibia)	69.294	27.281
	(f)	1.728 (humerus + radius)	71.429	28.112
	(g)	1.422 (femur) + 1.062 (tibia)	66.544	26.198
	(h)	1.789 (humerus) + 1.841 (radius)	66.400	26.142
	(i)	1.928 (femur) + 0.568 (humerus)	64.505	25.396
	(k)	1.442 (femur) + 0.931 (tibia) + 0.083 (humerus) + 0.480 (radius)	56.006	22.050
Female	(a)	2.317 (femur)	61.412	24.178
	(b)	2.533 (tibia)	72.572	28.572
	(c)	3.144 (humerus)	64.977	25.581
	(d)	3.876 (radius)	73.502	28.938
	(e)	1.233 (femur + tibia)	65.213	25.674
	(f)	1.984 (humerus + radius)	55.729	21.941
	(g)	1.657 (femur) + 0.879 (tibia)	59.259	23.330
	(h)	2.164 (humerus) + 1.525 (radius)	60.344	23.757
	(i)	2.009 (femur) + 0.566 (humerus)	57.600	22.677
	(k)	1.544 (femur) + 0.764 (tibia) + 0.126 (humerus) + 0.295 (radius)	57.495	22.636

span is about the same as the height. Where only smaller remains are available a single long bone can provide remarkably reliable evidence of stature. Formulae exist for relating the long bones to the height, and those of Dupertuis and Hadden are probably the most reliable for general use (Table 3.1).

Where several bones are available the mean of several estimations should be taken. A proper osteometry board is essential to such precise work.

Age

The fetus   The age of the fetus may be fixed with near mathematical accuracy by direct measurement and the appearance of the ossification centres.

First to fourth months:
First month—1.25 cm long embryo enveloped in villous chorion. Limb buds only present.
Second month—2.5 cm long. Head well formed. Ears and hands already well formed.
Third month—9 cm long. Placenta formed. Nails appear.
Fourth month—15 cm long. Sex clear. Hairs appearing on head.

Fifth to ninth months:

Length*	25	30	35	40	50 cm (vertex to heel)
Month	5	6	7	8	9
Weight	350–	700–	1.2–	1.5–	2.5–
	450 g	900 g	1.4 kg	2 kg	3.5 kg (less cord, etc.)

*The length in centimetres equals five times the number of months gestation (after 4 months).

 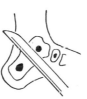 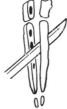

At the seventh month (legally viable): 35 cm 1.2 kg. Lanugo all over. Nails just short of finger tips. Centres of ossification in os calcis 5/12, astragalus (talus) 7/12 and manubrium 6/12, and first segment of sternum 7/12.

Ossification centres of importance month by month: 1.5/12, clavicle; 2/12, all shafts of long bones, metacarpus and tarsus; 3/12, ischium; 4/12, superior ramus of pubis; 5/12, os calcis; 6/12, manubrium sterni; 7/12, astragalus (talus), first segment of sternum; 8/12, last segment of sternum; 9/12, cuboid, lower femur.

Immediately after birth   there are functional changes in the circulation, but the ductus arteriosus does not close for some weeks. The 'fetal' form of haemoglobin gradually decreases until, at 6 months, only the adult form is to be found.

For 24–36 hours the umbilical cord dries. At 36–48 hours a ring of demarcation begins to form around its root of attachment. At 5–6 days it sloughs off and in about 10 days the scar is healed.

A period then intervenes until the lower central incisor teeth erupt at about 6 months. The variable increase in weight (about 0.5 kg per month) provides the only basis for estimation of age during this time. Prematurity must be allowed for.

In youth   the age may be estimated with fair accuracy from the eruption of teeth and the development and fusion of centres of ossification.

Eruption of teeth (6 months to 25 years):

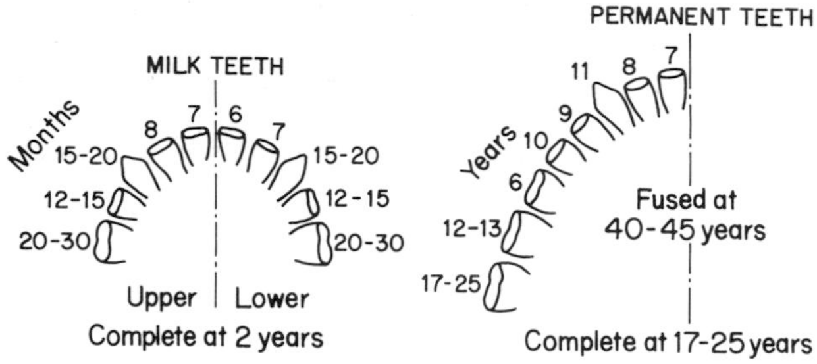

Fig. 3.7 Eruption of teeth.

The dismembered remains of a child were found upon search in the back garden of a London house after suspicion had been aroused over the disappearance of a child of 2 years, a daughter of the woman living there. Neighbours, who knew her to be living there with another man in the absence of her husband overseas, had not seen the child for some months, and the mother's story that she had sent it to an address in a provincial town to be away from enemy air attack was not substantiated on inquiry. The jaw, which showed a just erupted second milk molar tooth, provided evidence of the age of the remains; but there was no possibility after the prolonged period of burial—some 12 months—of establishing the cause of death. No criminal charge could be made.

Centres of ossification and union of bone (1–25 years)   Reference must be made to textbooks of anatomy for full details of the ossification of bone, but a summary of the more reliable centres and fusion data will provide an initial guide to age. Females are as a rule about a year ahead of males in maturing their skeleton.

Year

by 1   Head of femur, humerus, and tibia.
2   Lower tibia and radius.
3   Patella.
4   Upper fibula, greater trochanter of femur.
5   Lower fibula.
6   Head of radius, lower ulna.
7   Scaphoid of hand, rami of ischium, and pubis.
8   Int. epicondyle of humerus, olecranon.
10   Lesser trochanter of femur, os calcis epiphysis.
11   Trochlea of humerus.

12 Acetabular 'Y' cartilage union.
13 Ext. epicondyle of humerus appears—and unites.
14 Coracoid united to scapula.
16 Olecranon united to ulna.
18 Head of radius and femur fuse with shafts.
20 Lower radius, ulna and femur to shafts. Iliac crest to body.
21 Appearance of a centre at inner end of clavicle.
22–24 Fusion of secondary epiphyses of inner end of clavicle and articular facet of ribs.

After 25 years the accuracy of age estimation deteriorates sadly. For some 15 years, until about the age of 40, there is little but the general appearance to give any guidance. At about 40 the skull vault sutures begin to close, and at about the same time the ziphisternum unites with the body. Teeth show a progressive apical (root) translucency irrespective of wear and tear (Fig. 3.8).

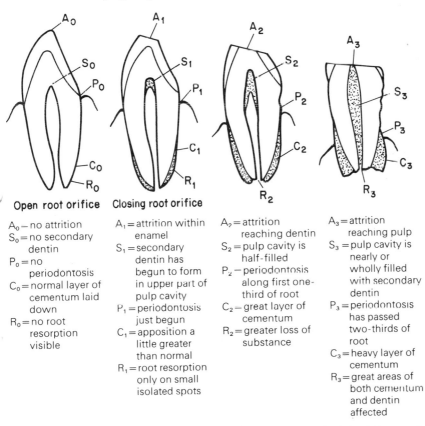

Open root orifice | Closing root orifice

A_0 — no attrition
S_0 = no secondary dentin
P_0 = no periodontosis
C_0 = normal layer of cementum laid down
R_0 = no root resorption visible

A_1 = attrition within enamel
S_1 = secondary dentin has begun to form in upper part of pulp cavity
P_1 = periodontosis just begun
C_1 = apposition a little greater than normal
R_1 = root resorption only on small isolated spots

A_2 = attrition reaching dentin
S_2 = pulp cavity is half-filled
P_2 — periodontosis along first one-third of root
C_2 — great layer of cementum
R_2 = greater loss of substance

A_3 = attrition reaching pulp
S_3 = pulp cavity is nearly or wholly filled with secondary dentin
P_3 = periodontosis has passed two-thirds of root
C_3 = heavy layer of cementum
R_3 = great areas of both cementum and dentin affected

Fig. 3.8 Diagrams showing point values allotted as a standard in determining age in teeth. Changes in attrition secondary dentin, periodontosis, cementum and root resorption according to degree of development. (Reproduced, with permission from G. Gustafsen, 1950, *Journal of the American Dental Association*, **41**, 45.)

After 60–65 years the angle of the lower jaw begins to open out and its alveolar ridges to subside until, in very old age, it once again acquires the obtuse angle and the toothlessness of infancy (Fig. 3.9).

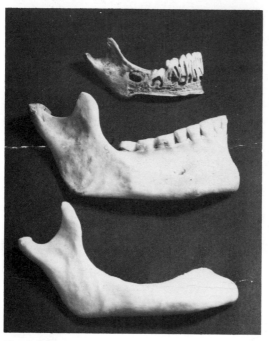

Fig. 3.9 Varying shape and dentition of lower jaw at 2 years, 22 years and 82 years. Note the atrophy of alveolar ridge and muscle attachment markings accompanying increasing age. Lack of proper dental care encourages 'ageing'.

Colour of skin, eyes, hair

The natural colouring of the skin in its fresh state may give a clue as to race, and anthropological measurements (called cranial indices) of the skull by an expert may narrow the issue to certain world types. Care must be taken that the eye colouring is not misread. When decomposition enters the eye the iris becomes greenish brown whatever its original shade. It has also been known for the eye colour to be taken from a glass eye without its being recognised as artificial. Eye defects such as casts and lens operation defects are important to note, for many people have their attention caught by them.

Hairs provide important clues in crime investigation, for they remain identifiable on both the body—even in states of most advanced putrefaction—and on alleged weapons in crimes committed perhaps long before. They often provide the only connection between a weapon, or even the accused, and the victim of an assault. The most minute examination of the body at the scene of a crime for attached foreign hairs often repays

Hairs from static

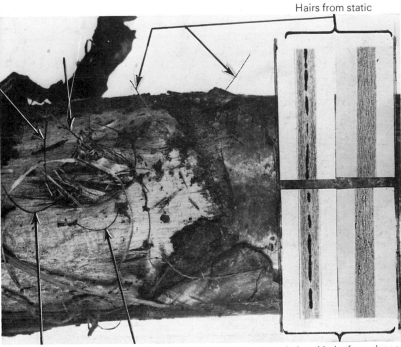

Sample head hairs from deceased

Fig. 3.10 Comparison of hairs found on blunt weapon alleged to have been used for murder and sample hairs from dead girl. Weapon found several weeks after crime was committed and some 360 metres from the body (see also Fig. 3.3).

the time consumed, providing clues of a striking, though circumstantial, kind likely to influence a jury strongly in the event of a case depending on such evidence.

In the Godalming 'wigwam' murder, outlined at the commencement of this chapter (p. 21), a birch stake was found lying in long grass some 360 metres from the body, dead from blunt injuries to the head. The stake could clearly have inflicted the principal head wound and careful examination showed (Fig. 3.10) nine hairs adherent to it a short distance from its heavier end. They were identical with head hairs taken at the time of autopsy from the dead girl, and had kept in perfectly good condition on both the body—covered with slime and seething with maggots after 3½ weeks' burial—and on the weapon in spite of rain and wind.

Reconstruction of the vermin-riddled remains of the head of a body discovered concealed in a copse in a railway siding at Bedford showed that one of several heavy blunt injuries sustained had been to the left eyebrow region— likely to have resulted in soiling of the weapon with both blood and possibly also eyebrow hairs. A sapling bough, found upon search in some nearby bushes, was found (Fig. 3.11) to have both head and six eyebrow hairs jammed between crevices on its surface in addition to its being stained with blood. The hairs were identical with samples taken from the dead body at the time of autopsy.

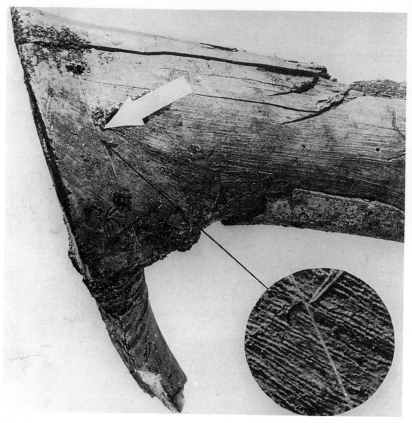

Fig. 3.11 Sapling bough found near scene of crime, showing on close examination long hair (magnified inset) suck to surface near end. Comparison showed it to be identical with head hair sample taken from dead body at autopsy.

The phrase 'identical with samples taken from the deceased' is a sad confession of the limitations of hair evidence. Colour, texture, form, approximate age—even the pattern of the cuticular scale—cannot enable the scientist to say to whom the hair belonged. He may be able to say at once if the hair is *not* human, or perhaps that it is some animal or vegetable fibre mistaken for human hair. He may also be able to state firmly that a hair is, or is not, similar to that in a sample from deceased (or accused), and to point out its site of origin from the body (see below). Activation analysis has greatly increased the individuality of hair.

In the case of a murdered WAAF girl, found in a ditch in Suffolk, certain hairs, found on the clothing of accused, were shown to be identical with the dead girl's head hairs, a strong circumstantial connection between the two. Samples from women with whom deceased had lawful associations provided a complication. Accused's wife's hair was found to be identical with that of the victim of the crime. Accused (Heys) was convicted on other evidence.

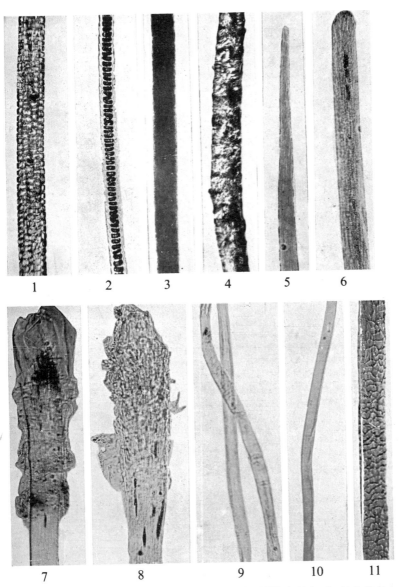

1 2 3 4 5 6

7 8 9 10 11

Fig. 3.12 Hairs and fibres by photomicrography (× 200). 1. Hair of rabbit. 2. Hair of cat. 3. Hair of dog. 4. Wool of sheep. 5. Human eyebrow tip. 6. Human body hair tip. 7. Human hair pulled out. 8. Human hair fallen out (dead). 9. Cotton (American warp). 10. Silk 11. Cellulose acetate impression of cuticular scale pattern of human hair.

Hair may be dyed, bleached, curled or singed, and thus add to the details of identification. Cells at its root may be sexed.

Firmer evidence may be given on the location of hairs from the body. Head hairs are commonly square cut, or, when healed, disc-ended. All body hairs are bluntly 'pointed', and eyebrow hairs are tapering and more sharply pointed (Fig. 3.12). Pubic hairs, often found on search of the victims of rape, or murder during rape, are curly or wiry. Microscopy will distinguish fibres of various kinds from human hairs (Fig. 3.12).

Section shows head hairs to be rounded, pubic oval, and moustache more or less triangular.

Dental data

No unidentified body should leave the mortuary without a record of the teeth being made. Details of residual dentition and fillings, of dentures, or gaps suitable for dentures, and other information must be recorded — or, even better, the jaws preserved intact after excision.

> In R. *v.* Haigh, the 'acid-bath' case, the victim had been shot and the body immersed in commercial H_2SO_4 for 2–3 days. Most of the body had dissolved to a charred fatty residue, but acrylic resin upper and lower dentures were found upon search of the remains, and identified by a London dental surgeon as made for the missing woman.
>
> In R. *v.* Manton, the 'Luton sack murder', the strangled victim was found naked, trussed up in potato sacks, in a river. Identity was established by sex, age, colour, height, an appendix scar, a pregnancy, finger-prints — and edentulous jaws (containing residual roots). A local dental surgeon produced records identical with the victim's residual dentition and denture casts identical with those prepared from the dead woman.
>
> Much progress has been made by Gustafson in Sweden on ageing individual teeth, but the technique is one for the dental expert.

Occupational stigmata, scars, tattoos, etc.

This is no place for a list of occupational stigmata, but their study has the fascination of Conan Doyle's Sherlock Holmes tales, and they should be stored in the mind as they are seen for the day when identity proof might make use of them.

Scars have many forms from the stitch-marked line of a surgical scar to the broad deforming expanse of a burn scar. Fresh scars are reddish, age gradually whitening, and usually contracting, them. Continued stretching, as in the abdomen, may cause them to bulge or alter their shape.

Tattoos provide entertaining study, reflecting travel, history, war, occupation, sex interest and love of the older-fashioned kind, with an array of anything from bold manly dragons and serpents to lewd indecorous female forms and open sexual invitations. Initials and dates, regimental or nautical details, and, sometimes, identity numerals provide more scientific basis for identification. Carbon, indigo and vermilion are the common pigments used, and as they are injected beneath the cutis they are more or less permanent; they are often revealed in striking detail when the slimy detaching cuticle of the decomposing body recovered from water is wiped away.

Disease

The doctor is in a particularly good position to help the police with regard to the probability of signs or symptoms of disease found upon examination of a dead body, and the likelihood of medical attention and treatment, of which records might exist. Such detail was present in the Dobkin case outlined below, a fibroid tumour being present, records of which showed that surgery had been refused.

No detail is too trivial for note among the data preserved for identification purposes; much that is noted may prove to be of little value, but better so than to have no record of some vital detail produced after the body has been disposed of.

As an example of the application in criminal practice of the foregoing principles of identification a short summary is appended of the classic Dobkin Baptist church cellar murder which occurred in 1941–42.

The Baptist church cellar murder. *R. v. Dobkin.* In July 1942 the dismembered, partly burned remains of *a woman*—identified at once as such by the uterus (enlarged by a fibroid tumour) which lay in the exposed pelvis—were discovered by demolition workers under a cellar floor at the rear of a disused bombed Baptist Church in Vauxhall, London. The conditions, bearing in mind the character of the debris in which the body was found, suggested *burial for 12–18 months.*

The head was detached from the trunk, but complementary with it, and parts of the arms and legs, together with the lower jaw, were missing (Fig. 3.13). A minute fragment of scalp with hairs lay stuck to the back of the head, but search of some 3 tons of the debris in the cellar floor failed to reveal any other human material. A yellowish powder, which proved subsequently to be slaked lime, lay over the tissues, which were almost dry, especially in the head and neck regions; it had been sprinkled over the body to keep down the smell or accelerate the disintegration of tissues, but had, of course, preserved them.

Reassembly of the body showed it to be about 153–154 cm (60¼–60¾ in) in *stature.* Allowance had to be made for missing lower leg and foot bones and for soft tissue. Pearson's formulae, used with the remaining intact long bone (humerus) as a basis, gave an estimated height of 1.50–1.55 m (60½–61 in): the Dupertuis and Hadden tables were not then available (see p. 26). It was later given in evidence by a sister that the dead woman, then identified, was 1.55 mm (5 ft 1 in) or 'about her own height' (which was 1.55 m (5 ft 1 in)).

Colouring was provided by the tag of hair (Fig. 3.13), which was dark brown, ageing, going grey. *Age* was estimated from the condition of closure of the skull vault sutures, and the palate suture (closing at 45–50 years) as being about 40–50 years.

At this stage the police were therefore informed that the remains were those of a woman, 1.53 m to 1.55 m (5 ft to 5 ft 1 in) in height, with dark brown hair, going grey, aged 40–50, *with fibroid tumour of the womb* (Fig. 3.13), who was likely to have met her death some 12–18 months previously; *teeth were*

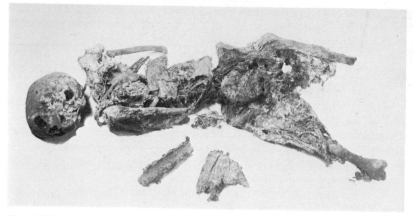

Fig. 3.13 Remains as found in Baptist church cellar murder (R. *v*. Dobkin). The head had been severed from the trunk and partial dismemberment and burning had taken place before final burial in lime-strewn earth. A fragment of hair was found on the back of the head. The womb (which contained a fibroid tumour) can just be defined. Upper jaw teeth remained (see Fig. 3.15).

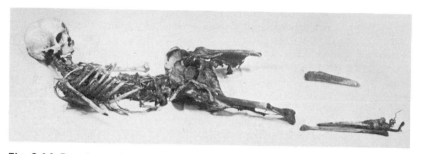

Fig. 3.14 Remains partly reconstructed.

available in the upper jaw to further the identification if dental records could be traced.

The police had ascertained, in the meantime, that the wife of the fire-watcher to the Baptist church premises had disappeared without explanation 15 months previously (11th April 1941). She had last been seen in the company of her husband whom she was pestering for arrears of maintenance. She was 1.53 m or 1.55 m (5 ft or 5 ft 1 in) in height, with dark brown hair going grey, aged 47, and had refused medical attention at two London hospitals (where records were traced) for a fibroid tumour of the womb. Her dental surgeon was traced and produced a record of the condition of the upper jaw as he last saw it. The upper jaw of the victim (Fig. 3.15) was identical in respect of shape, residual teeth, fillings and denture fitting marks: it showed, on x-ray, residual roots in the correct regions.

Superimposed photography as first practised in the Ruxton case was presented to complete the identity data (Fig. 3.16).

Dobkin, who as fire-watcher was the only person with access to the cellar in question, had had a fire there during the night of 15th April, 4 days after Mrs Dobkin had disappeared. It had been *drawn to his attention* after some

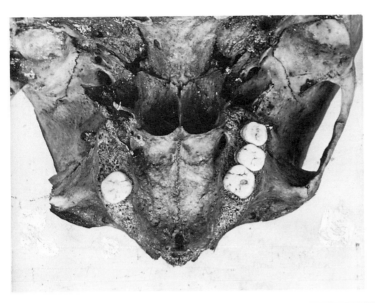

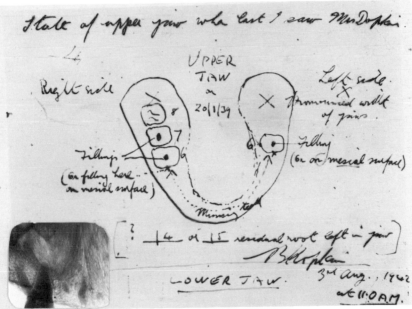

Fig. 3.15 Comparison, for proof of identity, of details of dentition of upper jaw of victim of murder (R. *v.* Dobkin) and diagram made by dental surgeon from records of attendance upon woman supposed to be victim. The photograph (with x-ray insert) is exact counterpart of mirror-form diagram (which refers to possibility of residual roots).

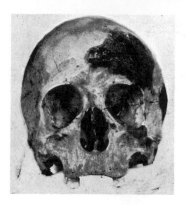
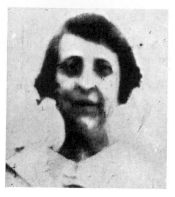

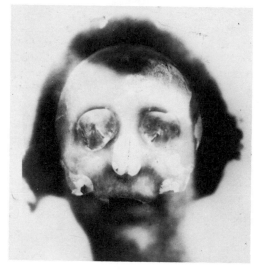

Fig. 3.16 Superimposed photography for comparison of full-face features of missing woman with skull of remains. Baptist church cellar case.

2 hours by a passing constable, and the prosecution suggested that Dobkin had been endeavouring to dispose of the dead body of his wife and that the fire had got beyond his control. The remains showed fire burns at several centres. Bags of lime similar to the sample on the body were found in the fire-watcher's premises next door. Dobkin had no proper explanation for the fire and later tried to deny knowledge even of the existence of the cellar.

Among the tissues preserved by the lime were the thyroid cartilages, which showed dried bruising around a fractured superior cornu of the right ala. This provided the only evidence on which to suggest that death was due to strangulation by the hand, the only likely cause for such a stray fracture, and the opinion was not strongly contested by the defence. Dobkin was charged with murder, convicted at the Old Bailey and executed.

In R. *v.* Haigh (the 'acid-bath' murder), a well-to-do Kensington widow was lured to Crawley, shot, stripped of a fur coat and jewellery, then immersed in a drum of strong commercial H_2SO_4. A few fragments of skeletal bone, three gallstones, and intact upper and lower dentures of resistant acrylic resin were recovered from surface soil in a yard on premises rented by Haigh in Crawley. The dentures were identified by a London dental surgeon as those made for the missing woman; this evidence of identity was not contested. Haigh, who confessed to five other similar crimes, was convicted and executed. Had he exercised a little more patience, the identity of this woman might have been almost impossible to establish, for experiment showed that, given a rather longer period of immersion in H_2SO_4, both the teeth and the acrylic resin gum basis would have disintegrated. Of the fragments of skeletal bone recovered, only one—part of an os innominatum—could be sexed (by a preauricular groove), and there was nothing by which an estimation of age, height, colouring or other identity data could be established.

This does not, in law, preclude the Crown making a charge of murder—as it did in a case where a woman was pushed through the porthole of a liner at sea (R. *v.* Camb)—or when an Eastbourne doctor, who had benefited by the will of an elderly patient, later cremated, was charged with her murder in 1957. Where there is no body or remains of a body, the Crown is entitled to lead a charge of murder if the circumstantial evidence points that way sufficiently strongly.

4

Blood-stains and grouping

The design of blood-stains on clothing is a subject for elementary deduction. Blood soaking into a cloth runs by viscous spread locally, but tends to gravitate downwards, and may help to indicate the lie of an injured or dead person—either of whom may bleed. Blood spurting from an artery tends to spray finely, and, welling up from veins, to run down over the body on to the undersurfaces, or the knees when a subject is sitting, for example, cutting the wrist.

Clothing smeared by wiping has only surface smears, often on wrinkled or folded surfaces: sometimes the shape of even a small stain has special significance (Fig. 4.1); a rape seen in Suffolk was followed by wiping the blood-stained penis on the inside of the then dead victim's greatcoat.

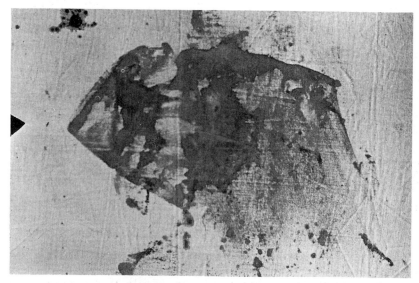

Fig. 4.1 Imprint of blood-stained hatchet on bed-linen at scene of murder by multiple head wounds.

A blunt weapon dealing a blow which splits the tissues is often un-stained—until second, third and further blows are delivered, for the blow causes momentary crushing of vessels and several seconds may elapse before bleeding commences. Further blows may then splash blood in any direction.

In a murder on a railway siding in the Midlands five blows were struck to different parts of the head with a bough, splitting the skin, knocking out teeth, fracturing skull, face and skull bones; yet since each blow had a new location the weapon was but slightly stained (see Fig. 3.11).

A public toilet in Hythe, the scene of a savage 'beat-up' in which the bleeding head of a man on the floor had been repeatedly kicked, had blood splashed on the undersurface of a handbasin, all four walls and the ceiling. Blood had pooled and run away on the floor (see Fig. 1.2).

Blood splashes often indicate the direction in which the blood has been ejected from a wound or thrown off a weapon. The spots are preceded by tiny globules, and so on oblique impact with a flat surface the stain resembles an exclamation mark with the narrow end striking first (Fig. 4.2).

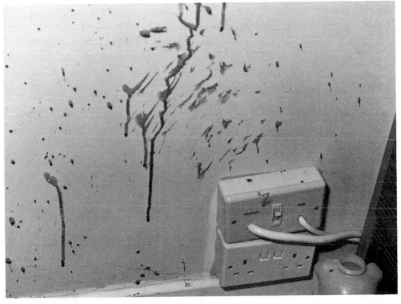

Fig. 4.2 The pattern of blood-stains coughed against a wall by a man who had been stabbed in the chest . . . and was coughing blood.

Nail-scrapings have sometimes given positive tests of distinctive blood groupings similar to persons suspect on other grounds, and the hair of a man who had shaved his beard and taken a bath after a murder was found 'positive' for blood.

Tests for blood

Stains may be plainly those of blood, requiring proof only for legal purposes, or may, because of their small size, or age, or rusting on a weapon, or because of washing—a precaution most 'wanted' men take at an early stage—be so obscured that only laboratory examination can distinguish them from other stains. Washing or bleaching may prevent even this. Samples may be scraped off—with some non-ferrous scraper—or soaked away from fragments of cloth cut out for test. The precise situation and size of any stain must be recorded before it is removed. Physiological (normal) saline in a watch-glass left under cover for a half to as much as 24 hours, is as good a solvent as any, and will bring out the oldest blood-stains.

Preliminary tests for blood

Peroxidase tests for blood detect the power of haemoglobin to oxidise—a colourless reduced compound of phenolphthalein in alkali turning bright pink (Kastle–Meyer test). A filter-paper rubbing of a suspect area will detect the merest trace of blood in quite old stains.

The phenolphthalein test, accurate to 10-15 million dilution and almost specific (except only with traces of copper), is performed by placing several drops of the test extract in a watch-glass with a drop or two of:

> 130 mg phenolphthalein
> 1.3 g potassium hydroxide   } boiled till clear—
> 100 ml distilled water

adding 20 g powdered zinc during boiling, and adding several drops of 20-volume hydrogen peroxide. A pink colour indicates a positive result.

Such tests are preliminary tests for blood. A negative result excludes blood; a positive test is no more than an indication that the stain may well be blood. Further—conclusive—tests are indicated.

Conclusive tests for blood

These include microscopic and microchemical.

Microscopy for red cells may be successful even after the stain has become dry. A diameter measurement will be necessary to avoid confusing, say, small sheep cells with human erythrocytes. Agglutination species or group tests may also be applied to intact cells.

Camels have oval or elliptical non-nucleated cells, and birds, fish, reptiles and amphibians have similar, but nucleated, red cells. Precipitin tests will confirm the species of the blood (see below).

Microscopy will sometimes indicate the blood to be menstrual, when endometrial cells are present in some quantity; such evidence is sometimes of help in establishing the association of a suspect with a menstruating victim of a sexual assault. The nuclear shape in some white cells has definite male or female form, but the blood must be quite fresh for this test of the sex (see p. 26).

Microchemical tests   depend upon the composition of blood, and demand an elementary knowledge of the subject. Blood is a compound protein with an iron-containing pigment (haematin) bound to a protein (globin). It has a characteristic spectrum containing well-defined absorption bands and can be changed in composition or broken down to form subsidiary compounds by the action of simple chemical agents.

Carboxyhaemoglobin   has a spectrum so like that of oxyhaemoglobin that the scaled spectroscope is necessary to define the degree of shift to the right (towards the violet); it is unaffected by reducing agents, but otherwise behaves like oxyhaemoglobin.

The haemochromogen test   —which is more certain of success with dilute blood than the haemin test—is performed with a solution (Takayama's) of:

Sodium hydroxide (10%) ⎫
Pyridine   ⎭   3 ml of each

Grape sugar (sat. soln.) ⎫
Distilled water   ⎭   7 ml of each

Several drops of this fluid are added to powdered or dissolved suspect blood-stain and examined by low power under a cover-slip. Fine sheaves of feathery pink crystals of haemochromogen (alkaline reduced haematin) will settle after some 5 minutes at room temperature.

In practice the demonstration of haemochromogen, a delicate decisive test, and confirmation by spectroscopy leave no possible doubt that a stain consists of blood.

Identification of blood as human

Though the shape and size of fresh red cells may give some guide to the species, most blood-stains are dried and the question whether they are human must depend on the detection of human protein by immunological techniques. Anti-human-globulin test sera are preferable.

The precipitin test   which uses antisera prepared from rabbits by injection of human protein is highly sensitive, a cloudy reaction appearing at surfaces of contact (interface) between test and human tissue suspensions. Other species fail to react at all, or, as with the nearer related higher apes, demand sera made more sensitive by absorption techniques. The use of electrophoretic methods has much improved the delicacy of these precipitin tests.

The individuality of blood

Since Landsteiner first identified the ABO blood groups in 1900, further groups such as the MN and rhesus (Rh) systems, the Lewis, Kell, and Duffy antigens, and more recently the protein complexes (Gm and Gc) and the haptoglobins (Hp), have added vastly to the individuality of blood. Haemoglobin also has types (HbF and S(ickle)).

The fact that such differences of character can be detected, and the knowledge that they are all inherited on mendelian principles, has given blood grouping great medico-legal significance.

Blood-grouping tests can be used:

1. to show whether blood-stains on weapons, clothing or elsewhere could—or could not—have come from suspect or from victim, provided, of course, they did not have identical groups;

2. to assist in apportioning or fitting together human parts disintegrated in air and rail crashes;

3. to 'mark' newborn infants, thus forestalling mistakes in clinics and hospitals—as finger-prints would;

4. in inheritance disputes; in disputed paternity problems—in affiliation and divorce actions.

The basis of these forensic applications of blood testing is as follows.

The blood of all persons falls within one of four primary groups (phenotypes), O, A, B or AB, as a result of their cells containing neither, either or both agglutinogens. Lattes has said: 'The fact of belonging to a definite blood group is a fixed character of every human being and can be altered neither by the lapse of time nor by intercurrent disease.' Blood, like finger-prints, is an unalterable primary character. The ABO types occur in England (whites) with the frequencies shown in Table 4.1.

Table 4.1

Group	Agglutinogen in red cell	Agglutinin in serum	Frequency (white) England
O	Neither	Both anti- $\left\{\begin{array}{l}A\\B\end{array}\right.$	47 per cent
A	A	Anti-B (beta)	42 per cent
B	B	Anti-A (alpha)	About 8 per cent
AB	A and B	Neither	3 per cent

Further group complexes (see Table 4.2) have continued to make their appearances, and their distribution has been found, as might be expected, to depend partly on racial and geographical factors. The Rh (CDE/cde) antigens in some 85 per cent, the M (30 per cent), N (20 per cent), and MN (50 per cent), the Lewis (75 per cent), and more recently the haptoglobin (Hp) and gammaglobulin (Gm) complex—both universally found—have proved particularly useful.

Antibodies to all but the ABO groups have to be prepared: they do not occur naturally. Recognition of the specific protein components of blood has rested on electrophoretic methods of separation.

Another feature of interest was the discovery that about 75 per cent of people secrete water-soluble group substances identical with their blood groups—in saliva, sweat, semen, gastric and other body fluids. All 'secretors' also secrete a strange substance called 'H' substance, the real nature of which is as yet not understood.

Inheritance of blood groups

Bernstein, elaborating the Mendelian principles of inheritance, formulated two major 'rules', depending on the inheritance of one gene from each parent.

    1. A blood group gene cannot appear in a child unless present in one or other (or both) parents.
    2. If an individual is homozygous (e.g. AA) for the blood group gene, it *must* appear in the blood of all his/her children.

    A further principle also holds. Each group agglutinogen (a 'phenotype' emerging on serological test) carries paired genes, one derived from each parent. Group A may be homozygous (the genotype AA) or heterozygous (AO); and B also. So the only mating that could produce all four genotypes AB, AO, BO and OO is a heterozygous A × B (i.e. AO × BO).
    A simple table of 'possible' and 'impossible' groups is shown in Table 4.2.

Table 4.2

Parents mating	Children possible	Groups impossible
O × O	O	A, B, AB
O × A	O, A	B, AB
O × B	O, B	A, AB
A × A	O, A	B, AB
A × B	O, A, B, AB	—
B × B	O, B	A, AB
Law 2 results in further possibilities.		
O × AB	A, B	O, AB
A × AB	A, B, AB	O
B × AB	A, B, AB	O
AB × AB	A, B, AB	O

The phenotype A may have the genotype structure AA or AO, and similarly the phenotype B may be genetically distinguished as BB or BO. Each individual inherits one gene from each parent, and so the comparatively simple phenotype structure of Table 4.1 may be elaborated genetically:

Mating of O with O cannot produce cells with A or B or AB, but A mating with B has the following gene type possibilities:

1. AA × BB		1. AB
2. AA × BO	with possible	2. AB and AO
3. AO × BB	children	3. AB and BO
4. AO × BO		4. AB, AO, BO or OO

and an A × AB can result in AA, AB, AO or BO, but not of course OO.

Subgroups of A—A₁ (78 per cent), A₂ (22 per cent) and even weaker A agglutinogens—can only be detected by using the more sensitive anti-A agglutinin of sera of group O. The anti-A of group B persons is generally weaker and may result in an AO being classed as O. The job is one for the expert—and the Family Law Reform Act 1969 gives the court power both to order blood tests and to designate the experts who shall do them.

Grouping tests can never *establish* a paternity; they may show that an alleged paternity is impossible. Using the full range of blood groups can now exclude 93 per cent of wrongly accused men. Naturally the larger the number of identifiable data examined, the greater the probability of exclusion. It is the addition of Gm Gc, haptoglobins, and the newer red-cell enzyme variants such as phosphoglucomutase (PGM) that has raised falsely accuseds' exclusion rate to over 90 per cent (Table 4.3).

Table 4.3 Percentage chance of exclusion by individual systems

Red cell antigens	
MNSs	32.1
Rh	28.0
ABO	17.6
Duffy	4.8
Kidd	4.5
Kell	3.3
Lutheran	3.3
Serum proteins	
Haptoglobin (Hp)	17.5
Gc	14.5
C3	14.2
Gm	6.5
Red cell enzymes	
Erythrocyte acid phosphatase (EAP)	21.0
Glutamate pyruvate transaminase (GPT)	19.0
Glycoxalase (Glo)	18.4
Phosphoglucomutase (PMG)	14.5
Esterase D (EsD)	9.0
Adenylate kinase (AK)	4.5
Adenosine deaminase (ADA)	4.5
6-Phosphogluconate dehydrogenase (6-GPD)	2.5
Total combined chance using all systems	93.0

Nickolls–Pereira test   A method of identifying dry stains, even when so tiny that ordinary methods of agglutination are useless, relies upon the principle of 'mixed agglutination'. The stained cloth fibrils are teased out in anti-A or anti-B sera, washed and then treated with test (indicator) A, B and O cells to detect the absorbed (or attached) aggluitnins, as shown by an adhesion of the indicator cell to appropriately soiled fibres.

Errors in grouping may arise owing to:

1. *Pseudoagglutination*, the result of aggregation or formation, usually from drying, or because the suspension is too concentrated.

2. *Cold agglutinins* of a non-specific character, due to working at too low a temperature. Heat agglutinins are of less importance.

3. *Low titre or weak agglutinogen*   The former is an obvious defect. The latter is likely to arise in testing for the subgroup A_2 and A_2B, the A_2 component of which is weak.

4. *Infancy*   The agglutinins are not present in the serum at birth, becoming developed during the first few months.

5. The difficulty of preparing good M and N sera; they are also unstable.

6. The presence of an extremely rare 'suppressor' gene (the 'Bombay gene') that suppresses A or B antigen, giving the blood an O reaction.

Absorption methods require considerable technical skill and should not be undertaken lightly; where the results are likely to carry grave consequences, the tests *must* be left to the expert, who is constantly performing such tasks and will be unlikely to commit the errors outlined above.

5
Types of injuries and wounds

The law of wounding

The code of conduct which has gradually come to be written as law from common usage since early times is called the *common law*. It has been added to by Acts of Parliament which has enacted *statutory law*. Both forms of law may be applied:

1. For the preservation of civil rights of individuals or of companies, in compensation for damage, in control of business, trade, etc.—*civil law*.

2. For the punishment of public offences and crimes, offences against the person, etc.—*criminal law*.

The student of forensic medicine need know very little of the intricacies of civil law in practice, but he must know something of several sections of criminal law—notably those dealing with assaults, wounding, homicide, sex offences and abortion—and these will be described briefly as the sections on these subjects are set out.

The terms 'injury' and 'wound' are used without any material difference of meaning except, perhaps, for injuries sustained by an assault with some weapon. It would be more natural to refer to a split eyebrow which resulted from a fall to the ground as an 'injury' and to one which followed from an assault with a beer bottle as a 'wound', but the distinction is unimportant in a medical sense.

The law on wounding is very clear, and the student should be familiar with it in its broad terms rather than in its precise legal wording: it is set out under the Offences Against the Person Act 1861 which in effect qualifies the older common law on killing.

Apart from 'assault', as from the throwing of a brick at a man, and 'battery', which would apply only if the brick hit the man, the law sets out certain classes of 'wounding', and, in the event of death within a year and a day, caused or accelerated by wounding, several types of homicide.

Wounding

1. Inflicting 'actual bodily harm' (common assault) or 'unlawfully and maliciously wounding or inflicting any grievous bodily harm', which includes harm suffered while trying to escape from threatened hurt.

2. To wound, or cause grievous bodily harm, or shoot at any person, or attempt to discharge a loaded firearm—'with intent to maim, disfigure, disable any person, or do other grievous bodily harm'.

3. By attempting 'to choke, suffocate, or strangle any person ... with intent to commit or assist any other person to commit any indictable offence'.

The law has never defined a 'wound', but any legal provision that 'the whole skin must be broken' plainly cannot hold.

In Scotland the word 'wound' is not used, any asssault upon another person constituting a crime at common law irrespective of injury being sustained. Any wounding merely aggravates the 'assault'.

Homicide

The killing of a person may be:

1. *Justifiable*—as in judicial execution, by a police officer suppressing riots, or effecting arrest; and in self-defence or defence of another person against a dangerous assault, or in preventing some crime such as rape or burglarious entry into a dwelling-house.

2. *Excusable*—as in self-defence or a sudden quarrel (a chance medley), or in defence of one's own home or family, or when it follows from some misadventure beyond the control of the accused, as following upon an operation of a lawful character, or from lawful and moderate punishment, or in sport such as boxing.

3. *Murder*—which is homicide accompanied by 'malice aforethought'. It must be unprovoked intent to cause death (or grievous bodily harm likely to cause death), or arise out of an attempt to resist an officer of justice, to avoid arrest or to escape from custody.

The Homicide Act 1957 abolished the concept of 'constructive malice'—unintended killing in the course of committing some other offence—previously regarded as murder. It designated certain types of murder as 'capital', meeting sentence of judicial execution. But the death penalty was abolished by the Murder (Abolition of Death Penalty) Act 1965 for a trial period, and this still operates.

The 1957 Act also defined 'impaired responsibility' (see p. 244), and this improved the older yardstick of the McNaghten Rules (see also p. 245), though not disposing of the defence of 'insanity'. Either defence might be put forward. A child under 10 is incapable in law.

'Wilful murder' requires the intent to kill, or a reckless indifference as to whether death ensues from the act, *except* where:

    (*a*) accused was insane, or suffering from diminished responsibility (see p. 244), (*b*) acting under gross provocation, or

(*c*) the act was part of a suicide pact, or

(*d*) the crime was infanticide.

4. *Manslaughter*—which is unlawful killing 'not amounting to murder' because:

(*a*) death was the unintended result of an unlawful act, e.g. a fight or an unlawful abortion, or

(*b*) death is caused by criminal negligence, as from the misuse of a firearm, or

(*c*) the killing was occasioned by gross provocation.

The older offence of manslaughter by dangerous driving has been replaced by Section I of the Road Traffic Act 1972 which makes it an offence punishable by a maximum of 5 years' imprisonment to 'cause the death of another person by the driving of a motor vehicle on a road recklessly, or at a speed or in a manner dangerous to the public'.

Most 'excusable' homicides are in practice treated as 'manslaughter' owing to absence of the intent to kill.

The degree of negligence required to bring any act of a doctor into the category of 'criminal negligence' is so gross that it rarely occurs except when the doctor is drunk and, in spite of this, operates, performs some obstetric procedure, or drives a car—and kills some person. A surgeon who negligently performs a 'colostomy' on a stomach, excises 20 cm of femoral artery in mistake for the vein, nibbles his way through the rear wall of the bladder doing a perurethral 'prostatectomy' during a New Year's Eve party, or excises bowel or prolapsed uterine vault in mistake for umbilical cord or placenta, is likely to place himself in jeopardy of a manslaughter charge—and, as in most of the cases quoted, is likely also to be drunk at the time. As a medical man is considered more capable than the layman of recognising his inability (because of drinking) to perform some act requiring skill and care, the fact that he was drunk at the time only aggravates the offence.

Types of wound

Abrasions

These are grazes of the skin, and although the fact that they are confined to the cuticle prevents their being grave or serious, there can be no question that they are among the most highly informative and forensically important of all injuries.

The skin may be injured by the direct impact or pressure of some object which, crushing the cuticle, stamps a reproduction of its shape and surface markings upon the skin. The noose in hanging (see Fig. 7.9), the bite of teeth (Fig. 5.1), the finger-nails in strangling (Fig. 5.2) or the impact of a weapon (Fig. 5.4) may all leave tell-tale marks of their shape.

Sometimes nail impressions are drawn away and long- or short-drawn scratches result. The depth and breadth of these may be compared with the nails of a suspect (in which blood may lie) and their direction will

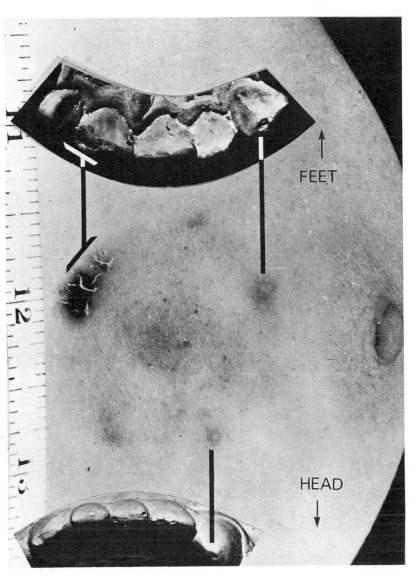

FEET

HEAD

Fig. 5.1 Scaled photographic comparison of bite-marks with models of upper and lower front teeth.

often show twisting or other evasive movements of the victim. Teeth may also leave a patterned bite-mark (see Fig. 5.1).

In a charge of murder (R. *v.* Loughans) a man accused of strangling a woman licensee at Portsmouth with a right hand (according to the interpretation of the medical evidence) produced a right hand deformed by the loss of three finger-tips. The reach of the thumb to stumps was, however, ample to effect the grip found, and scratches between the finger-marks were

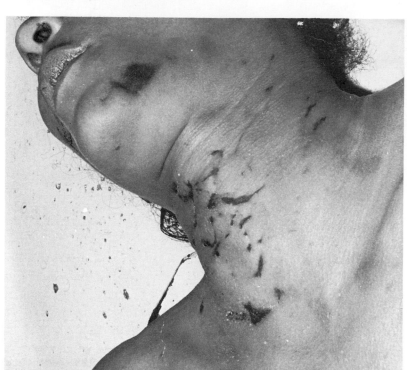

Fig. 5.2 Abrasions and bruises. Strangulation finger and finger-nail marks on the neck, together with abrasions on the lower lip, and under the chin, consistent with efforts to loosen the grip (left hand).

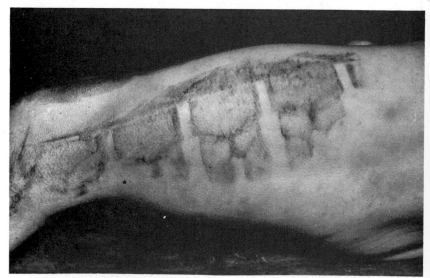

Fig. 5.3 Pattern of tyre crushed into the skin surface of a youth run over by a non-stop lorry—an important clue, to be photographed, preferably to scale.

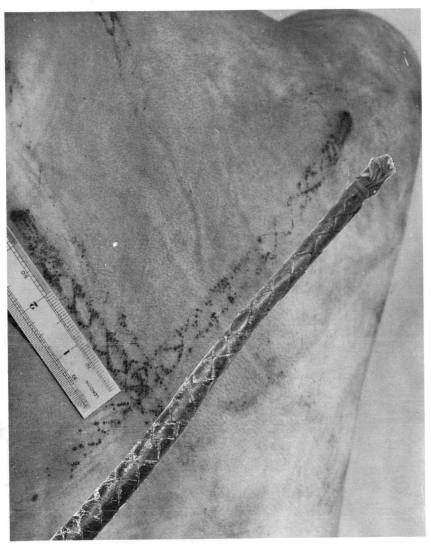

Fig. 5.4 Direct skin abrasion by whip. Reproduction of surface of switch with steel wire ferrule tip and diamond pattern leather finish used to whip girl bound and gagged in bed (R. *v.* Heath).

interpreted as the results of attempts by the victim to release herself from the strangling grip. Loughans first made a confession, then withdrew it, pleaded an alibi, and that the hand was too weak to strangle, but finally admitted his guilt.

When the abrasions result from grinding or sliding on the ground, as often occurs in street accidents, the direction of the slide may be important. It is shown by the presence of a bevel descent into the graze on the starting edge of the injury and of minute tags of cuticle-like fringes along the finishing edge. Any swerve in the motion is reflected in curving of the gritty lines of scratches. The distinction between direct impact impressions (Fig. 5.5) and the linear sliding abrasions following a fall to the ground is not difficult and should always be one of the primary aims of autopsy in a street accident, for it will form an unbiassed basis for a reconstruction of events by which witnesses' and a driver's statements may be corroborated or questioned.

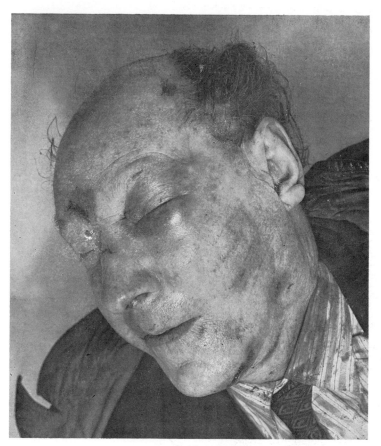

Fig. 5.5 Beat-up murder. Multiple facial and jaw injuries, including a 'black eye' and a jemmy-bar-shaped crush graze of the cheek.

Bruises (contusions)

These consist of spreading escapes of blood into the tissues from areas crushed by blunt injury. A blow from a fist or a fall against a piece of furniture may leave the cuticle apparently unharmed when, beneath the skin, the connective tissues have been crushed with sufficient violence to tear the capillaries and smaller veins coursing through them. Blood escaping from these will spread along any line of either traumatic or natural cleavage and the area will become discoloured purple. The shape of a bruise seldom gives an indication of the size of the object responsible for the injury. The toughness or flabbiness of the tissues bruised, their vascularity, the density of surrounding tissues, and the time lapsing, determine the rate of growth in the size of a bruise, and only where death can be said, from some other finding, to have supervened quickly can the shape of a bruise have any significance.

In the case of a girl pinned down by one soldier on a cricket ground in Kent while another raped her, death followed rapidly from asphyxia and a change in position on the part of the two assailants was effected after death: the second had intercourse when the girl, thought to have fainted, was in fact dead. Finger-marks on the throat and over the right thigh from pinning holds were unusually localised for this reason.

Bruising develops more easily in soft, vascular, lax tissues such as the eyelids than in tough and less vascular ones such as the palm of the hand or the sole of the foot. A boxer can 'harden' or 'toughen' himself to sustain, without bruising, blows which would leave an alcoholic 'black and blue'. Infants and old people bruise more easily than adolescents, or

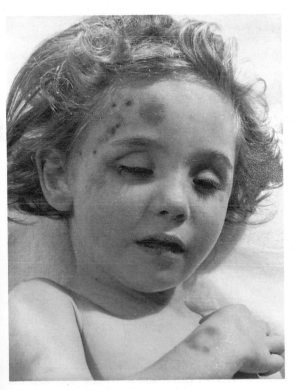

Fig. 5.6 Multiple bruises. Battered baby case showing head, arm and wrist injuries arousing suspicion of ill-treatment. (See also Fig. 11.9.)

a boxer in the prime of life. Diet and disease also have their effects on bleeding and clotting times, and may alter the consistency of the fats in supporting connective tissues; doctors must bear these facts in mind when expressing views on bruises.

Colour changes take place as the haemoglobin breaks down, and the bruise gradually fades as absorption of its pigment proceeds. From the crimson colour of fresh blood, a bruise passes during succeeding days through brown to a greenish yellow, and finally fades away from a pale straw colour. The length of time required for this varies a great deal according to the natural drainage of the part affected and the vitality of the circulation as a whole. For instance, bruises seldom resolve at all when situated under the dura, and are notoriously slow to resolve in the aged.

While the process of resolution is going on the bruise may shift as a whole under the influence of gravity. A bruise of the temple may sink down into the eye, and a deep bruise in the hip may, some days later, make its appearance at the knee.

For evidential purposes bruises are so variable owing to these many controlling factors that they are less reliable than, and seldom indeed as accurately informative as, abrasions.

It is sometimes asked whether bruises can be caused after death, and the answer can be in no doubt, for so long as fluid blood lies in the capillaries and veins any injury that crushes the vessels may free blood to percolate into surrounding fascial planes. After death, pressure of blood is only physical and the extent of blood spread can only be very limited. The problem does not arise often and should give little difficulty. It is very seldom difficult to distinguish between injuries with vital bleeding from a vehicle running over a live body, and the tearing and crushing of dead tissues.

Lacerations

These involve a splitting or tearing of the whole skin, and are likely to develop in company with surface grazes and deeper bruising. The extra force which splits the skin is usually aided by:

1. The projection and partial fixation of skin in certain areas over bony prominences, as over the skull, cheek, nose, elbows or knees. The skin is pinned and split on unyielding bone beneath.

2. A rolling grinding movement as when a vehicle runs over a body. Skin may be ground loose over underlying connective tissues or split where the tension by dragging or stretching exceeds the limits of its elasticity.

The edges of such splits are always ragged, as they have been literally torn apart from each other. Hair follicles and bulging fat cells lie along the edges of the wound (Fig. 5.7) and, under the skin, nerves and other more tough tissues, may be avulsed and hang loosely in the depths of the wound.

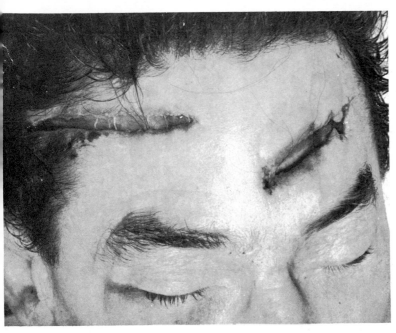

Fig. 5.7 Split lacerations of the brow caused by blows from a poker. Note the ragged character of the margins of the wound.

It is not difficult to distinguish between splits and incised wounds owing to the features just described. Local bruising is a feature of the split for the wound is really a blunt one, pinning and crushing rather than cutting into the tissues. A blow from an axe may crush only along a line, and the ragged splits from hammers and other blunt instruments on the head may be accompanied by only local bruising. When the victim survives a few hours, or tissues have been split apart, bruises may spread or become coalescent, and their significance must fade accordingly. Skull vault fractures may carry bruises away from initial sites of impact.

Lacerations are commonly seen in rape, where forcible entry splits and tears the hymen, or in indecent assaults upon young children, whose tight perineal tissues may suffer grave injury.

Blunt impact may split the skin over some local bony prominence so that a doctor mistakenly reports that death appears 'undoubtedly to have resulted from a bullet wound of the head'. A little more care reveals the true character of such injuries. In that case a woman had been struck more than once on the side of the head with a stool (subsequently burned) and, stripped of all clothing, had been sewn up inside four potato sacks and toppled from a bicycle into a stream. The case was one of murder and a misleading firearm diagnosis was a poor start for the criminal investigation which followed. (Luton sack murder. R. *v.* Manton.)

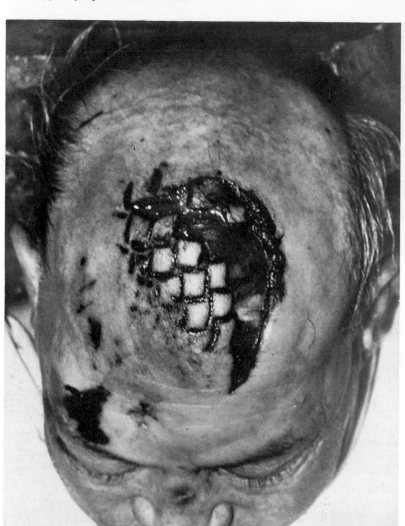

Fig. 5.8 Lacerated wound of high centre brow, raising suspicion of foul play. The 'squared' pattern crushed into the flap of skin that has been torn away matched the wire mat under the body. He had pitched downstairs on to it.

Incised wounds

These are made by cutting instruments, and may vary in sharpness according to the character of the weapon and the nature of the stroke made. For instance, a chopping blow with an axe causes a wound ragged enough to deserve the term 'cleft', whereas a cutting movement with a sharp razor (Fig. 5.11) effects a clean-cut surgical type of wound whose

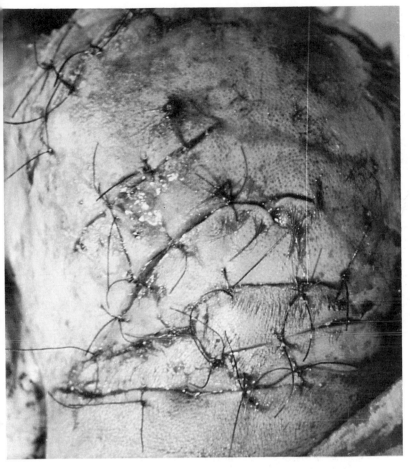

Fig. 5.9a A photograph produced by the police for the purpose of obtaining a pathologist's opinion as to the nature of a weapon used to assault a club watchman: the detail (after surgical repair) is useless for this purpose.

edges are sharp, and offer striking comparison with the split edges of a laceration.

Incised wounds are common both in suicide and in homicidal attacks, but the two forms differ in such striking respects that they must be considered in detail.

Suicidal incised wounds are of a classic pattern, certain to follow tradition whether or not the subject has read a treatise on forensic medicine. Let the student take a knife in his own hand and make some mock 'wounds' upon himself with the (imaginary) intent to take his life.

The would-be suicide is almost certain to do either of the following.

1. Make innumerable superficial stroking cuts over wrists and neck, and maybe also over chest, abdomen, groins or legs where he knows

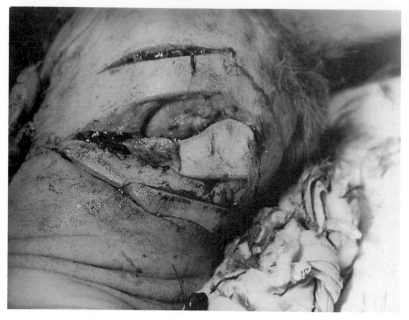

Fig. 5.9b The same head injuries before repair. The surgeon happened to have secured a photographic record before repair for his own purposes: excellent detail for opinion is available.

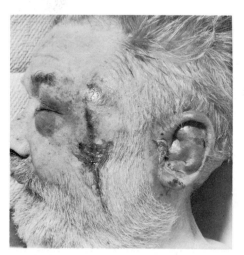

Fig. 5.10 Murder. Linear crush impression on cheek of man hit by piece of wood from door frame. The prominences of the temple and cheek have borne the brunt of injury and blood has spread into the eyelids.

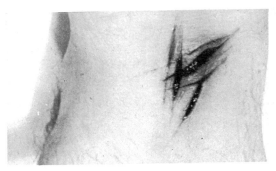

Fig. 5.11 Self-inflicted wounds of the left wrist by a razor. A series of tentative superficial wounds inflicted prior to a classic cut throat.

vital arteries lie. The strokes are 'finicky', deliberate but half-hearted, and for the most part merely divide skin. One case had 74 such wounds.

2. Cut the throat. This is a traditional suicidal method: the knife commences by several 'feeler' strokes of a 'tentative' character high up on the side of the neck opposite to the hand usually used—right- or left-handed on left or right sides respectively. Some six to twelve such 'tentative' scratches in the skin are common, set parallel to each other and close together (Fig. 5.12). One or more, commonly several, deep

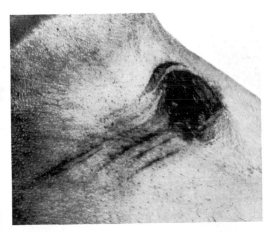

Fig. 5.12 Tentative suicidal incised wounds of the throat inflicted (right to left) by the left hand, starting superficially and deepening before withdrawal.

incised wounds then sweep across the neck, curving first down, then across the midline, then towards the opposite ear. The wound gradually deepens and then becomes shallow again, being sloped up towards the floor of the mouth throughout (Fig. 5.13).

It is remarkable how constantly suicides repeat the classic character of this wound: it almost always crosses the midline through the thyrohyoid ligament, and may be remarkably determined after the preliminary hesi-

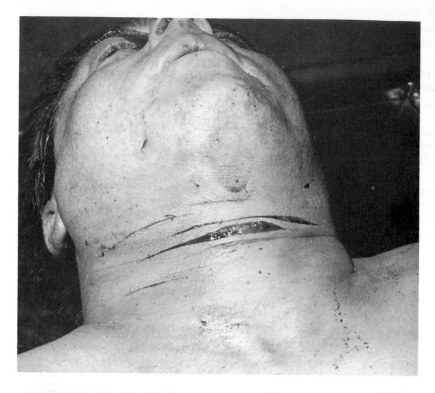

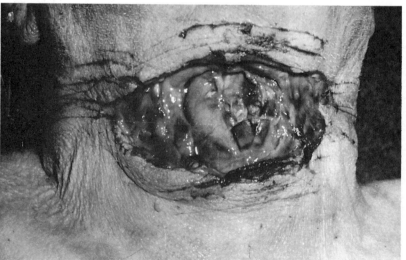

Fig. 5.13 Two examples of the classic suicidal cut throat. (*a*) is more superficial and tentative than (*b*).

tancy, cases often being seen in which everything from skin to spine has been severed, often with repeated hackings deep in the first principal wound. It has been known for a man virtually sever his head by transverse incisions of great width and depth—yet remain conscious enough to resist interference a few minutes after, kicking a St John's Ambulance man downstairs to sustain a Colles fracture.

As the head is usually tilted back before the wound is made, the carotid arteries, slipping back on each side of the spinal column, often escape injury, so that bleeding is venous and loss of consciousness slower. Air embolism may occur.

Homicidal incised wounds are so often directed to the throat that a

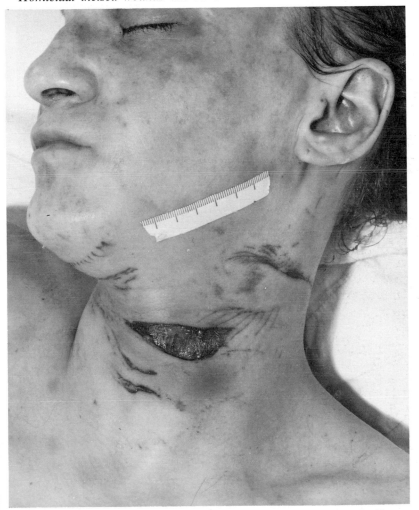

Fig. 5.14 Slashed cuts in a murderous assault with a saw-tooth bread-knife. They are widely spread, aiming at the vital part of the neck, but lacking the careful selectivity of the suicide.

comparison of their character with suicidal throat wounds will have practical importance. *Unless the victim is asleep they will present a slashed rather than a careful incised character*, often consisting of a group of wild slashes directed at the throat, but missing the precise elective situation of the suicidal wound. Even when the subject is asleep, drunk or drugged, the wounds have none of the tentative hesitancy of the self-inflicted cut throat; clean-cut wounds of a deep deliberate character (Fig. 5.14) are to be expected.

In comparison with suicidal cut throat, homicidal wounds:

1. lack the unhurried election of site;
2. lack the tentative scratches;
3. lie both higher and lower on the neck;
4. run in parallel straight lines, often diagonally;
5. deepen rapidly, often being slashed;
6. are not repeated in the depths of the principal wound;
7. slope back or downwards;
8. are often associated with protective injuries to the forearms or hands.

Consideration of the circumstances will enable the student to enumerate these differences. The cuts on the hands are also classic. The hand that holds the knife is often injured between thumb and forefinger, and may still hold the weapon, whereas the hand raised in protection is often cut across the gripping aspect of the palm (Fig. 5.15), or between the fingers, or across the forearm, wrist or knuckles.

Self-inflicted and homicidal incised wounds sometimes have a sexual flavour. The former are rare: the only self-inflicted penis wound I (KS) have seen was a self-performed amputation for a vast cancer. Erotic sex murders may be accompanied by injury to the sex organs, breasts, vulva, penis and scrotal sacs sometimes being slashed in a sadistic frenzy.

Stab wounds

These have a penetrating quality that the wounds so far described have lacked; it is their depth which acquires for them the descriptive 'stabbed', whatever the character of the surface wound of entry. Stabbing is a movement which may be made with sharp-pointed weapons such as knives and bayonets, or by blunter-pointed instruments such as pokers or closed scissors. The entry wound is a slit if the weapon is sharp-bladed with any kind of point, and it may sometimes be apparent from the slit whether a knife with single or double cutting edge was used. Rocking of the weapon or twisting of the victim may tear open such slits (Figs. 5.16 and 5.17) and repetition of a stab without complete withdrawal may 'double' the entry wound, so that opinion with regard to the width of the blade must be judged with great care. The deepest wound is a guide to the minimum length of the blade, and the least rocked or split entry to a deep stab can be taken as an approximate guide to the maximum

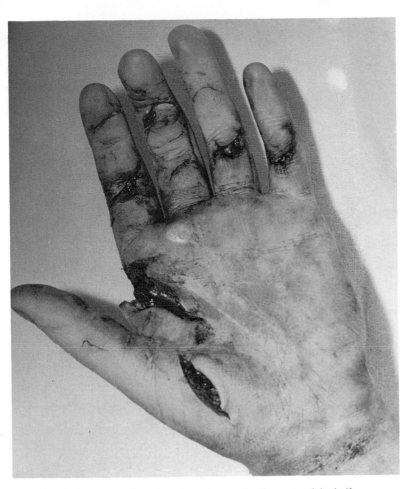

Fig. 5.15 'Defensive' slicing of the hand intervening in an attack by knife, attempting to ward off wounds.

width of the blade. When a stab is shallow only the point of the weapon may have entered, and no reliable information can be given as to the measurements of the weapon. Never insert a weapon alleged to have been used 'to see if it will fit', for it will at once become soiled with new blood.

Stab wounds with blunter instruments, such as pokers, closed scissors or chisels, tend to graze the cuticle, split as well as cleanly penetrate, and often bruise the ring of tissue surrounding the entry hole. The more blunt the point of the weapon the more likely is the entry hole to become a ragged, often cruciate, split.

It is the penetrating character of stab wounds which makes them so dangerous. The most vital injury may lie beneath a trivial-looking entry wound.

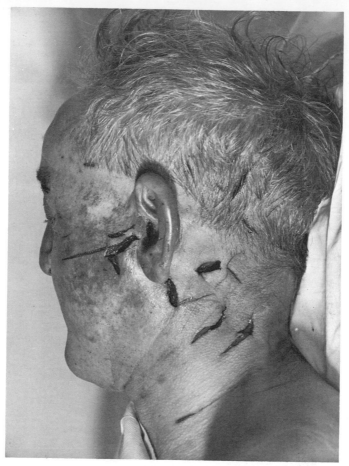

Fig. 5.16 Murder by stabbing. Some twelve stab wounds set close together on the left side of the head. Wounds inflicted with a bayonet with the victim held on the ground: some 'rocking' and change of direction are evident.

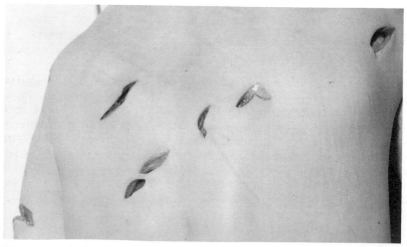

Fig. 5.17 Multiple stab wounds of the back, showing the effects of twisting and reinsertion of the knife.

A girl, sitting on a settee with her fiancé at a table, was taunting her sister, who was cutting bread with a table-knife on the opposite side of the table, with her lack of success in achieving boy friendship. The sister, exasperated, seized the knife and threw it hard across the table. Her victim had turned away her head, but the weapon buried 'a part of its blade' in her neck through an entry wound behind the ear. The knife was snatched out, but the girl fainted and died some 40 minutes later. The blade had penetrated under the floor of the skull, through the posterior auricular branch of the jugular vein (causing minor air embolism), passing through the neck muscles between the arches of the first and second cervical vertebrae (dividing vertebral artery and vein), to reach with the tip of the blade the very centre of the lower medulla. The gravity of this stab wound could not be conceived from the apparently trivial character of the entry slit.

Stabbed wounds are common to both suicide and homicide and, as with incised and slashed wounds, their features are so different that they must be separately described.

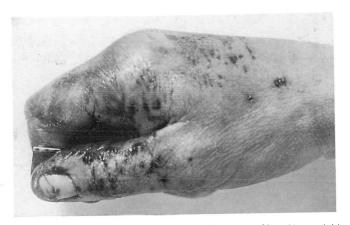

Fig. 5.18 *Post mortem* changes. Cadaveric spasm of hand in a suicide. A safety-razor blade is gripped tightly between thumb and first finger as at death.

When some penetrating weapon is used for suicide, the clothing is likely to be pulled aside and the way to some vital spot selected so as to avoid obstruction. The way to the heart, unlike homicidal stabbing, is sought under the ribs, in the 'pit' of the stomach, sometimes with trial 'feelers'.

A site even slightly removed from this 'elective' situation should arouse suspicion of homicide, and this even more so if the clothing is in place.

Stabs in the back (Fig. 5.19) are always certain to be homicidal, and when stab wounds are repeated in any part of the body, the larger the number the greater the certainty of murder.

Lastly, the hands (see Fig. 5.15) may be cut in attempts to ward off homicidal wounds, shielding or grasping the weapon.

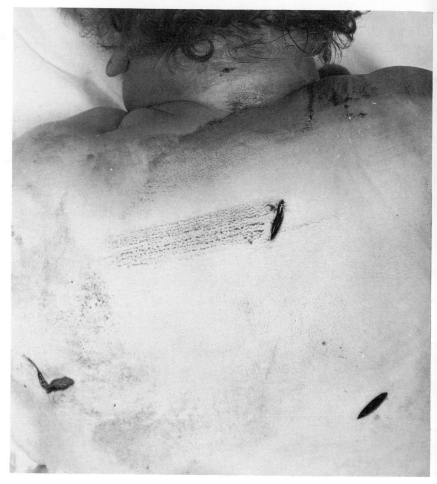

Fig. 5.19 Stab wounds of the back in murder. The lower right wound shows the features of a single-edged knife with a blunter upper end; the wound on the left is V-shaped due to twisting.

Wounds sustained by accident

Little can be said about these except that whereas suicidal and homicidal wounds follow certain traditional rules and recur, like the characteristic throat wound of suicide, with striking repetition of all the details, accident is just what the word itself implies—it is something unforeseen. It is not planned and does not, therefore, develop along orthodox lines. Accident may do anything, and the only rule which can be applied is that wounds which do not naturally conform to the types described are *likely* to have been accidental.

The immediate effects of wounds, shock and haemorrhage will naturally influence the ability of a victim to 'go on'—either inflicting or ward-ing off wounds—and also affect consciousness and the ability to move about. It is, however, exceedingly difficult, if not impossible, to say, even after seeing a wound, how long consciousness would remain, how long some voluntary movement could be made, and when death would have been likely to have occurred. There have been cases where a man survived five stab wounds of the chest, including two of the heart, where a man cut both jugular veins and many small vessels after taking a quantity of lysol, yet managed to climb three flights of 18 stairs each to leap from the flat roof of his tenement, and where a stab in the axilla caused death within a few seconds. Caution is the only guidance it is safe to give, and one's opinion should clearly be prefaced by the covering qualification:

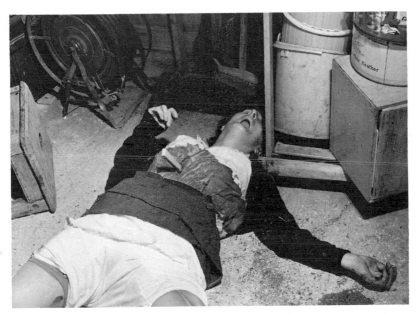

Fig. 5.20 Murder or suicide? The situation and direction of this single stab wound could fit either. The garden shed in which she lay was not locked, but the clue lay in a vice fixed to a work-bench above the stool seen on its side by her arm. It was set to the width of the knife handle she had deliberately impaled herself on the knife.

'It is *likely* that death will have taken place within a period of ...' etc. Nothing is certain with medicine and the variability of reaction to injury is astonishing. The circumstances often help to evaluate the medical findings.

A British Army soldier serving in Klagenfurt during the occupation of Germany was found dead, slumped in the easy-chair of his bedroom. He had been stabbed on the top of the left shoulder and through the heart: only the shoulder wound had bled externally and, as blood-stains led from the window-bay to the chair—some 3·5 metres—the prosecution argued that he had sustained the shoulder wound whilst by the window, made his way to the chair, and sustained the fatal wound into the heart as he sat there. The heart wound was likely—but not certain—to have caused instant incapacity, and it had only bled internally. A defence by wounding during a scuffle was not sustained, the charge of wilful murder by stabbing being found proven.

6

Firearm wounds

The study of firearms and ammunition—ballistics—is sufficiently complex to demand specialists. No doctor in ordinary practice will ever be asked to express, from inspection of a wound, weapon or bullet, more than an elementary opinion of matters which are properly the province of the firearm expert. Whenever the issue is a serious one, such an expert will undoubtedly be summoned to give technical assistance in the reconstruction of events.

But the doctor will be shown firearm wounds and must be prepared to recognise them, to define entry from exit wounds, to express some preliminary view as to range and direction, and to distinguish the characteristic features of suicide. He will also be expected to say whether a given weapon could have caused the wounds he found, and for this he must know something of the common types of firearm and be roughly familiar with their mechanism and fire-power. He cannot afford to be altogether ignorant of the subject.

Elements of ballistics

Types of firearms

Usually only small firearms are used for crimes of violence, and it is with these alone that the doctor need acquaint himself. There are two types:

1. In *smooth-bored weapons* the bore, or inside of the barrel, is perfectly smooth from end to end. The diameter of the bore may become narrower or 'choked' towards the muzzle, a design which holds the shot together longer. These weapons fire round lead pellets, usually scores of small lead shot of the kind used for specific gravity measurements, and are ordinarily used only for sporting purposes at ranges of under 50 metres.

2. In *rifled weapons* the bore is scored internally with a number of spiral 'grooves' which run parallel to each other, but twisted spirally, from breech to muzzle. The projecting ridges between these grooves are called 'lands'. Rifled arms fire a single bullet which is forced down the

barrel on discharge and given a spiral motion by the twist of the lands which grip—and mould—it, scoring a series of parallel lines on the body of the bullet. It thus acquires a gyroscopic steadiness, and may carry 'true' for over 1000 metres.

Smooth-bored weapons are called 'shotguns', a term which should be limited to firearms discharging shot, and are now all long-barrelled (guns). Their mechanism is designed to fire a cartridge loaded with lead pellets, and twin barrels, differently choked, are usually mounted side by side. The hammer which strikes the percussion cap on the base of the cartridge is an integral (usually internal) part of the breech block, and the weapon is made to 'break' or open on a hinge across the breech-facing so that the empty cartridge cases may be extracted or spring ejected (Fig. 6.1).

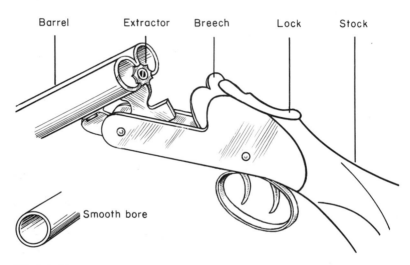

Barrel   Extractor   Breech   Lock   Stock

Smooth bore

Fig. 6.1 Diagram showing close-up details of twin-barrel (smooth-bore) shotgun revealed by 'breaking' the gun.

Rifled weapons may be either long-barrelled (rifles) or short-barrelled (pistols). The mechanism of these is designed to fire a succession of single bullets from live rounds fed into the firing chamber from a magazine. In the rifle this is a steel box clipped into the under-aspect of the breech, and in pistols it is either a similar spring-loaded magazine fitted into the interior of the butt (automatic pistol), or a revolving chamber (revolver) built into the barrel frame and turning to bring a fresh live round into line with the breech-face and barrel as the trigger is pulled (Fig. 6.2).

The rifle is designed for effective fire up to some 2000–3000 metres, using a cartridge with a long charge of powder and given a long barrel to enable the discharge to give the bullet a powerful 'send-off'. The pistol, built for close-range work, carries only up to some 350–550 metres. On discharge, the breech pressure in the rifle (and the force of discharge of flame and gases at the muzzle) may be as much as 20 tonnes,

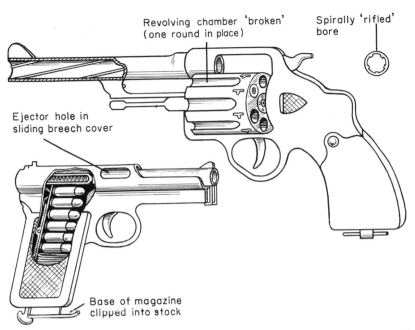

Revolving chamber 'broken'
(one round in place)

Spirally 'rifled'
bore

Ejector hole in
sliding breech cover

Base of magazine
clipped into stock

Fig. 6.2 Diagram showing general characteristics of the two common types of pistol, the 'revolver' (above) and the 'automatic' (below), each with rifled bore.

whereas in the pistol the smaller charge may only achieve some 4–6 tonnes. Either is sufficient to split clothing and skin and shatter underlying tissues, even bone.

The empty cartridge case may be extracted from the chamber by a bolt action, ejected by a cam mechanism on 'breaking' the weapon or, in automatic pistols, thrown out mechanically by an extractor operated by discharge gases. Such empty cases bear marks individual to the weapon which has fired them—from the chamber, hammer, breech-face and ejector. The expert can, by comparing a 'crime' shell-case with trial cases fired from a suspect weapon, say whether that weapon fired the 'crime' shell, for the innumerable scores and scratches imprinted on it are repeated every time a round is fired from the weapon. Any shell-case found either ejected at the scene, or still in the breech or chamber (see Fig. 6.14), must be preserved with care.

Calibre or gauge is measured by the internal dimension of the barrel and used to be given in decimals of an inch in Britain (e.g. .22, .303, .45 inch). The metric system is now in use (e.g. 6.35, 8.0, 9.3 mm). The dimension in the rifled weapon is measured between 'lands', not grooves. In smooth-bored shotguns the method of measuring calibre is the same up to a maximum of .5 inch (1.27 cm). Bores larger than this are expressed by a more old-fashioned method: the number of spherical balls of pure lead, each exactly fitting the inside of the barrel, which go to weigh one pound is given as a figure expressing the bore. If twelve go to the pound the weapon is called a 12-bore; a somewhat smaller bore, needing more shot to the pound, might give a figure of 20, an 'elephant' gun, a 6 or 8.

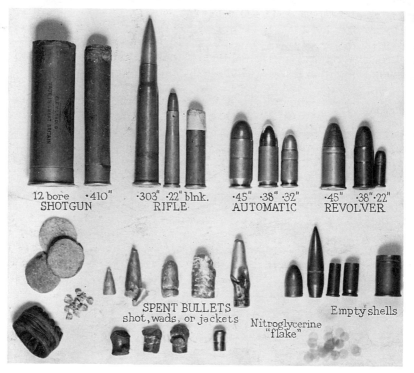

Fig. 6.3 Types of small firearm ammunition (above) and specimens of disc, wad, spent shot, bullets, shell-cases, etc., recovered from bodies or scenes of crime.

Cartridges consist of a cartridge case with a central firing cap at the base, the propellant powder, and the projectile, which is either a charge of shot or a bullet. The cartridge case is made of brass, or a brass base and plastic tube, with a plastic tube carrying the shot. In all except automatic pistol cases the base of the cartridge projects as a rim, ensuring that it does not move forward into the barrel on closing the weapon: it is upon this flange that the ejector obtains a grip. In automatic weapons the fit is by the taper, and there is a groove round the base for the extractor.

The cap contains a small amount of priming powder ignited by the heat generated by the sudden blow of the trigger hammer. This fires the main propellent charge which, burning all the way, drives the bullet or shot down the barrel. In the case of shot a flat disc or wad lies between the propellent and pellets, acting as a kind of piston driving them out bunched close together. The main charge ignites instantaneously with a bang, but is still burning on projection out of the muzzle, and still contains some particles of unburned powder. Hot explosive gases, flame, smoke, unburned powder and the projectile (bullet or wad and shot) all become shot out with tremendous force. At close ranges, say within 15 cm, all will cause injury to the body, giving the entry wound many special characteristics which the exit wound will lack.

Modern powders consist of nitroglycerine or nitrocellulose 'gelatinised' and often impregnated into gun-cotton or some other vehicle. 'Cordite' is nitroglycerine, gun-cotton and mineral jelly, cut as small sticks, often tubular. Many powders are chopped into flakes which the expert will recognise at sight. Unburnt particles of powder may remain adherent to clothing or skin, or are shot into it, forming a speckling called 'tattooing'.

Bullets consist of solid tin-hardened lead or, in modern ammunition, a core of lead covered by a jacket of tough cupronickel-coated steel or brass with cupronickel or gilding metal (nobeloy). Some cores are composite, containing an aluminium tip or softer nose, and packed with incendiary (phosphorus) or explosive charges, sometimes burning 'tracer' during flight. The bullet is held in the case by a grooved indentation round the neck—a cannelure.

If the student and doctor will familiarise themselves with these elementary ballistics they will not feel ignorant in dealing—even if only in an elementary way—with firearm wounds, with the cartridges and projectiles found during their examination, and with weapons handed to them. An understanding of the weapons and their projectiles is essential to the medico-legal interpretation of firearm wounds.

Characteristics of entry and exit wounds

The entry wound

At close quarters this is likely to bear the marks of everything which bursts with such explosive force out of the muzzle (Fig. 6.4). Its dimensions will vary with the calibre of the weapon.

A *'contact' wound* (Fig. 6.6) will be split, scorched (the hairs singed), maybe slightly blackened, and with the muzzle area alone soiled with particles of partly burned powder. The tissues beneath the skin will be bruised by blast and often blown away from their supporting structures. They may be tinted cherry-red by the carbon monoxide of the gases forced in. Up to 5–8 cm with a small weapon or as much as 12–15 cm with a larger one such as a rifle these features will continue, fading away until only tattooing remains.

A *near discharge* within arm's reach but over 15 cm, will show only a split entry hole and scattered tattooing by powder markings. The latter may be found up to arm's reach, about 1 metre (1 yard), a most fortunate coincidence from the viewpoint of reconstruction, as will be clear when considering self-inflicted wounds.

A *more distant discharge* anything over 60–90 cm from the body will remain the same for ranges up to some 55 (pistol) to 180 (rifle) metres (Fig. 6.8); the entry hole up to these ranges is split by 'tailwag' of the bullet before it settles down to a true gyroscopic 'nose-on' course.

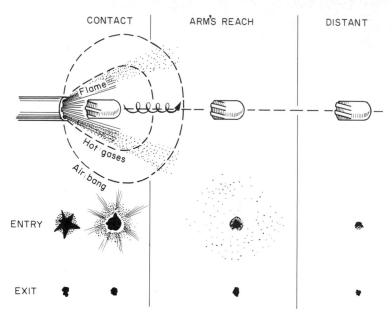

Fig. 6.4 Diagrammatic representation of effects of discharge of firearm with body surface in contact, up to arm's reach, and beyond. The character of the entry and exit wounds at these distances is shown below.

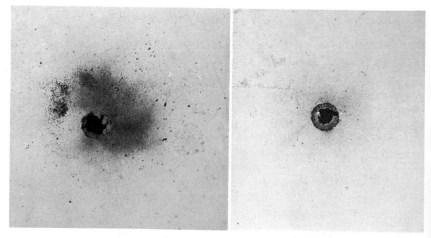

Fig. 6.5 Entry wounds of .22 rifle: left at 5-cm range; right at 20-cm range. The drilled in entry of the fast-spinning bullet and faint powder markings are both visible.

Entry wounds are also soiled by the spin of the bullet, which, revolving at 2000–3000 times per second, wipes its surface grime on the 'doormat' of the skin before passing into the body. The entry wound, even at ranges beyond 'tailwag' effects, still shows this tell-tale soiling.

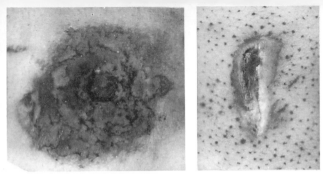

Fig. 6.6 Entry (left) and exit (right) wounds from contact discharge of a heavier weapon, a .303-inch service rifle. The bullet struck the spine and emerged sideways. The speckling around the exit is dried blood lying in the skin pores; it simulates tattooing, but washes off.

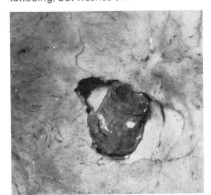

Fig. 6.7 Bullet lodged in skull—to be removed *with bone*, not dug out, owing to danger of spoiling rifle marks.

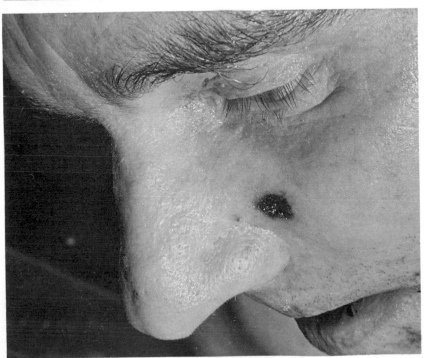

Fig. 6.8 Small-calibre bullet entry hole from outside powder marking range. When in the scalp, or covered by blood, such holes can easily escape detection.

The exit wound

On the contrary, the exit wound will show none of these features. It will consist merely of a hole in the skin—torn to a degree dependent upon the momentum of the bullet leaving the body, its lie (nose-on, wobbling, or turning over and over), and the amount of bone splinter it carries away with it.

In cases of distant wounding only the soiling ring may distinguish entry from exit, unless some deflection by striking bone gives away the bullet's direction. Where the momentum of the bullet is reduced as at the end of its course or after striking bone, there may be no exit wound.

At close range the entry wound, being split by blast, is larger than the exit, unless the bullet comes out sideways, or carrying bone with it. At more distant range the entry and exit are the same size (again unless the bullet is deflected by bone). Most extensive tears in the skin take place when splintered bone is carried out with the bullet at exit, and these may be mistaken for lacerated wounds due to blunt injury.

X-ray will facilitate a search for a 'lost' bullet, though patience in tracing its track will lead to the same end, and, further, show its course. The bullet must not be defaced in its recovery, or its rifling pattern will be spoiled.

The course of the projectile

This is traced by a line commencing at the entry wound and running into the body along the track of the missile so long as it continues on a straight course. As soon as the bullet meets dense tissue, such as bone, capable of deflecting it, the projectile may suffer a violent change of

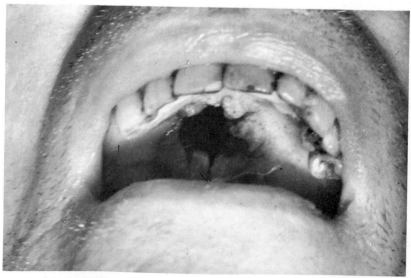

Fig. 6.9 Suicide. Very close (inside the mouth) discharge of .32-inch pistol, showing restricted powder markings.

direction. Portions of bullet jacket may be torn off in striking bone or teeth, and these may be flung in different directions. They are most damaging fragments.

Further evidence on direction may be obtained where a bullet has traversed bone, for in doing so it bores a hole which widens out. The exit side is almost always bevelled, the dimensions widening as the disintegrating force of the bullet spreads out into the bone. The skull shows this particularly well, but any wall of bone which is holed by a bullet shows the same tell-tale feature.

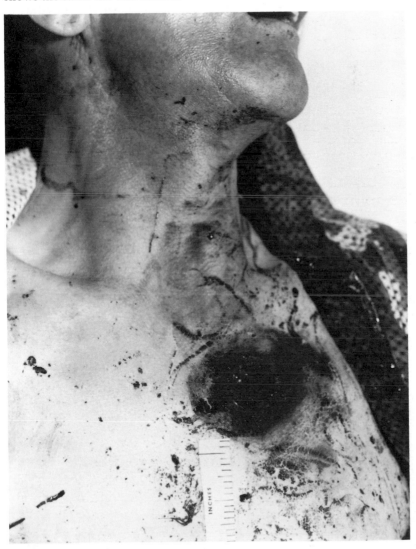

Fig. 6.10 Twelve-bore shotgun entry wound at close, but not contact, range. The victim was challenging an intruder carrying a sawn-off shotgun.

In one case seen, only a dry skeleton remained, a nest of rats having settled down round the body and eaten away all the soft tissues. The vault bone showed a bullet wound passing from the interior through the top of the head. The hard palate and skull base were shattered at the site of entry indicated by this direction. Such findings provided classic evidence of a suicidal act—in the site of election (the mouth), and in the direction of discharge.

Something more must be said of shotgun wounds with regard to range. The contact wound, though likely to be large and much disrupted owing to the large calibre of the popular 12-bore shotgun, differs in no material

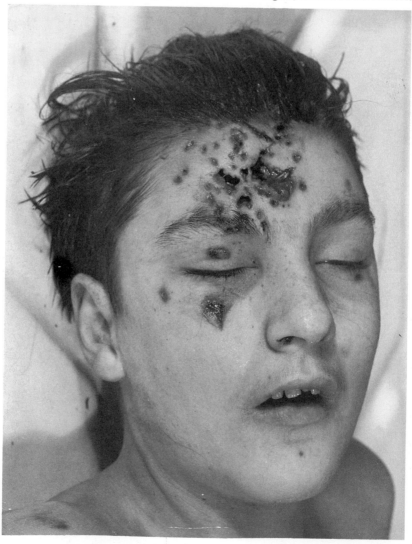

Fig. 6.11 A .410-inch shotgun wound at a range of 2.5–3 metres. The wad entered the skin below the eye. The main charge broke through the skull.

way from any other entry wound (Fig. 6.10). Unless the part of the body sustaining the force of the muzzle blast is split open, as is common only in head wounds, there is not likely to be an exit wound. The wads and lead pellets have little penetrating power and usually come to rest, spent, as soon as they meet any tough tissue, particularly bone.

A flat piece of bone which had been found on a country road by a police officer told almost the whole story of a suicidal wound. It was vault bone freshly blood-stained, and marked on its internal surface by a number of lead shot. Such conditions could only follow a shotgun wound sustained by placing the muzzle in the mouth (a common suicidal site of election) and blowing off the cranial vault. The body of a young man was found 14 metres off the road, lying on its back with a 12-bore shotgun across the legs gripped near the muzzle by the left hand. The face, brow and top of the head were split open by discharge through the roof of the mouth.

As the range increases, the charge of shot begins to spread, stray pellets coming to lie outside the main bunch of shot. At a range of as little as 2–2.5 metres the entry wound may show these marginal pellet holes, and over this range the spread in centimetres may be taken roughly as equal to two and a half to three times the distance in metres. Shot spread over 50 cm will have been fired from a range of about 18 metres. Much, of course, depends on the 'choking' of the bore, the narrowing near the muzzle which helps to keep shot together for a greater distance, and no exact opinion is possible until trial rounds are fired from a particular weapon. However, the shotgun does give this further information at ranges over the tattooing distance of about 1 metre, whereas

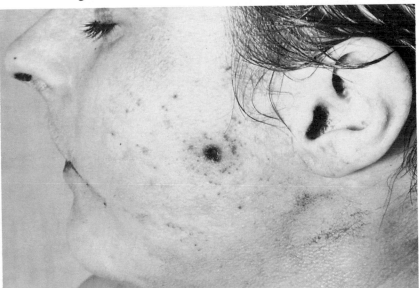

Fig. 6.12 A close discharge entry from a .32 pistol, showing a ring of powder 'tattooing'. A second entry wound—in the scalp above the ear—was seen only after blood was washed away.

even the expert is incapable of deciding the range for single bullet wounds between the extreme of tattooing and the last few score metres of the trajectory when the bullet has begun to 'stumble'. Some tail wobble, having a tearing effect owing to the lateral waves of pressure it sets up, may help to define the range up to some 55–75 metres with a pistol, and as much as 180 metres with a rifle. It is these lateral waves of pressure which may disrupt tissues so far around the actual track of a bullet. Thin plates of bone, such as orbit roofs, may crack when the bullet passes through the brain, and 'black eyes' may follow.

Reconstruction. Suicide, accident, murder

The principles outlined above will enable the inexpert to give sound and useful views on a firearm wound without delay—always a valuable asset to the police. It will be wise of the doctor to make it clear that these preliminary views on the type and calibre of the weapon and on range and direction are subject to the small corrections that a particular weapon may demand, and that he must be shown any firearm as soon as it is found.

The questions the doctor will be suspected to answer are:

1. Could the wound have been inflicted with that weapon?
2. At what range was it fired?
3. From what direction?
4. Could it have been *self*-inflicted?

The answers to the first three questions are based on the characteristics of wounds set out above; the last question becomes evident when the

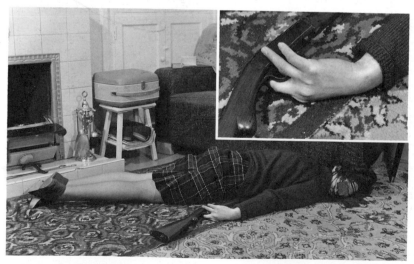

Fig. 6.13 Suicide by firearm, the finger still inside the trigger guard. Entry wound in 'elective' site behind the right temple, a very close discharge. *Insert*. Thumb still pressing on trigger after discharge and collapse from settee to floor. The use of a firearm is rare in women.

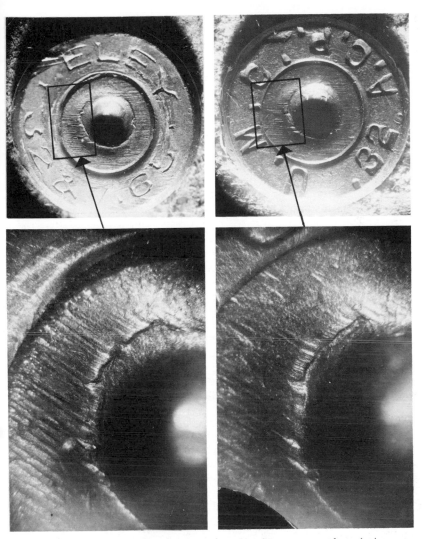

Fig. 6.14 Comparison of 'crime' cartridge (found on floor at scene of murder by shooting) with 'test' cartridge (fired from suspect weapon) showing identical breech-face markings.

first three have been settled. A wound can be self-inflicted only from a range within the subject's reach (except where some string or cord is rigged up to pull the trigger—when it will be found—the victim being neither desirous nor capable, after injury, of undoing his apparatus). This range is, for practical purposes, the limit also of tattooing (1 metre is about arm's reach), and within this range any kind of firearm wound is possibly self-inflicted, though as the length of the barrel of the weapon increases, so does the difficulty of reaching the trigger. A string trigger pull may be rigged up, or a pencil or a pen-holder, sometimes broken,

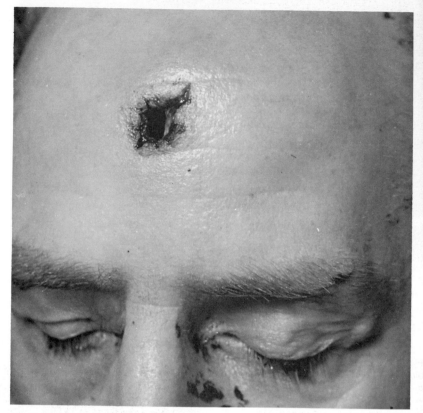

Fig. 6.15 Suicidal .32 pistol bullet wound in centre brow. The muzzle, pressed in contact, has pinned the force of discharge on to the scalp, splitting the entry wound.

may be found lying near the gun: it has been used to push away the trigger to fire the weapon. The significance of these objects may escape the inexperienced police officer, and the doctor should ask about them. The experienced police officer will probably remind the doctor of them.

Self-inflicted wounds of a deliberate suicidal character are almost always contact or virtually contact wounds. They have certain classic sites of election (see Figs. 6.9, 6.13, 6.15)—the right temple (or left in left-handed persons), centre brow, the roof of the mouth and over the heart. An entry wound situated off an elective site like that in Fig. 6.16, neither centre brow nor temple, or an entry in the face (never chosen by a suicide), or an inaccessible part such as the back of the body (Fig. 6.17), should always arouse suspicion of foul play. When, in addition, such a wound is inflicted from a range outside arm's reach, suspicion grows stronger.

Circumstantial evidence usually solves the problem of the single wound *not* bearing the stamp of suicide. It is rare for a suicide to be able

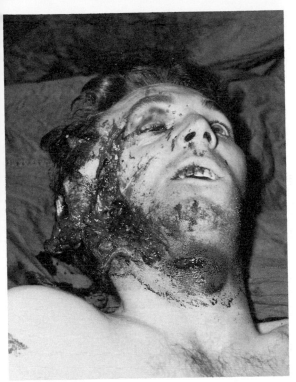

Fig. 6.16 Close-range suicidal wound beneath the chin, showing marked powder-blackening around the entrance. The slightly elliptical shape indicates that the direction of the blast was from the left side (confirmed by the large ragged exit wound on the right of the face).

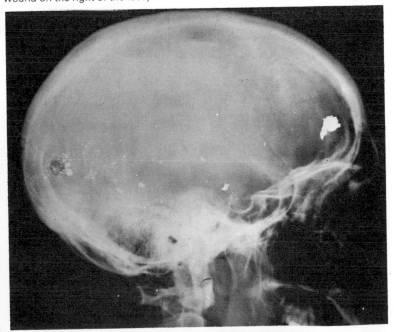

Fig. 6.17 X-ray showing track of .22-inch (6.35 mm) bullet through head from midline entry at back of head (left) to 'spent' bullet, deformed by passage through bone, in brow region.

to fire twice in any of his sites of election, for they are vital. Two or more wounds like those seen in Fig. 6.18 spell almost certain homicide. When any such entry wound is beyond reach, it can only be accidental or homicidal.

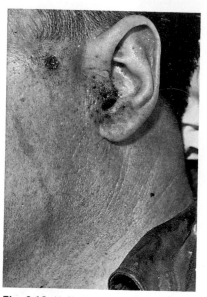 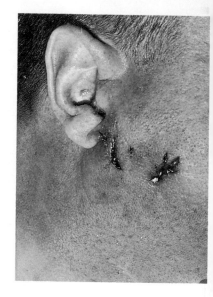

Fig. 6.18 (*left*) Entry wounds of two discharges from a .38 (6.68 mm) pistol at a range of about 10 cm (A6 murder). (*right*) Exit wounds in the same case. Bone has come through with the bullets, splitting the skin.

7
Asphyxia

The essential substance of asphyxia is the struggle to breathe against some kind of interference with respiratory movements (Fig. 7.1). Hypoxia or anoxia, a reduction in the oxygen tension in the blood and tissues, and cyanosis, due to accumulation of reduced haemoglobin and an increase of CO_2, rapidly ensue and, by stimulating the respiratory centre, quicken the struggle to breathe. In the turmoil that ensues cyanosis deepens, intense congestion develops and, unless the obstruction to respiration is removed, the veins become turgid, and showers of petechial haemorrhages begin to break out in the skin, under the conjunctivae, over the lungs and heart—anywhere that engorged capillaries find room to burst. These form a characteristic feature of asphyxia.

Many scientists also use the word asphyxia for forms of respiratory difficulty which do not arise from mere obstruction to the mechanics of breathing—conditions such as HCN poisoning in which the blood is carrying plenty of oxygen but the cell enzyme's capacity to use it has been poisoned, and CO poisoning where the oxygen-carrying capacity of the blood is cut down so drastically by the greater stability of Hb for CO. But these conditions are merely forms of hypoxia. Cyanosis, venous congestion and petechial haemorrhages are not features of these states, whereas they are common to all forms of interference with the mechanics of breathing. Forensic medicine is more concerned with such mechanics than with academic distinctions between types of anoxia, and when, as is undoubtedly so, the whole range of accidental and criminal forms of asphyxia—suffocation, choking, drowning, hanging, strangulation and 'traumatic' asphyxia—are strongly characterised by the features described above, there are strong reasons for groupong them together.

The development of fatal asphyxia passes through three phases:

Phase 1   Marked by hypoxia and slight cyanosis, accumulating CO_2, quickening and deepening of respirations.

Phase 2   Livid congestion develops from venous and capillary stagnation, and respirations become laboured. Petechiae break out, consciousness becomes confused, convulsions occur.

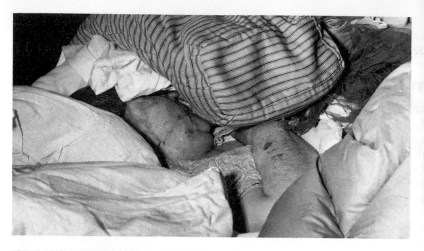

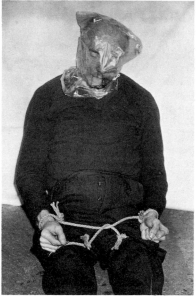

Fig. 7.1 (**a**) Murder by suffocation of old lady surprised in her bedroom by an intruder. The white top pillow and long bolster had been folded over her face to suppress her screams—but with fatal results.
(**b**) Unintentional suffocation inside a plastic bag placed over the head during masochistic exercise. The loosely bound wrists and thighs led to a loop encircling the scrotum.

Phase 3 Twitchings, decrease, respirations become infrequent, shallow, gasping, loss of consciousness is complete, and the pupils dilate; death ensues. Terminal vomiting is common.

The time factor in asphyxia

When asphyxia is uncomplicated and pursues these classic phases to a fatal termination, it is likely that some 2 or 3 minutes elapse before unconsciousness supervenes, and maybe 4–5 minutes before death takes place. It is not possible to state the lapse of time more exactly, for many factors in addition to simple mechanical interference with respiration are likely to operate. Struggling, by increasing the oxygen consumption, will hasten death.

Many happenings such as strangling, or immersion in water, which might precipitate such a course of events, terminate suddenly, often within a few seconds of their commencement, in quite unexpected death before the classic changes of asphyxia can become established. The reason for this is that a vagal inhibitory mechanism supervenes and its effects leave the face pale, lacking the classic changes of asphyxia.

A woman of 63 died suddenly 'the moment her husband put his hands on her neck—perhaps to threaten to strangle her'. Autopsy showed no evidence of asphyxia and the medical evidence for the prosecution went far to support the defence that death was sudden, unexpected and quite unintended.

Persons gripped by the neck in a struggle to effect a pinning hold often die unexpectedly in the passion of the moment, and autopsy may give good reason to believe that death ensued suddenly. Phrases such as 'I gripped her by the throat and she suddenly went limp' ... 'I tried to bring her round, but she was dead' afford good evidence of the rapidity with which death may occur. Asphyxial changes in such cases are of a trivial character, or absent altogether.

Many masochistic experiments in binding and hanging in erotic youths end tragically in sudden death as a cord slips and tightens on the neck. A vagal reflex may also cause sudden loss of consciousness so that death follows from asphyxia. Erotic self-suspensions, tying-up, gagging or 'experiments' with plastic bags may end unexpectedly quickly.

A boy of 15 who had been warned by his father to stop 'experiments in the unconscious world' was found nearly dead on a first occasion, quite dead on a second, suspended by a cord from the stair rail at his house. The changes of asphyxia were slight.

The hallmarks of masochistic activity, which may end fatally, include trasvestism and bondage (see Fig. 7.10).

A student of 18, dressed in girl's tights, a sweater, 'bra' and sponge 'falsies', was found dead on his bed. A plastic bag was tied with a slip-knot fairly tightly round the neck. There were only a few petechiae in the scalp.

Sudden deprivation of oxygen can initiate much the same reflex. Miners entering a zone of concentrated methane or workers entering an atmosphere of gas concentration may become instantly unconscious, and die within seconds unless the inhibitory reflex that arrests respiration is relieved. The reason for the suddenness of such deaths is not yet clear. The reserves of oxygen are slender, and struggling or convulsions may quickly use them up and thus shorten the course of events in a more classic asphyxia.

The intrusion of such factors into the causation of death may so shorten the course of events that reliable timing is a matter of great difficulty. My experience has suggested that although 15–20 seconds of a strong strangling or effective suffocating grip *can* dispose of a healthy adult while causing pronounced asphyxial changes showing this to be the main cause of death, several minutes is more usual.

> In cases examined from the great London Tube shelter disaster of 1943, several hundred persons hurrying down some ill-lit stairs to take shelter from an air-raid stumbled and fell into a vast heap of bodies, and autopsies showed that many factors—traumatic, mechanical, anoxic, vagal and asphyxial—had been operating in various degrees.

This question of time is of the greatest importance in law. When a grip must be held for several minutes to cause death, the court may reasonably think it a long and significant period. If the time can be as short as a few seconds and death may come as something of a surprise, then the intention of killing may well have been absent.

Post-mortem appearances in asphyxia

The outstanding features of all forms of asphyxial death are (1) intense venous congestion and cyanosis with pronounced lividity, and (2) the presence of innumerable petchial haemorrhages—in the skin and conjunctivae, and beneath the serous membranes of the lungs and heart. The degrees to which these may become developed at death may vary, but their presence is essential; if not established, the cause of death is certain to include other factors.

> Two children of 18 and 38 months were found dead in a pram concealed in the bushes at Bognor. Comparatively slight asphyxial changes were found, and, in the absence of signs of violence, attributed to suffocation. Their trivial character raised suspicion of an adjuvant factor, and later inquiry (and analysis) showed that each child had been given 6 or 7 carbromal tablets prior to suffocation.

The first feature, *cyanosis*, resulting from accumulation of reduced Hb in increasingly stagnant capillary and venous blood, becomes most pronounced where, for mechanical reasons, congestion has become most intense. In hanging and strangulation it is most marked in the head and neck above the level of constriction, and in traumatic asphyxia its lower level may indicate the site of pressure across the chest. In suffocation and choking it is more general in its distribution, and in drowning it is often less marked owing to the special conditions of this form of asphyxia. Such is the degree of peripheral stasis that in clear-cut cases the *post mortem* livid stains are pronounced, a deep cyanotic tint, and are sometimes coarsely spotted with asphyxial petechiae. When the subject lies on the face, suffocating, this lividity will be prounced over the front of the body, and the presence of white pressure marks over the nostrils and mouth, set in sharp relief against the livid background, may provide the only evidence of the cause of the asphyxia found. Hanging for some hours will, on the contrary, cause the lividity which might otherwise have been spread through the trunk to appear most strikingly in the legs.

The right side of the heart and the veins returning blood to it are, in asphyxia, turgid with dark blood, and an intense venous congestion and cyanosis become established in almost all organs.

The second feature, petechial haemorrhages, is a classic obsevation, and a striking characteristic of all forms of congestive asphyxia. Tardieu, the French police surgeon, who originally described them on the visceral pleura, has his name perpetuated in them, for it is as 'Tardieu spots' or petechiae that they are still described. This immortality was easily achieved, for they are a striking feature and common to all forms of true asphyxia. Indeed, without them it would be doubtful whether a diagnosis of asphyxia could be supported. They, like the livid stains, are most marked where, for mechanical reasons, capillary congestion is most pronounced. They appear commonly (Fig. 7.2) as a fine shower in the

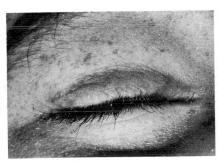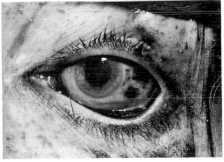

Fig. 7.2 Asphyxial petechiae in (*a*) the eyelids and (*b*) the conjunctiva in strangling.

scalp, brow and face in hanging and strangling, and in the zone above the level of compression in traumatic asphyxia. Where the capillaries are least firmly supported they are likely to be most numerous—as in the subconjunctival tissues and under the pleural and pericardial membranes; but they can appear almost anywhere if the degree of congestion and cyanosis is sufficient—in the substance of the brain, the lungs and the heart muscle, in mucous membranes of the glottis or pharynx, and, less commonly, in mesenteries and intestines, sometimes under the mucosa of the renal pelves. Vessels may burst in the eardrum and in the nose, causing bleeding, and the intense congestion of the lungs which causes frothed fluid to accumulate so quickly in the air passages may also include petechial blood.

Two factors are concerned in production of petechiae. One is simple mechanical obstruction to the venous return of blood from the parts, increasing capillary pressure to bursting-point. The second is hypoxia, which, by increasing the capillary permeability, encourages the escape of whole blood into the tissue spaces.

These features, varied a little according to the mechanics of the form of asphyxia in each case, will provide sound primary evidence that death was due to asphyxia.

One of the effects of asphyxia is to cause vomiting—a consequence of medullary hypoxia. As a result, the air passages may be filled *at the end of the asphyxial event* by inhaled vomit, the subject being already unconscious. It is important, especially in infants, that this finding should not tacitly be assumed to be the cause of the asphyxia: it is more likely to be the result.

Lastly, subjects cut down from hanging or infants relieved from strangling (e.g. by the cord) 'just in time' may nevertheless fail to regain consciousness—dying shortly after from the consequences of irreversible cerebral hypoxia—often with petechiae and oedema.

Suffocation and gagging

The purest forms of asphyxia are seen in suffocation by closure of the nostrils and mouth, as when the face is buried in bedding, or deliberately closed by gagging (Fig. 7.3). It is not essential that the mouth and nostrils should be completely closed at the start, for obstruction will increase as congestion develops, and saliva, mucus, oedema fluid and traces of blood will pour out into the mouth to further the obstruction to breathing. Indeed, aged and very young subjects may die although the mechanical cause of the obstruction is removed before they succumb. They cannot clear the bronchial tree of accumulated fluids soon enough to avert a fatal issue.

Epileptic and inebriated subjects are sometimes found dead face downwards with white pressure marks on nose and mouth or set in relief aginst the general lividity of the front of the body, giving evidence of suffocation whilst unconscious.

Infants provide a serious problem of the same kind: in the past the Registrar General's returns included disturbingly high figures for 'accidental mechanical suffocation' in infancy, but better criteria at autopsy and an understanding of the real complexity of the problem have caused a substantial reduction in these figures.

A better understanding of the obscure nature of the majority of 'sudden deaths in infancy', and the danger of assuming that the presence of many petechiae implies some mechanical obstruction to breathing, introduces an air of caution into the interpretation of such cases.

Gagging is a form of suffocation encountered in housebreaking and sex-adventure tragedies. It is a kind of asphyxiation which must have caused many a burglar and not a few rapists to find—to their dismay—

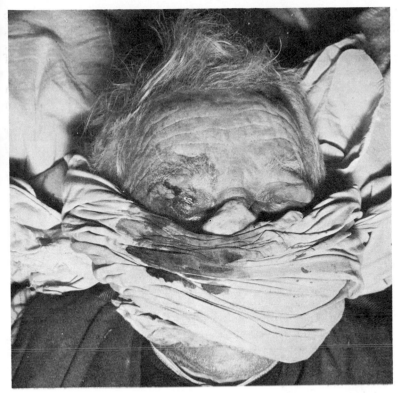

Fig. 7.3 Suffocation by gagging. Old shopkeeper found gagged and bound, face down, on bed above ransacked shop. A second tie and a mouth-plug were found under the cloth gag. The bleeding comes from a wound over the eye.

that a murder lay on their hands. Heath lay in this category (see Fig. 5.4).

A housebreaker at Maidenhead broke into a house packed with an elderly woman's accumulated 'treasures', and ransacked the place whilst the old lady sat bound and gagged on a chair downstairs. She was dead on his return, and before leaving the house he bundled her into a trunk. He was found at St Alban's a few days later, wearing a scarf belonging to his victim: he had left a tell-tale finger-print in the house and was convicted of murder.

An elderly grocer, surprised by two men, was left bound and gagged on his bed (Fig. 7.3), at Chertsey, whilst the till was rifled. He was dead when entry was forced next morning, a triple gag having caused suffocation—aided by saliva and mucus. His two assailants were convicted of murder.

Choking

As already mentioned, a death from choking may be so sudden that its nature is quite unknown until autopsy reveals something impacted in the air passages, usually across the glottis.

> After a New Year's Eve party four people tottered home the worse for drink. One, a man of 36, sank into a chair and appeared to fall asleep. Twenty minutes later he showed no response to an invitation to 'have another'. He was dead. Autopsy revealed a whole onion impacted in the glottis: he had not been seen to take one though a jar of onions was on the sideboard.

> In another case a child playing in the street ran away from an approaching car, but fell dead in the gutter. Autopsy revealed a toy balloon (which it was later said to have been blowing up) deflated and impacted in the larynx. In neither case was asphyxia developed, for death had occurred quite suddenly from vagal inhibition.

Where this reflex inhibition does not intervene, the classic signs of obstructive asphyxia will be developed at death.

'Choking' is the correct term for impaction of an unswallowed bolus of food or some other object that gets 'stuck in the throat'. The fouling of the glottis by vomit—such a very common terminal event—is better termed 'vomit fouling'. Drunkenness, drug-taking, head injury or partial asphyxiation often end this way.

Choking is, with the rarest exceptions, always accidental. It is most common in children and the aged—expecially if simple-minded and gluttonous, bolting the food without thought, or drunk.

> A mentally impaired child of 6 years died with the glottis completely blocked by a mass of unmasticated bread. The mother had watched it feed every day since infancy, cutting the food into small scraps for fear it would bolt too big a mouthful and choke. She had turned her back for a few seconds whilst the child sat eating some chopped brown bread. When she turned back it was blue in the face and making a few final choking attempts at breathing.

Immersion and drowning

The *post mortem* changes that develop when the dead body lies in water have already been described (on p. 14). This section is concerned with the process of drowning: it is by no means a simple asphyxiation due to filling the airways with water.

As in choking, death may also in immersion be precipitated by vagal inhibition originating in the nasopharynx or glottis. This was likely to have operated in the 'Brides in the Bath' deaths. Sudden immersion in very cold or very hot liquids may also cause immediate cessation of breathing and precipitate death by cardiorespiratory inhibition.

> A man who slipped off his barge in the Pool of London fully dressed, hat on head, into ice-cold water, showed no evidence of drowning, and a night-watchman who fell into a vat of scalding oil showed no signs of vital reaction to this. Both were healthy.

Where no such factor operates, the signs of drowning should be present. Fine froth will swell up out of the nostrils and mouth (Fig. 7.4), and it will seldom be tinged with blood, for intrapulmonary petechiae are uncommon when the lung is full of water. The same froth fills the glottis and main air passages, water descending deep into the principal bronchi and thrusting the residual air beyond it, causing gross overdistension of the lungs described as 'ballooning'. So compressed is the vascular bed of the lung owing to filling of the air passages with water and tense overdistension of the sacs with air, that there is little room for dilatation of the vessels, and few become distended enough to repture. Drowning is the one form of asphyxia in which Tardieu petechiae are almost always absent altogether.

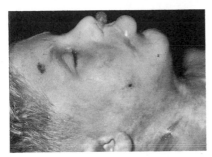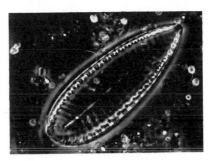

Fig. 7.4 (*left*) Characteristic fine froth at lips and nostrils. A sample must be obtained—and compared with a control from the water in which the body lay.
  (*right*) Laboratory microscope photograph of a minute diatomaceous organism. Many thousands of varieties exist.

During the agonal struggle to survive, air and water are likely to be gulped into the oesophagus, and both are usually found at the cardiac end of the stomach—sometimes with silt, weed or other foreign matter. Silt or grit will be found in samples of bronchial fluid to distinguish it from the fluid of acute pulmonary oedema, or beer or other fluids fouling the air passages, and microscopic diatomaceous matter rapidly enters the circulation in a live victim of drowning. Microscopy of spun acid digests of brain and bone marrow tissues will often provide this laboratory proof of immersion alive. A dead body thrown into the river shows no such changes, though water may run into the dead throat or upper air passages.

In the case of a woman strangled on the parapet of the new Waterloo Bridge whilst under construction, and who fell or was pushed over the then unrailed edge on to a river-bed exposed by low tide, there was no evidence of drowning though the body was, when found, half-floated by the rising water and rolling in it. She had died before the water covered her. A murder charge followed.

Drowning is not just an asphyxial event. Serious disturbances of fluid balance and blood chemistry ensue immediately upon inhalation of water. It if is highly salted, as is sea-water, an osmotic concentration of the blood in the capillary bed of the lung ensues, and its salt content rises. The chloride (or other electrolyte) concentration of blood returning to the left side of the heart is raised.

If, on the contrary, fresh river or bath water is inhaled, the circulating blood is diluted and electrolyte concentration is reduced. The red cells may swell or burst, and haemolysis may ensue. Chloride and potassium concentrations are initially lowered, but hyperkalaemia later ensures owing to haemolysis.

Swann and others have shown that fatal drowning in salt water is as

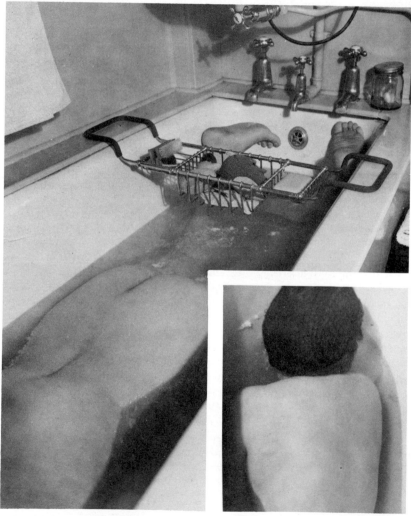

Fig. 7.5 Drowning. Woman face down, dead in domestic bath, alone in house. A bruise of the centre brow raised suspicion, but autopsy revealed a several-day-old infarct of the heart. Inhalation of water was terminal—on collapse.

much as four or five times slower than in fresh water—haemodilution being far more dangerous. These physical changes, like those of diatom absorption, can develop only when the victim is alive. Drowned persons may nevertheless be drugged, drunk or disabled by injury before immersion. Autopsy must be a searching one.

The sooner the body is recovered after drowning the better the evidence of drowning. When putrefaction is established the water in the air passages will have shifted, the lungs rotted with gases, and the chemistry of the blood disturbed. Only circulated diatoms in intact tissues may show the cause of death.

The classic changes of drowning may also be lacking when victims, weakened by exposure and cold, finally lose their will to survive and slip quietly into deep water.

Divers occasionally get into trouble from hyperventilation, from vertigo due to pressure changes, and from vomiting. The 'Valsalva manœuvre' known to physiologists may also be created by a long 'crawl' with fixed inspiration tending to promote peripheral venous pooling. Unconsciousness may supervene from central hypoxia.

Lastly, it must be remembered that rescue is no guarantee of survival: even if the hypoxia and electrolyte disturbances are reversed, pneumonitis may ensure from fouling of the lung by filthy water.

Suicide, accident and murder in drowning

These often present difficult problems. However the subject came to drown, the actual process of drowning will take much the same course. The bulk of the evidence which serves to distinguish one case from another will be circumstantial.

Epileptic subjects, or those who have collapsed for other reasons, may be found drowned in quite shallow water or in a bath, and accidental drowning may also befall those heavily affected by drink. The minor injuries which may be found as the result of collapse or fall under these circumstances must not be allowed to arouse suspicion of foul play.

Clothing often affords help. Persons found dead clothed in a swimsuit or entirely unclothed are likely to have been accidentally drowned, whereas persons recovered fully clothed may fall into any of the categories. A suicide may have filled the pockets with stones to ensure drowning. When the top clothes are left in a neat pile close to water, suicide is certain; indeed, a note will frequently have been left with the clothes. The hat is particularly tell-tale, for a suicide seldom leaps into water without tearing off his hat and any other clothing he feels may prevent him making a clean end of his life. He may tie his hands or feet together for fear he may lose his nerve and struggle to keep afloat.

A man tied a 5.6 kg (14 lb) weight round his waist and attached a floating buoy to which attention was drawn by a note pinned to the warehouse doors at the side of the dock into which he jumped.

Common sense also applies. During night-raids on London in the icy cold weather of February a nurse was noticed to have disappeared from ward duty at about 2 a.m. She was found only 15 minutes later, face down, dead of drowning in a bath filled with 'stone-cold' water. The act was clearly suicidal.

Those accidentally falling into water may, on the contrary, be not only fully clothed but likely also to wear the hat which may, by floating away, draw attention to the occurrence. Victims of accident may make despairing clutches to prevent their falling into water and objects may be found grasped in the hand (see Fig. 2.1b); or they may scratch and tear the hands or finger-tips. Minor injuries may be present in keeping with their having slipped and fallen. More serious injuries or ominous evidence of foul play will have to be present before a question of murder arises, and open verdicts, for lack of evidence, are common in persons 'found drowned'. The tight collar, it must be remembered, will cause a band of whitening constriction around the neck. Great care must be used in evaluating blunt injuries to the body, for they may be sustained by bumping into an obstruction or toppling over a wall or parapet, striking the body or head in falling, hitting craft or floating objects on immersion, or being struck or cut by the screws of small craft. Nothing short of injuries incapable of such an explanation would by themselves justify real suspicion.

Strangulation

This is one of the most fascinating chapters in forensic medicine, for with the comparatively rare exceptions of accidental strangling in revolving machinery, by driving bands or by clothing, and of suicidal strangulation by a ligature, strangling is a deliberate killing, usually by the bare hands. Strangulation by ligature or the hands is common in infanticide (see p. 167).

It is, of course, impossible to strangle oneself manually, for as unconsciousness supervenes the hands will relax and the grip will become released. With ligatures drawn round the neck the same argument applies except when wound round many times and tied or held tight by some mechanical device like a pencil used as a tourniquet twist, and wedged between jaw and collar-bone.

> In the 'chalk-pit' case, a man, lured to an address in Kensington, was set upon and died. Very little mark remained to show how, but an ill-defined line of constriction (as by rope or cord) encircled the neck, rising a little on one side: asphyxia had followed. Whether he was strangled, trussed, suspended or slumped in a chair remained in doubt. His body was dumped in a Surrey chalk-pit.

Strangling should be assumed to be homicidal until the contrary is shown to be more likely under the circumstances. Violent rape or plainly homicidal injuries are sometimes present to show the nature of the strangling. It may have been effected to facilitate rape, or to stifle cries for help during a robbery with violence. Indeed, death may not have been intended, for sudden vagal inhibition or cerebral anaemia may precipitate death from a grip which would not be capable of causing asphyxia. Prostitutes will say that their clients often 'nearly strangle' them, and deaths from strangling by the hands do occur in such circumstances. It will be for the pathologist to assist the lawyers to understand the mode of dying, and to fit the medical facts to the law as justly as possible. Criminal intent is what really matters.

The large majority of strangulations are effected by the hand, and it is likely that marks of the grip will be found on the neck (Fig. 7.6). They are not always distinct, nor is there always some kind of finger-nail impression or scratching to assist in locating them. But bruises of a finger-tip kind, small rounded bruises up to 1.2 cm (0.5 in) diameter, are common; if not sufficiently clear to define on the skin they may be revealed in the tissues immediately beneath. Curved nail impressions or tearing nail scratches, made either by the victim endeavouring to loosen the grip or by the gripping hand being torn away, are likely to be present on the skin.

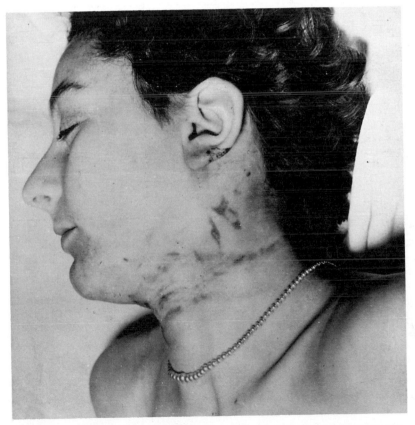

Fig. 7.6 Strangling by the hand and ligature. Nail marks from the repeated pressure of strangling fingers on the neck, together with the linear impression of of an encircling ligature (of electric flex).

The situation of these is important: a grip from a right hand, made from in front, will be likely to leave a thumb impression on the right side of deceased's neck, usually high up, often under the lower jaw over the cornu of the thyroid, and several finger-marks on the left side of the neck, from the counter-pressure of opposing fingers. These are usually a little lower down, lying in a line along the left side of the thyroid cartilage. It is important to remember that the grip may be relaxed and then reapplied, so repeating these marks—often with the fingers stretched a little farther round the neck.

Under pressure between thumb and fingers the voicebox is squeezed. Bruising may occur behind it as it is rubbed over the spine, and fractures are common, especially in elderly persons with calcified cartilages. The most frequent of these is a fracture of the superior cornu of the thyroid at its base; a little extravasation of blood around it, exposed by dissection, will serve to distinguish it from sesamoid joints in the cornu. It is strictly local pressure of a finger or thumb which causes this localised fracture, and only where the grip has been of great violence is it likely that more extensive fractures of hyoid and thyroid cornua and alae will be found. In one case of an assault with rape committed by a soldier upon a woman met causally in the street and dragged into a front garden, there were six fractures and most extensive bruising over and behind the voicebox. In twenty-five successive cases of manual strangulation fractures were present as follows:

None	1 thyroid cornu	2 thyroid cornua	Cornua and ala	Hyoid
2	17	3	2	1

In the Baptist church cellar murder, R. *v.* Dobkin, the victim, dismembered, burned, and buried for 15 months, had been strewn with builder's lime—which had preserved a solitary fracture of the superior cornu on the right side, together with adjacent soft tissues containing the dried blood which

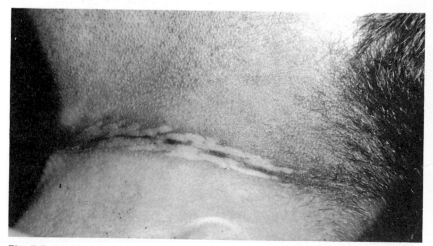

Fig. 7.7 Doubled-rope twist mark of constriction of the neck, with vital flushing of the skin.

showed that the injury had occurred in life. It was the strictly confined nature of this significant little fracture that justified the assertion that death was due to strangling with the hand.

Less frequently two hands are applied and thumb-marks are found on each side in front, with the marks of counter-pressure from fingers over the back of the neck: the skin here is thick and the tissues so tough that only very considerable violence will be likely to leave any mark. The hands may also be applied from behind, reversing these marks.

Strangulation with a ligature is rarely suicidal. Such deaths, though

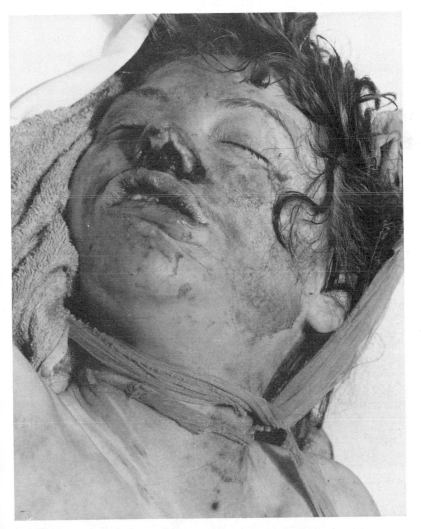

Fig. 7.8 Murder by strangulation with a nylon stocking. There are signs of resistance in scratches around the chin and near the tie in the neck. Nose-bleeding is common in asphyxiation.

nearly always homicidal, are not always intended by the assailant, for here, too, death may come suddenly. A scarf, rope, piece of bedding, strap or stocking is turned once or twice around the neck, drawn tight and—twisted or held or tied—is kept tight until death follows, usually in an extreme asphyxia. If there is no knot the ligature may subsequently come loose or be taken away, leaving only impressions.

> The body of a Polish woman was found hidden behind the hedge bordering the famous Wrotham Hill, Kent, 'beauty spot'. Broad cloth-type pressure marks were drying out brown in the skin across the front of the neck and asphyxial changes were present—but no ligature. It was later found that a lorry driver strangled her with a woollen vest held tight from behind.

The line of the tie is usually about the level of the mid-voicebox and is commonly uniform and horizontal, as distinct from the marks of a hanging ligature which lie higher, mark the skin deeply on one side, and rise to a suspension-point on the other.

Hanging

This form of asphyxial death, unlike strangling, is almost always suicidal. The ligature, which is placed loosely around the neck, becomes tightened as the body hangs or sags in it. Complete suspension is not essential, for death will inevitably take place so long as the noose is sufficiently tight to cause:

1. *vagal inhibition*—by pressure on the vagus sheath;
2. *cerebral anoxia*—by compression of the jugular veins (and rarely of the carotid arteries); or,
3. *asphyxia*—by lifting the glottis and tongue into the pharynx and obstructing the airways.

The neck breaks but rarely. Only where a drop with the noose already round the neck is suddenly ended by a jerking movement as the rope, or whatever it is, draws tight, may the cervical segments suffer a separation fracture or be dislocated obliquely. This is the method of judicial execution by hanging, where a drop of about 2–2.5 metres (6 ft 6 in to 7 ft 6 in) is arranged according to the weight of the subject. The cord gives way. The story that the odontoid process is tipped back into the cord, crushing it, is an 'old wives' tale' dating from older-fashioned methods of execution.

> In one interesting case a man who had cut his throat, opening the larynx and severing the local veins, bled freely and coughed and spluttered blood through his wound, but did not die. In great pain, he hanged himself on a tree by a rope. The noose lay at about the level of the hyoid so that breathing was still possible through the severed larynx. Death followed from cerebral anoxia due to compression of the neck vessels.

The level of tightening of the ligature is always much higher than in strangulation and less likely to encircle the neck horizontally. It is commonly set at about thyrohyoid level in front, rising to a suspension-point

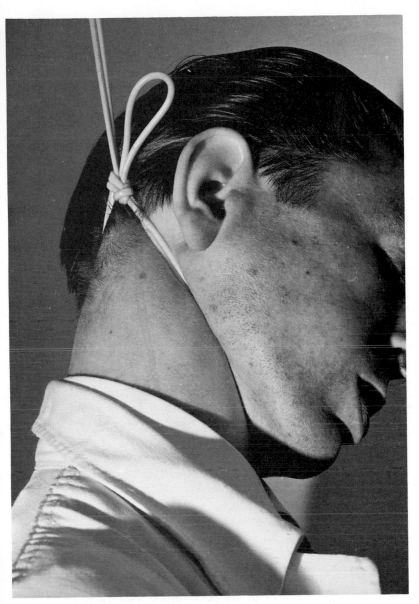

Fig. 7.9 Suicide by self-suspension. The doubled cord is 'slip' knotted so that the body weight draws it tighter. The 'open angle' is drawn up behind the right ear.

behind or under the ear on one or other side—or at the back of the head. The impression caused by the noose will naturally be deepest opposite the suspension point.

The usual autopsy changes of asphyxia may be present, congestion and cyanosis with petechiae being variably marked above the level of construction of the neck. This may bear the fine impression of the weave or cloth folds of the ligature. The skin later dries over these, causing the skin lines whitened by pressure to become brown. Small petechial haemorrhages often break out on the cuticle between folds of the ligature or in the flushed skin above it to give evidence of its application in life. The tongue, lifted up at its base and made turgid, may be protruded and the eyeballs prominent. Fractures of the bones of the voicebox are most commonly limited to the cornua of the thyroid. The pale lines of collar impressions, set in relief against the livid stains of skin, and the natural folds of skin, especially the deep creases of podgy babies, must not be confused with ligature marks.

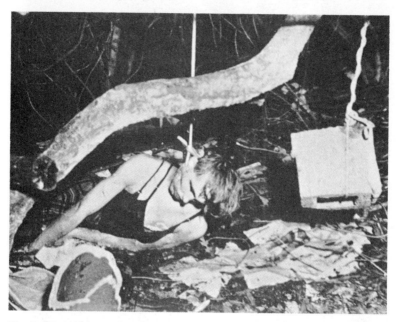

Fig. 7.10 Accidental death during masochistic exercise: a youth dressed in female attire, suspended from the neck by a counterpoising weight slung over a bough in a wood. Erotic literature lies on the ground.

Exceptions to suicidal hanging occur in young men as mishaps during experimental tying-up or suspension for the masochistic enjoyment of simple restraint or pain, or in sex perversions. Such subjects are often found naked, or may be clothed in women's attire, chained, padlocked, bound with straps or adhesive plaster, and found with pin-up types of alluring female nudes set out within view. Girls do not indulge in this dangerous perversion.

A naked youth was found in a lavatory hanging half off the edge of the seat, the penis turgid and dribbling semen, suspended from the neck by a rope to the inlet pipe of the cistern above. Several front-page nudes from a picture newspaper were laid out in a half-ring in front of him on the floor. Death was due to vagal inhibition and must have taken place suddenly, without warning.

These cases must not be mistaken for suicides; they are misadventures—the verdict used by the coroner.

Only one other form of accidental hanging is seen: infants wearing restraining apparatus may wriggle partly out of it and become asphyxiated by its tightening around their neck as they try to crawl away or fall over the side of the bed. The neck or a part of one shoulder and the neck may be found constricted.

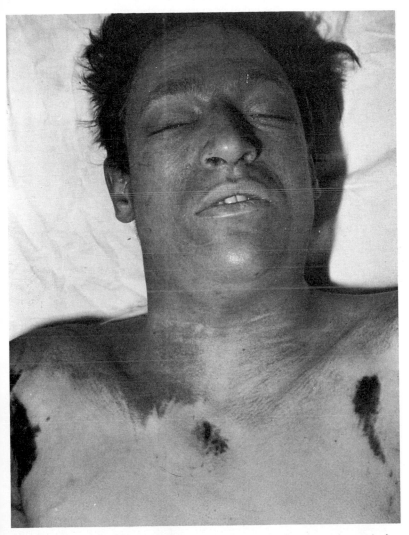

Fig. 7.11 Traumatic asphyxia. Crushing chest injury, pinning the neck vessels; face suffused and cyanosed.

Traumatic asphyxia

This is a form of asphyxia which is seen most clearly in heavy roll crushes of the chest or upper abdomen and chest, as in slow running-over by heavy vehicles or pinning and crushing beneath weights. Pinning alive must be maintained for some seconds for its full effects to develop.

A tractor levelling out a field was rocking itself in reverse and forward against a convenient lump in the ground, and had done three such movements when the driver decided to make a note of this spot for future use. It was a tramp who had lain asleep in the hedge, and had thrice, thus, been roll-crushed by the tractor. The entire chest was buckled and heavily crushed, the tractor wheels having run up across it obliquely from below. The head, neck and shoulders were deep violet, and shot with coarse and fine haemorrhages into the skin.

The classic features of traumatic asphyxia are due to simple mechanical pressure causing the compression of blood under increasing tension in the veins of the head and neck, reaching bursting point, and at the same time preventing breathing. The classic Burke and Hare murders in Edinburgh, designed to supply much-needed bodies for anatomical dissection, provided examples of mixed suffocation and traumatic asphyxia, Burke sitting on the chests of their inebriated victims covering their mouth and nostrils while Hare pulled them round the room by their feet.

8
Regional injury

The medico-legal aspects of blunt injuries to the head, spine, chest and abdomen are so important, and their correct interpretation so vital to accurate reconstruction, that attention will be devoted to them at the expense of setting out an encyclopaedia of blunt injuries to all parts of the body, many of which have little more than surgical interest.

Head injuries

Some knowledge of the mechanics of force and of the architecture of the skull and its content of brain are essential to a clear understanding of head injuries.

The amount of injury a blow can cause to an object it strikes depends upon both its weight and its velocity; this power, called the kinetic energy, is resolved thus:

$$\text{Kinetic energy} = \frac{m(\text{ass}) \times v^2(\text{elocity})}{2}$$

A prod from an iron crowbar is effective chiefly because of the weight of the weapon, and an impact from a bullet because of its velocity. The latter's influence is the greater, being squared. The other factors concerned are:

1. the extent to which the tissues can absorb the momentum of the object striking them; and
2. the movement as a whole of the part that is struck.

Local absorption of kinetic energy

The effect of a blow also depends upon the size of the area bearing the weight of impact. When it is all absorbed into a small area, as with a bullet wound, much of the tissue may disintegrate, the skin, soft tissues, even bone, disrupting along the track of the missile. Disintegrated fragments will become scattered in the neighbourhood to an extent depending upon their newly acquired momentum. Fragments of splintered bone may sometimes be found scattered through the brain when a sharp local impact has dislodged them from the skull vault, even though the object striking the head does not itself enter the cranium.

Skull injuries   As the energy of a blow is being absorbed the skull disintegrates in a characteristic way. The outer table of the skull gives way over an area corresponding often very closely with the shape of the body striking it (Fig. 8.1). It is thrust into the diploë, which is compressed

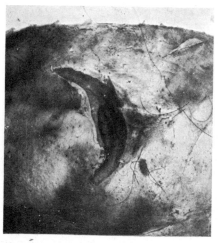

Fig. 8.1 Significantly shaped depressed fracture of vault of skull sustained by a workman who fell, head down, from a scaffolding on to the top of an upright member of the tubular steel scaffold frame.

then shattered. The force, by now spreading into surrounding bone, becomes borne by the inner table which bulges, then gives way over an area rather larger than that in the outer table. As a result any hole is bevel-edged, larger on its exit aspect: any shaped fracture is best studied at the point of impact on the outer surface (Fig. 8.3).

Secondary fissures run into the surrounding bone (Fig. 8.4), mainly away from the direction of the force—indicating the direction from which the blow has been struck—and along routes dictated to some extent by the architecture of the skull.

Broad impacts to the vault send multiple fissures radiating away from the main site of the blow. These are sometimes equally numerous and extensive in all directions as from direct impact at right angles, and in addition, occasionally show concentric ring fractures. Sometimes, as the direction of the blow becomes more angular, longer fissures run in one direction more than in another (see Fig. 8.4). These fissures develop along the lines through which the force is dissipating itself into the skull and away from its source. As they reach the sides of the vault and turn down towards the base they become directed into channels between the thicker buttresses of the floor of the skull. These buttresses are mid-

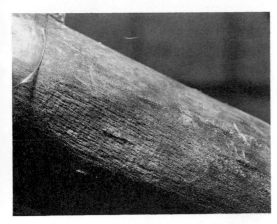

Fig. 8.2a Mark of cloth cap on ash stake found near murdered man, struck on head with blunt weapon

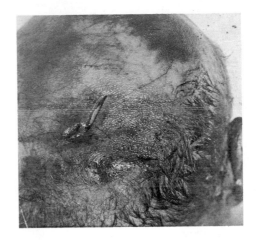

Fig. 8.2b Relatively slight surface wound on scalp—split on skull beneath.

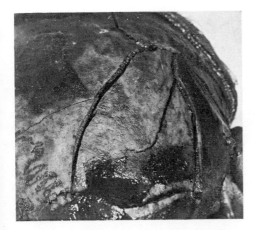

Fig. 8.2c Shaped fracture of skull vault, indicating approximate width of blunt weapon and slope of blow struck from behind.

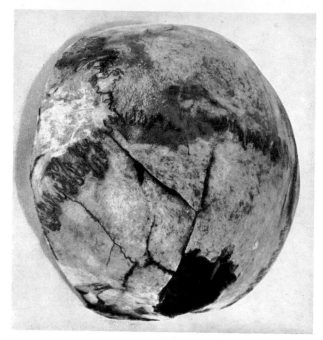

Fig. 8.3 Depressed fracture of skull from child murdered by beating on head with butt (stock) of a service rifle. The local sutures are loosened.

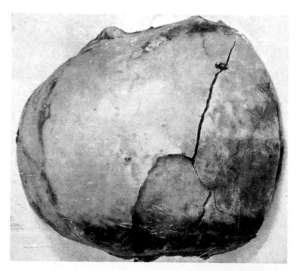

Fig. 8.4 Fracture of skull showing significant shaping of depressed area bearing brunt of impact, and main fissure running away along principal line of force.

frontal, mid-occipital, sphenoid wing and petrous processes on each side. They are exceedingly strong as compared with the plates of bone intervening, and lines of fractiure will usually:

1. course down the sutures or through the thinner bone between the buttresses; or
2. encircle the ring base of the occiput; or
3. cross the base in front of the petrous bones, side to side.

In order to cause this ring base type of fracture, the violence applied must either force the head down as a whole on the spine, as when a sack of grain falls vertically on the head (or the subject pitches on to the head), or, conversely, thrust the spine up into the skull, as when the

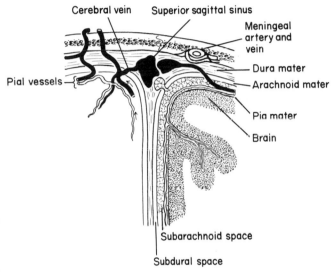

Fig. 8.5 A coronal section through the vault of the head, showing relation of skull to membranes and brain (after Gray).

subject falls vertically on to the buttocks or heels. A heavy blow directed underneath the occiput or the chin may occasionally do the same, lifting the skull from the spine violently enough to break it away from its strong ring base attachments.

The brain and its covering membranes are commonly injured locally, and it will be well to consider these local effects before discussing the more general effects of movements of the head as a whole.

Membrane injuries are common and have a very great forensic interest. Whether or not fracture of the skull takes place, injury may tear the membranes and cause intracranial haemorrhage. accumulating in the epi- or subdural or subarachnoid spaces according to its source.

Extra(epi)dural bleeding occurs both with and without fracture, and is commonest in youth. The sites are elected by the position of the principal (extra) dural arteries, more commonly the middle (54 per cent) or posterior (21 per cent) meningeal arteries. Haemorrhage is started by the tearing or splitting of one of these vessels by violent transmitted force, as with a boxing punch on the chin, or a local blow, or by fracture crossing the line of the artery (Fig. 8.6). The dura is lifted locally by the rising pressure of blood, bulging into the interior of the skull cavity and displacing the brain. Intracranial tension is increased.

A 'latent period', during which this blood accumulates, occurs in two-thirds of the cases. After the head injury has merely dazed or temporarily concussed the subject, an initial 'recovery' appears to take place. This may last long enough to cover the period of some further activity which may mislead lay persons as to the actual cause of the haemorrhage.

> A man fell from his bicycle on to a concrete path, but appeared to suffer no immediate harm other than bruising of the scalp. Some 2 hours later during drinks at a public-house to which the deceased had walked, he grew quarrelsome and ended by fighting another man, exchanging only several blows of little weight—all to the face and chest—before collapsing and dying. Autopsy showed a clot of about 100 ml (3½ oz) accumulated beneath a fractured skull at the site of the bruise due to the fall from the bicycle. The circumstances had naturally appeared to the police to throw responsibility on his adversary at the public-house.

Subdural bleeding is rarely purely subdural, though tearing of perforating veins over the vertex or of one of the venous sinuses by a fracture may limit it so. More often it is associated with subarachnoid haemorrhage. One striking 'latent' form of subdural haemorrhage which has come to be recognised as invariably traumatic in origin is the subdural haematoma, or blood cyst. It is most commonly seen over the cerebral cortex and undoubtedly develops by leakage from torn perforating dural veins which lie in this region. Leary has pointed out that comparatively slight blunt head injury may, especially in the elderly, tear these veins, but as leakage of blood is slow the symptoms of a grave mishap may not develop and it may be at autopsy after a long and uneventful life that evidence of such trauma comes to light. The subdural space has no mesothelial lining and can do very little to resolve blood clot. It remains much the same for months or years, except for ageing of pigment and a gradual thickening of the encysting membrane. It can enlarge if bleeding recurs from mural capillaries, but rarely does so.

It is remarkable how rarely any symptom complex follows from the development of these subdural cysts: the elderly, in whom they occur so much more commonly, are merely a little more confused and forgetful than before.

Subarachnoid bleeding is, unlike other membrane haemorrhages, more likely to be due to natural causes than to trauma. Common causes are listed in Table 8.1.

The most easily missed cause is the developmental (congenital) aneurism, for it may be no more than a pinhead swelling. Symonds reported 41 out of 124 published cases of spontaneous subarachnoid haemorrhage

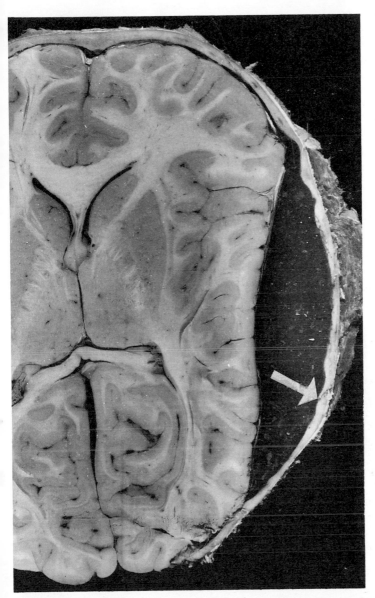

Fig. 8.6 Fracture (arrowed) of the temporal bone, tearing the middle meningeal artery and causing extradural haemorrhage. Boy struck on the head with brick, apparently little hurt, lapsing into unconsciousness 4 hours later.

Table 8.1

Natural causes	Traumatic forms
Ruptured developmental aneurysm	Contusion or laceration of brain
Ruptured atheromatous arteries	Explosive blast
Leaking cerebral haemorrhage	Trauma to the vertebral artery
Purpuric states, leukaemia, etc	Blunt injury to neck

in which the cause remained undiscovered. Detection of these small aneurysms demands the most painstaking dissection, but this usually brings its reward: their finding may, for instance, absolve a suspect from responsibility.

> An ageing father, fighting with his son, struck several well-directed but comparatively light blows with his fists, and then had the mortification of seeing the younger man collapse and die. A ruptured developmental aneurysm was found at autopsy, and the father was discharged after a sympathetic police court hearing at which the probability of spontaneous rupture, especially on exertion or excitement, was explained.

Subarachnoid bleeding in the brain stem region can also result from hard blows such as 'chopper cuts' with the side of the hand across the

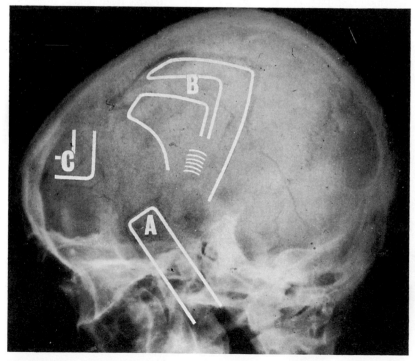

Fig. 8.7 Head injuries. Three skull fractures (said to have resulted from fall of boulder from a height into mine shaft) fitting a wrench found at the scene, suggested an assault.

back of the neck. Failure to find a local cause such as an aneurysm or angioma should arouse suspicion of injury—possibly of foul play.

The brain may be locally bruised or torn by penetrating force. It may also suffer more diffuse jolting, and this is the cause of concussion. Little may be seen by the naked eye, but microscopy may show fatal perivascular haemorrhage and neuron damage. Repeated injuries of this kind, as in boxing, may cause the progressive deterioration known as 'punch drunk'.

Epilepsy ensues in some 10 per cent of all blunt head injuries admitted to hospital, and, of these, about a half start to have fits within the first year. 'Open' head injury is more liable.

Movement of the head as a whole

Much more complex brain injuries follow from the sudden absorption of force as a result of which the head is either suddenly displaced or suddenly brought to a stop *as a whole*. The whole concept of injury of a more general kind to the brain was elucidated by some experimental work on the mechanics of head injury by Holbourn, an Oxford research physicist (1941). The principal physical facts are:

1. The adult skull is a very rigid structure; unless fractured it does not change shape. The brain, though not easily compressed, *is* easily displaced (as by intracranial haemorrhage) and deformed (as by twisting strains)—see Fig. 8.8.

2. The brain, circulating blood and cerebrospinal fluid are all of about the same density. They all tend to move together when the head is suddenly moved (or decelerated) along a straight line by a direct impact.

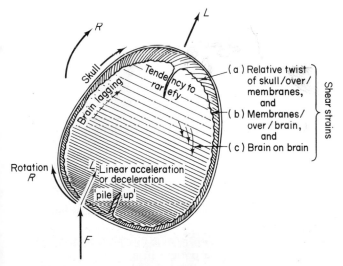

Fig. 8.8 Effect of force (*F*) on movable head, causing linear (*L*) and rotational (*R*) strains.

Only mild 'pile-up, occurs under the force of impact, and mild 'rarefaction' on the opposite surface (contre-coup).

3. Sudden rotation of the skull is more gradually imparted to the cerebrospinal fluid and the brain.

While their inertia is being overcome the rough interior of the skull-cum-dura drags over the surface of the brain and stretches, even tears, its arachnoid and perforating vascular tetherings. The *rate* of change counts most.

An analogy is obtained by rotating a bottle of water in which a piece of wool is suspended. Sudden twisting causes the wool (= brain) to lag momentarily inside the rotating bottle (= skull), chafing over its interior. A direct impact, on the contrary, causes no appreciable relative movements of wool and bottle (or brain and skull), though slight pile-up may occur momentarily under the force of impact. Damage is then only likely if the bottle (= skull) fractures.

Denny-Brown and Russell showed long ago that it is virtually impossible to cause concussion in the cat unless the head is free to move. Only when it is free can acceleration/deceleration and rotation (shear) strains develop: the latter cause by far the more serious harm. Not only does the skull chafe over the surface of the brain; the brain undergoes the sort of twisting that you feel when your tighten a roll of paper in the hands, each lamina twisting over that beneath, stretching, shearing, tearing the tissues from the surface to the very core (Fig. 8.8). The brain stem is especially liable to harm as the spinal column fixes it, acting as the pivot on which the head rotates.

These shear strains operate irrespective of the skull being fractured. Membrane tears causing haemorrhages, and surface or deep contusions of the brain occur *without fracture* in about three-quarters of all fatal cranial injuries.

'Contre-coup' can be explained on these physical principles. It is a form of brain injury in which an equally—even sometimes more—pronounced surface bruising of the brain is found exactly opposite the site of impact as under the blow itself. The whole surface of the brain suffers chafing injury, but this tends to be accentuated by piling-up of the brain under impact and rarefaction (with stretching of pial vessels and arachnoid tetherings) over the opposite surface. Occipital impacts may thus cause grave injury over the frontal poles, left-sided blows right-sided physical injury.

Alcohol and head injuries

When head injury is sustained by a person who has already had 'a few drinks' even the most experienced doctor may find it impossible to assess the relative importance of each factor. It is wise to watch such a complex subject for some time, preferably as a patient in a hospital (rather than as a suspected 'drunk' in a police cell). Even the experienced police sergeant can be misled, finding that his 'drunk and incapable' reveller is

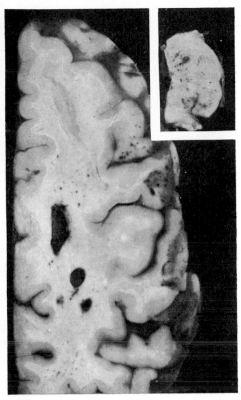

Fig. 8.9 Contusions of surface convolutions, white matter and (inset) brain stem, caused by violent impact of head with ground. The lobe shown lay opposite the site of impact with the ground, and the injuries seen are of contre-coup form, due to shear-strain.

in a deeper coma—occasionally dead of a cerebral lesion—when visited in the morning. Regular visits to the cell are a wise precaution, but a bed in the hospital is far safer for everyone. Better to watch a few 'drunks' sleep it off than to suffer the chagrin of a death in the police cell from an operable head injury.

It is well, also, to remember that a high blood alcohol does not exclude grave head injury, for the most hopelessly inebriated may totter into a lamp-post or fall downstairs. Caution is well repaid.

Of all distinguishing clinical features, those listed in Table 8.2 are alone likely to afford some safer indication.

The following are so equivocal as to have little diagnostic value: smell of breath, furred tongue, size of pupil, incoherence or slurring of speech, impaired co-ordination and orientation, tremors, restlessness or excitement, reduced blood pressure or subnormal temperature.

No examination would be complete without them, but to lean on them for diagnosis might mislead. It is on the sum, rather than on any one or two features of the clinical state, that diagnoses must rest. The clinical

Table 8.2

	Drunk	Concussed
Colour	Suffused, flushed, warm	Pale, clammy
Pulse	Fast, bounding	Slower, feeble
Pupils	Sluggish reaction to light	Brisk reaction to light
Breathing	Sighs, puffs, eructates	Shallow, irregular, slow
Memory of event	Confused memory, improving.	Retrograde amnesia often unrelieved by time
Behaviour	Unco-operative, abusive or sullen, insolent, loquacious	Co-operative. Quiet

assessment of 'drunkenness' without concussion is dealt with more fully on p. 327.

Spinal cord injuries

Three kinds of injury befall the spine—vertical compression, excessive bending (by flexion, extension or laterally) and dislocation. A forth, an avulsion or dragging apart vertically, is seen only in violent hanging; it is accompanied by a complete severance of the cord, which cuts short its forensic and clinical interests.

Diving vertically, or sustaining heavy impacts vertically on the top of the head, or, in reverse, sitting violently on the buttocks, can direct such force through the line of the spine as may compress and crush one or

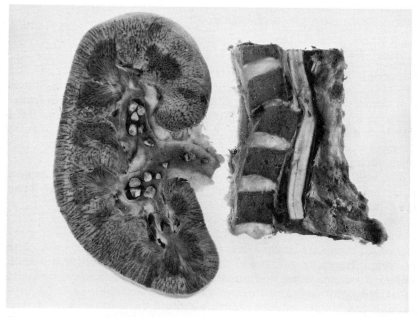

Fig. 8.10 Fracture dislocation of the cervical spine following a 'dive' on to the head in a game of rugger. The cord is crushed, and a calculous urinary infection ensued.

more of the vertebral bodies. The spinal cord may escape injury, but the roots of emerging nerves may become crushed or later become nipped by growing callus or scar tissue. Intervertebral discs may become displaced or crushed and the spinal cord may become nipped, crushed or torn across.

One very interesting type of fracture dislocation requires care in both clinical and autopsy examination. A blow on the brow or chin may tilt and throw back the head, causing a momentary dislocation of the neck—usually about C4 or 5—tearing prevertebral ligaments and injuring the cord, but reducing spontaneously into place. The dangers of regarding the paralysis which results from apparently trivial injury as hysterical and of overlooking the (now reduced) injury at autopsy are great. One such case concerned a man who, after a few drinks, fell, striking his chin on a letterbox, stumbled and seemed to lose the power of his legs, was regarded as drunk and helped home. He died early the following morning from progressive spinal cord swelling and haemorrhage due to self-reducing dislocation of the spine at C5/6. Only expert neurological examination or exposure and section of the cord after death can show the nature of the injury.

Twenty-five per cent of all spinal injuries are located at about C4-6, and another quarter at about T10-L3. The spinal cord is injured in about one-half of all cases of fracture of the spine.

Blunt injuries to the chest

The chest is far less complicated a structure in relation to trauma than the head, but its form is similar in many respects, for here, too, a semi-rigid bony case envelops vital structures of a softer, more mobile and deformable character. The chest, however, is a cage of far more malleable and easily deformed substance, especially in children whose cartilages and pliable rib-shafts give the chest a remarkable yield without fracture. Cases of heavy pinning which have virtually pinned the sternum to the spine, crushing the heart and lungs, yet recoiling without fracture to normal form, are commonly seen in children. Further, the heart and lungs though tethered in the mediastinum are freely mobile on their 'stalks' and these may stretch, tear and bleed. Lastly, the maintenance of an airtight intrapleural tension is essential to the function of each lung; without it the lung collapses and becomes an idle passenger prone to complicating diseases.

At the same time the chest and its contents can maintain a good functional output under stresses which would cause the brain to cease working. The effects of trauma to the chest are not so startling; indeed, many injuries are virtually symptomless. This fact must be remembered in assessing the importance of injury in relation to subsequently recognised disease of the lungs. Tuberculosis is commonly 'lit up' by injury. In a case examined 7 months after a symptomless prod in the chest with an oar, tuberculosis was found to be rife beneath the site of alleged injury, and the probability that trauma disturbed and extended or 'lit up' the disease was admitted.

Injuries to the chest can, like those to the head, be placed in two groups, according to whether the force is wholly absorbed locally or causes disturbance of the entire chest contents.

Local absorption of injury, when slight, may result in no more than some bruising of the chest wall, and perhaps fissured fractures of ribs without injury to deeper structures. But as the lung may be contused and air sacs torn, often beneath an intact pleura, so that subpleural bullae make their appearance flecked with blood from torn surface capillaries and veins. Occasionally, deeper cortical bruising of the lung results in the development of a haematoma which may be localised in the interstices or in air sacs closed by pressure of accumulated blood.

As soon as the weight of impact is sufficient to thrust broken ribs into the interior of the chest, far more serious injuries will result. Tears in the parietal pleura will admit blood into the pleural cavity, often in some quantity, and penetration into the lungs will admit both blood and air, the lung at once collapsing and thereby reducing the flow of blood to some extent. Rather less bleeding will take place at the same time into the lung, and some may appear at the mouth or in the sputum.

Rib injuries are less extensive and cause self-healing valvular pneumothorax more commonly than do penetrating wounds from weapons and bullets. They are also less liable to infection.

As the rupture of lung sacs is due mainly to their inability to empty themselves of air fast enough on rapid compression by impact, it also follows that trauma is the more serious if emphysema is already present. The already distended lung is thin and most vulnerable so that the air sacs readily burst.

The other complications of local injury—air embolism, haemothorax and lung infection—are of less forensic interest. One interesting result of trauma, the exaggerated reflex vagal response to trivial pleural stimuli, has been described. Sudden vagal inhibition and death may result, especially in highly emotional subjects.

The heart is sometimes crushed and torn by a buckled sternum—most often perhaps in car drivers impaled on the steering-wheel. Except where the pericardial sac is torn, a rare event without the heart also being injured, the heart appears to be able to stand remarkable trauma without faltering appreciably in its function. Even where the ventricles have been penetrated by ribs or a weapon, some kind of valvular closure may be effected and life may continue.

> In one case examined a man had stabbed himself over the heart five times; four of the wounds had penetrated the cavity of the chest, three penetrating the heart. Yet he survived and was recovering in hospital, to his chagrin, when on the fourth day he seized the water carafe by his bed, dashed it on the bed locker, and cut his throat with the jagged stem, dying of haemorrhage soon after.
>
> In another case a man in a London prison was found hanged by some torn sheeting in his cell. At autopsy two punctures were seen over the heart and

exploration revealed a mail-bag needle transfixing a rib cartilage and sticking into the heart. The stabbing had evidently had little effect and the man had resorted to hanging himself.

The association of chest trauma and coronary arterial spasm, or injury followed by coronary thrombosis, is acceptable only where the relation in time is close and there is evidence of injury to the affected vessel. Intramural splits and haemorrhages do occur in the coronary arteries, and when mural damage occurs thrombosis is undoubtedly encouraged.

Generalised trauma to the chest, such as that seen in exposure to blast, results in injuries comparable with those seen in the brain. A combination of rotational shear strain and of linear acceleration⇌deceleration causes innumerable tears of the connective tissue of the lung substance, usually confined to the interstices. The lung is flecked with petechiae, both on the cortex and deep in its substance where capillary vessels in the interstices have been torn and have bled: extension through torn alveoli into the air passages may fleck the sputum with traces of blood, but seldom more. Sometimes more serious intrapulmonary bleeding may ensue, or the lung may rupture, causing a pneumothorax or traumatic emphysema of the mediastinum or chest wall.

Explosive impact directed both at the chest, seen in many war cases in London in 1940–44, and through the mouth and air passages, seen, for instance, in a worker undoing an 'Irish' post-office bomb behind a chest screen, may cause these injuries. A form of contre-coup is seen in the lungs when the pressure wave hitting one side is succeeded by the negative phase. The subpleural surfaces of the lungs bear the brunt of the damage.

Blunt injury to the abdomen

With descent to the abdomen the increase in mobility of the casing becomes increased to the extreme degree possible in the human body; with the exception of the spine the entire wall is fascial and relies for its form on muscle tone. The abdominal contents are designed to move in relation to each other and, within variable limits, suffer no harm by this. It is only where displacement is restricted by short mesenteric attachments as in the duodenum or the caecum, or where a distended viscus suffers trauma as with the stomach after a meal, that injury is likely.

It is remarkable how often the loops of bowel slip away even from penetrating weapons especially when penetration is slow. I have seen a murder by a curved sword passing through the entire abdomen, back to front, without injury to its contents. A blunt local pinning or prodding blow, such as from the steering-wheel or handlebar, is the most common cause of rupture, but sometimes a flat impact, prone on the ground, will cause the stomach to rupture. Kicks from a horse provide a number of such cases, one in my own experience following a friendly slap on the haunches by a woman, unacquainted with the temperament of horses, visiting a sales stables. Evidence of the location of these blows is usually present both in the skin and around the injured parts; bowel, liver, spleen or kidneys are commonly crushed or split, and variable general or retro-peritoneal haemorrhage will certainly result.

Where the blow is of a broader character no surface injury may be visible, and grave danger of overlooking serious internal injury exists. The abdominal wall may yield before the impacting object, and mesenteries, gut, stomach and liver may be pinned and crushed across the spine, release of the pressure permitting immediate uncontrolled internal haemorrhage. In the case of the liver this splitting and haemorrhage may be deep seated, emerging only after a few days in the portal fissure. With slapping impacts of more sudden violence the only likely injury is rupture of an already distended stomach, sudden compression increasing the intragastric tension.

> A child of 5 who climbed over the sill of its first-floor play-room after lunch, to fall nearly 5 metres (15 ft) prone on to a flat concrete surface, died of rupture of the front wall of the stomach which contained a large meal. No injury was visible on the abdomen externally.

The same splitting, usually mucosal first and muscular and serous later, is sometimes seen in drowning where much air and water may be gulped down into the stomach. It has also been seen when an intended intra-tracheal anaesthesia has 'gone the wrong way' ... into the oeso-phagus. Rapid distension is the cause of disaster.

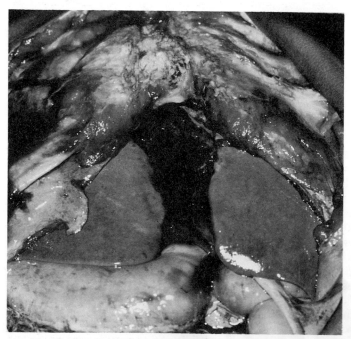

Fig. 8.11 An abdominal injury seen in battered babies as a result of punching, kicking or hurling the victim into furniture—a ruptured liver. It is likely to escape detection, merely bleeding internally.

It is not unreasonable to suppose that less serious mucous and sub-mucous lesions of this kind might encourage the development of ulceration; thus local trauma and later ulcer formation might properly be associated.

A relationship between head injury—to the infundibular region (around the hypothalamic attachment of the stalk of the pituitary)—and gastric lesions has long been known (Cushing), and experimental gastric necrosis has been shown to develop throughout the oxyntic cell-bearing area following injections of posterior pituitary extract. Any lesion or destructive injury in the tuber region may cause gastric erosions or acute ulceration.

Explosive forces, both on land and in water from depth charges, may cause injuries of the same kind as already described in the brain and the lungs. No significance other than their surgical interest attaches to them.

In the pelvis, anatomical conditions demand a little further study. The bladder behaves much like the stomach, being likely to rupture only in the event of a kick or prodding blow sustained when the organ is distended: rupture is the commonest in the dome region. It is only a reflection of probabilities that a large proportion of such cases occur in drunken subjects, men, for the same reason, preponderating, and children rarely indeed suffering the mishap. Injuries to the bladder and urethra are usually, however, the result of fracture of the pelvis, splintered bone crushing or tearing the nearest part of the urinary tract. The membranous or bulbous urethra is the part which most commonly suffers, rupture being extraperitoneal. Straddle injuries are more striking than frequent; falling astride a wall or fence is their commonest cause, the bulbous or membranous urethra being split by crushing against the under-aspect of the pubic arch or torn open with the perineum.

The crush syndrome

During the bombing of London in 1940–44, persons were sometimes found trapped under heavy masonry or debris and could not be released, in spite of strenuous effort, before some hours had elapsed. After release alive, crushed limbs were noticed to become swollen, often tensely so. Shock developed, and at a later stage, in spite of successful combat of shock, the renal output of urine dropped; the urine became dark, smoky, contained albumin and gave a positive spectroscopic test for myohaemoglobin. Death might take place from uraemia owing to oliguria or anuria by the end of the first week, or, at about the same time, a flush of diuresis, a falling-off of pigment excretion and a transient 'show' of cellular casts might preface recovery.

The renal lesion clearly depended upon the presence of swollen pale necrobiotic muscle and involved the entire nephron, but the most serious lesions were a 'catarrhal' form of swelling and necrosis of the epithelium of the convoluted tubules, the second convoluted tubules containing granular casts pigmented by excreted myohaemoglobin. These, due to concentration of glomerular filtrate, were rather like those seen in 'transfusion kidney'. It is probable that the lesion is due to the attempted excretion of acid metabolites absorbed from the damaged muscle (Bywaters).

9

The ultimate effects of injury

Doctors and lawyers must be careful to define what they mean by the word 'shock'. Emotional disturbances, the effects of a blow across the throat, rupture of the uterus, a bleeding wound, crushing pelvic injuries, burns, corrosive poisoning, overwhelming bacterial infection, electrocution, can all cause shock of some kind. The common factor is injury—to emotional stability, to the delicate vasovagal or electrical control of the circulation, to tissues. It is these traumas that bring about the consequences wrapped up in the word 'shock'—haemodynamic, physiological and biochemical disturbances that betray a state of shock. Grant and Reeve, who studied the effects of injury during the 1939-45 war, wrote a classic account of the general effects of trauma (in 1951) without using the word 'shock' at all, and it is important to use the word with care among lawyers—to whom semantics mean so much.

Traumatic shock

The reaction to injury may be complex and prolonged, changing its features as time passes. The instant reaction to any hurt is largely a vasovagal reflex response, a 'neurogenic' kind of shock. A blow across the neck, in the 'solar plexus' or the scrotum may cause an instant vasomotor collapse—a disturbance of heart rhythm or breathing that may be fatal. An electric discharge through the body may also cause instant or near-instant arrest of heart action and breathing, or of brain function. If not fatal, these functional disturbances may set in train the classic features of circulatory failure—hypotension, peripheral capillary stasis and anoxia, described by Moon in 1943 as:

'a disturbance of fluid balance resulting in a peripheral circulatory disturbance which is manifest by a decreased volume of blood, reduced volume flow, haemoconcentration and renal functional deficiency'.

There have been fuller but no more concise descriptions of the basic effects of shock. No one denies the importance of vagal inhibition, but it is the other effects of injury—loss of blood, damage to the tissues,

125

liberation of histamine or cytotoxic substances—that build up the general features of shock. The failure to maintain an adequate blood pressure, and the reflex constriction of the peripheral capillary system, are the most damaging features. Shock results largely from:

1. *hypotension*—or a reduced cardiac output;
2. *anoxia*—from loss of blood pressure or output volume or oxygen-carrying capacity; and
3. *endothelial permeability*—increasing so as to cause loss of fluid, electrolytes and protein.

This section is most concerned with the effects of tissue damage, loss of blood and its consequences, and the later complications of injury. The 'Gram-negative bacteraemic shock syndrome' is a clinical emergency usually unconnected with trauma.

Few cases remain as simple as the experiments that are designed to explore the effects of these principal factors—blood loss, hypotension, anoxia, and the inevitable disturbance of fluid and electrolyte balance that follow.

A stabbing murder resulted in:
1. *Extensive penetrating injuries* to both chest and abdomen, accompanied by:
2. *Loss of blood, hypotension and a renal 'shut down'*, adding bacterial and toxic absorption, and
3. *Escape of intestinal contents* from the stab holes in the ileum added grave abdominal shock—both sensory and
4. *Biochemical*. It was controlled by:
5. *Surgery under anaesthesia*, adding inevitable trauma, further small loss of blood, partly replaced by
6. *Transfusion*, and anaesthetic toxic factors.
7. *Infection* developed along the track of two of the stab wounds.
8. *Chemotherapy* was set up in the endeavour to control the sepsis.
9. *Renal damage* ensued and the output of urine fell, a mild disturbance of electrolytes ensuing.
10. The girl, who was pregnant, had aborted early in the course of these successive events, adding the reflex trauma and minor, but now ill-spared, loss of blood incidental to this mishap.

   She died of what could collectively be called shock, complicated by successive events which added to a sum no damaged human machinery could survive.

So when doctors use the word 'shock' in court, they must be prepared to explain what they mean—simple emotional disturbance, vasovagal reflex, loss of blood, tissue destruction, an immune reaction, drug damage, or the consequences of these changes on the cardiac output, the blood pressure, the peripheral circulation and return flow; or the more profound and lasting effects of such changes—anoxia, capillary damage, histamine substance, bacterial or drug toxicity. The ultimate effects of injury may indeed be complex, but the law accepts a chain of events as linking cause and effect, however tenuous, both in criminal and in civil law. It is only when some entirely unexpected happening occurs that this chain is broken. When a man injured at work is being taken to hospital with good prospects, but the ambulance is struck by lightning or overturns in a ditch with fatal results, the chain of events is broken. The law calls this a *novus actus interveniens*.

Starvation, exposure and neglect

These conditions so often operate together that they may conveniently be considered together. The doctor sees two common forms of neglect:

1. *Self-neglect and starvation* in elderly or weak-minded persons who, irrespective of their means, choose to live in apparent poverty, dirty, unkempt, often verminous, and without adequate fluid or food.
2. *Wilful neglect of children*, often accompanied by starvation.

In both forms exposure to damp and cold, with trophic skin changes, often accelerated by infection, may play their parts in lowering vitality. Winter is likely to engender such circumstances more commonly than summer's warmth and sunshine, and poor living conditions naturally form the broad background against which these grim spectres emerge. War brings in its trail of devastation, mass starvation, exposure and neglect in which the health of whole nations may suffer gravely, and each winter may bring wholesale death from these causes.

In most cases of starvation seen in civilian life there is no complete deprivation of food, merely a grossly inadequate intake.

A man who had come to Britain to earn, in the shortest possible time, the money to buy a farm in Africa, had managed to save, from his employment at a dock-side gas-works at £4 per week, the sum of £52 in some 15 weeks in spite of paying for lodging and food and clothing. He lived in an unlit room in the Isle of Dogs, East London, without heat, eating white rice and stewed vegetables. He became thin and weak, but refused attentions of any kind, being found dead in bed one morning. Autopsy showed him to have reached an emaciated state with skin changes of pellegra and haemorrhages, both from the gums and around the knee joints, due to scurvy.

The conditions are more likely to present themselves as a mass vitamin defect or malnutrition with some superimposed infection than as a state of simple gross starvation. There is, however, a general loss of subcutaneous fat and dehydration, the body reaching states of emaciation akin to those seen in long-standing tuberculosis or carcinoma of the oesophagus or stomach (Fig. 9.1).

The skin is thin, dry, sometimes fissured and sore, drawn tight like parchment over the bony prominences, the cheeks hollow, eyes sunken, abdomen carinated, and legs and arms 'like broomsticks'. Pigmentation may vary from mere sallowness to distinct melanosis. The organs are atrophied and the walls of the stomach and intestines thin, almost transparent, from disuse. Only the gall-bladder is enlarged, filled with unwanted bile; the intestines lack the food matter and chyle which might have caused it to empty.

by sudden fall in blood pressure, the result of peripheral vasomotor relaxation and central circulatory failure. Interference with perspiration is likely to accelerate the process. The onset is sudden or preceded by a few moments of overbearing heat, dizziness, yawning, patchy flushing of the skin especially over the face, then sudden unconsciousness supervenes and the victim falls 'in a dead faint'. In conditions other than heat-stroke the subject is pale, sweating and breathing with long infrequent respirations, the pulse barely perceptible. In heat-stroke the skin may be flushed and dry, the pulse full, soft and rapid, and the temperature as high as 43°C (around 109°F)—like that of a cerebral catastrophe. This is, in fact, what heat-stroke is, the peripheral circulation and perspiration playing little part in its development.

The endeavour to separate sharply from each other those forms of heat-collapse which are due primarily to cardiovascular collapse (heat-exhaustion and heat-syncope) and those due to overheating of the brain centres (heat-stroke) are doomed to failure, for pure forms are rare. Drugs that inhibit sweating such as atropine and phenothiazine tranquillisers may also be involved.

Autopsy provides little evidence of the causation of death, for it is largely functional. The conditions are usually those of circulatory failure of central origin—cerebral or cardiac, with dilated chambers in the heart, pulmonary congestion and oedema with distended cyanosed afferent veins. Rigor comes on quickly and also passes away rapidly.

Hypothermia

Exposure to extremes of cold may result in freezing of the tissues which, if not reversed soon enough, will result in 'frost-bite' or gangrene of tissues or parts—especially the toes and fingers—which have lost their vitality. Severe cold, short of freezing, may cause capillary vascular stasis: red patches develop in the skin and 'blistering' may follow if stagnant anoxia continues. Men left for days exposed to extremes of cold adrift at sea or isolated with inadequate clothing in Arctic conditions suffer a painful *erythromelalgia* at first, but numbing soon follows and the dangers of frost-bite may well be overlooked.

As cold grips the body, metabolism is reduced and the body temperature falls below the minimum that can be registered on a clinical thermometer. The victim may cease to shiver, relapsing into a state of torpor which mercifully clouds the end.

In recent years, it has become recognised that the elderly, as well as infants, are particularly prone to harm from sustained cold. Hypothermia, that the young and fit can survive, can kill infants or the elderly in their own homes during winter months when heating or clothing is inadequate. There may be little to show for it, and the doctor who relies on an ordinary clinical thermometer to detect temperatures in the region of 20–30°C (or 70–85°F) is, of course, doomed to diagnostic failure. A termperature of 28°C (82.4°F) seems to be critical.

Prolonged hypothermia results in peripheral circulatory stasis, and anoxic 'blush patches' on the shoulders, knees, hands and feet may be the visible diagnostic feature. The vitality of the tissues may so deteriorate that gastric or intestinal erosions, pancreatic (fat) or hepatic necroses develop from autodigestion.

Burns and scalds

Local injury by heat may result from:

1. Dry heat, application of hot bodies and licking by flames—simple burns.
Moist heat—scalds.
Corrosive poisons—corrosive burns.
Electrical spark discharges, flashes and lightning—electrical burns.

Each has distinctive surface features, but the indirect results are virtually the same, for they involve capillary damage followed by fluid exudation, necrosis of dead tissue and shock. Electric injury carries the added danger of cardiac arrest.

Curling described duodenal ulcer complicating burns, but it is not very common. In a series of 250 burns and scalds, I found it only twice. Erosions of the gastric mucous membrane are far more common. Both conditions are due to the tissue hypoxia and capillary endothelial damage that ensue upon shock from burns. Any gastric lesion may develop, aided by peptic mucosal digestion and bacterial infection, to the full stature of an ulcer. Focal necroses are found in other tissues and fat emboli may occur.

The loss of fluid and of protein may become serious, both these and the vital electrolytes requiring careful balance. The mortality from extensive burns and scalds is high.

A burn, in law, is just a burn whatever its degree, from a mere patch of erythema or blistering of the cutis to the deepest charring of muscle and bone. But the special features of each form require description, as follows.

1. *Dry heat and fire* cause a graded series of changes from reddening and blistering due to capillary damage to soot-charred destruction of muscle and bone. The muscles may have a dry 'cooked' appearance and the blood in the vessels may be coagulated and dry for the same reason. The tissues are often pink from absorption of CO in the fire flames before death, and the blood may show saturations of as much as 40–60 per cent HbCO on test.

This finding is sound evidence that life was present at the time of exposure to fire, as is the presence of soot particles inhaled into the main air passages. The question whether a burn shows a vital reaction is one of great difficulty, for dead capillaries may be made to swell by heating—even boiling—the blood in them, and tissue fluid may be boiled to cause blistering after death. The muscles tend to contract as they are heated past protein coagulation level, and contractures of arms or legs result. The 'pugilistic' pose of clenched fists on bent arms is a common observation. The skin may also tend to split as it becomes dried, and such splits are sometimes mistaken for injuries.

2. *Moist heat*, as from steam or hot liquids, is, from its very nature, likely to be limited to the skin—or in the rare cases where boiling liquids are drunk, to the mouth and throat. In one case a woman knelt in front of a boiling kettle on a stove and tipping the spout forward drank the scalding water, as a suicidal act. The skin and mucosae are blistered and the cutis peels away sodden to expose raw inflamed subcuticular skin layers (Fig. 9.3).

3. *Corrosive burns* bear the special colour feature of their respective chemical; most common are the reddish (blackening) burns of spirits of salt (HCl) and vitriol (H_2SO_4), sometimes thrown at jilting or scorned lovers, or accidentally spilled over the body by burst containers. Nitric acid causes its characteristic brown burn, and carbolic its white insensitive skin wrinkling. Brown lysol stains were often seen round the mouth in suicides.

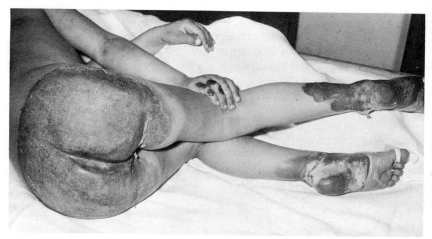

Fig. 9.3 Fatal scalds of the buttocks and feet of a child placed in a bath of scaldingly hot water.

4. *Electrical discharges* or flashes are characterised by a sharp local capillary spasm causing a local whitening, around which a zone of hyperaemia quickly becomes established. Sometimes the line of a discharge is raised as a chain of blisters, with the skin dried and wrinkled by the heat of discharge, and occasionally scorched or blackened by the flashes.

Lightning plays the most artistic pranks over the skin, causing leaf- and fern-like patterns, running over the body where steel clothing stiffeners and fasteners conduct it. Clothes may be explosively split.

Accident, suicide and murder by burns

Old people and children are the common victims of accidental fires by their careless manipulations of candles and matches or their inability to deal with sparks or clothing catching fire.

One old lady, found dead in bed after a fierce fire had been put out in her bedroom, was said to have been in the habit of poising a lighted candle on her bed-linen in a detached candle-socket in order to read her Bible.

An old gentleman, found in a Chelsea flat one Christmas with what appeared to be a pistol gripped in his hand, burned beyond all recognition had been manipulating a paraffin lamp over the gas stove, using the pistol-lighter to start a flame, when his clothing or beard caught fire. A woman in the flat below was awakened at 3 a.m. by crackling sounds, located a hot spot in her living-room ceiling—and went back to bed!

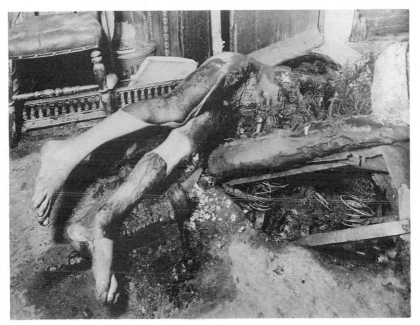

Fig. 9.4 Body of elderly man found with fore half buried in burnt-out armchair. A gas pistol was found in his hand and it appeared his beard may have caught fire in lighting a gas stove.

Children commonly play with fire with disastrous consequences, and infants sometimes fall into baths of scalding water or pull boiling fluids over themselves. The law has provided special protection for children under 12 years of age in the Children and Young Persons (Amendment) Act of 1952, section 8 of which enacts that:

'If any person who has attained the age of 16 years, having the custody, charge or care of any child under the age of 12 years, allows the child to be in any room containing an open fire or any heating appliance liable to cause injury to a person by contact therewith, not sufficiently protected to guard against the risk of his being burnt or scalded without taking reasonable pre-cautions against that risk, and by reason thereof the child is killed or suffers serious injury, he shall on summary conviction be liable to a fine not exceeding £25.'

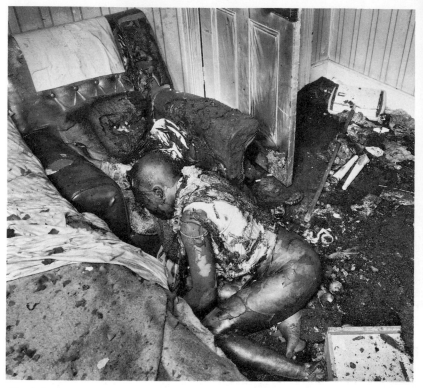

Fig. 9.5 Body of woman found after fire in bedroom had been extinguished. The fire was fiercest in the leather chair, and a scalp wound raised suspicion. A man was later charged with arson and murder.

Suicide is uncommon owing to the prospect of pain, but distraught persons sometimes pour paraffin or petrol over their clothing prior to setting alight to themselves. This self-immolation was more common in the East, but has spread to Europe in recent years.

Murder by fire is rare, but there have been a number of cases where attempts have been made to destroy the body of a victim of violence by setting fire to it. Post-mortem in fire cases should always keep the possibility in mind. Skin splits, bone flaking or fractures, and boiled blood masses, especially inside the skull must be accepted as normal fire damage and not allowed to start a scare of crime.

In 1930 a man named Rouse endeavoured to dispose of a man he had murdered by setting fire to the body. In the front compartment of a burnt-out car a body was found charred beyond recognition. The car was Rouse's, but the body was that of another man, and post-mortem examination showed that he had been murdered by some blunt instrument such as a hammer. Such a weapon was, in fact, found in a ditch hearby. Rouse, who would have benefited if the body were assumed to be his own, was subsequently arrested and convicted of murder.

In 1933 a charred body was found seated in a chair after a fire had been put out in a builder's premises in Chalk Farm. A note was found in the outer office of the building which read, 'Good-bye to all. No work. No money. Sam S.J. Furnace.' The premises belonged to a man called Furnace who was known to be in debt, particularly to a man called Spatchett. The police informed Mrs Furnace that her husband had been found dead, but autopsy next morning revealed a bullet wound in the back. Laundry-marks on the shirt indicated it to belong to Spatchett—who had also disappeared, and the dental data was recognised by Spatchett's dentist. Furnace was traced to Southend and arrested. He committed suicide while under detention awaiting trial.

It must not be assumed that the finding of smoke particles in the air passages and of carbon monoxide in the blood stream is enough to allay suspicion, for, of course, the drunk, drugged or disabled victim of crime may be enveloped by fire and burned. Only where fire charring is extreme is evidence of injury likely to become obscured; burns might obscure evidence of strangling with, say, a scarf, but not so readily fractures—or bullets.

It is also possible, of course, to die of exposure to fire without inhaling smoke, for the rapid consumption of oxygen by an intense fire may itself be enough to cause death. Raging fires leave little carbon monoxide in the atmosphere, and the body may just look pale.

Electrocution

The local character of an electric burn has been described already in the general section on burns. Death from contact with a source of electricity results from the discharge of current through the body rather than from burns; indeed, there may be no burns if the contact and earthing are good. The lethality of the discharge is related to current/time and the amount of current is determined by the relationship:

$$\text{amperage} = \frac{\text{voltage}}{\text{resistance}}$$

A girl dead in her bath, found as a result of a scream being heard, lay with the head still out of the water; a sister who ran to her received a shock as she touched the dead girl, and then saw an electric hair-dryer had fallen from a narrow window-sill on which it had lain into the water at the foot of the bath. Only the head, lying against a tap, bore any mark.

The voltage of the supply may be as low as 50, if the resistance is low and the amperage thus high, but a fatal result seldom ensues from sources of supply less than the 200–250 volt pressure on the domestic wiring system. A low frequency such as the 50-cycle domestic supply is more dangerous than a high-frequency current. It is likely to be more dangerous if:

1. The passage of current is not broken, as where a flex or unearthed metal apparatus is grasped and the wretched victim finds it impossible to unclench the hand.

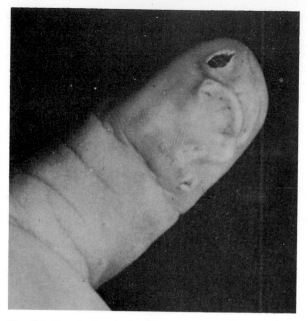

Fig. 9.6 Classic electric discharge burns of the thumb, with central charring of the cutis and raised white blistering.

2. The body contact, or earth, or both, are damp, so that the resistance of the skin is reduced or the effective area of contact is increased. Men working in damp premises or dug-out pits or shelters are frequently victims of severe, even fatal shocks, through handling damp connections while wearing water-sodden boots or shoes. The 'dry' skin offers many thousand ohms resistance—a wet skin no more than 200–300 ohms.

3. The victim is unprepared for a shock. The nervous element is a real one; everyone will testify to the difference between a shout, a bang or a slap on the shoulder which is expected or seen coming, and one which arrives like a 'bolt from the blue'. It is said that a man who used frequently to hold 240 volts for a bet in a public-house was killed instantly when he inadvertently leaned against the switch one night. He was unprepared to take the shock.

Post-mortem findings

Where there is a burn it will be likely to have the characteristic features already described—a dry cuticle, relatively insignificant weal, little burning, but striking local capillary contraction causing dead-white pallor of the surrounding zone. It may be so small as to be difficult to locate, especially in grimy tough-skinned workmen's hands, or not present at all.

An ice-cream merchant, preparing the next day's supplies in his wet stone-floored dairy, tripped over a flex leading to an electric fan and fell, clutching it across his chest. He was conscious but unable to release his grip and able only to utter feeble cries. Released after some 4–5 minutes, he died of fibrillation some 15 minutes later. Post-mortem examination showed a group of linear flex-patterned burns across the right hand and examination of the fan stand showed the wiring to be defective in its base.

Death in electrocution results from:

1. *Instant shock*, as with the sudden passage of high-voltage or high-amperage current, especially when the chest lies between contact and earth. The respiratory muscles 'seize up' and breathing ceases.

2. *Fibrillation and arrest of the heart*, usually the result of passage of a less powerful current. It can be as low as 0.1 ampere.

The autopsy findings in deaths from instant shock may be entirely negative, for it is only necessary for a current sufficient to arrest the heart (or medullary cardiac centre) to pass through the body. Burns may be absent. In fibrillating forms of death there is dilatation of the chambers of the heart, sometimes with petechiae under the pericardium and ventricular endocardium, and gross pulmonary and afferent venous congestion and cyanosis.

Electrocution by lightning

Deaths from lightning number about one-tenth those from accidents with industrial or domestic electric systems, but are important medicolegally, for they present certain causes for suspicion—disarranged torn clothing, split skin, fractured bones, and a variety of curious skin markings.

Spencer, reviewing lightning stroke and its treatment, emphasised that four elements are in operation:

1. The direct effect of a current of enormous voltage.
2. Burning by the flash.
3. The decompression⇌compression force of air displaced around the flash.
4. A 'sledge-hammer' effect of air compressed and thrust in front of the flash.

Streaked or leafy-patterned (arborescent) skin burns may be found. Skin wounds may be 'struck' by compressed or rarefied air effects, and bones may be broken by the same forces; these may arouse suspicion of foul play. Any metallic articles, such as buttons, keys, bracer parts, suspender buckles, are magnetised—a useful sign in the elimination of suspicion.

A man of 71 hurrying to shelter from a thunderstorm in Lambeth was in the act of putting the key into his flat door when the house was struck by lightning. The flash appeared to have come down a chimney through an iron grate and fender to an iron bedstead which reached close to the inside keyhole. The victim, still outside the door turning the key, was flung on to his back and appeared to have stopped breathing; he did not revive in spite of

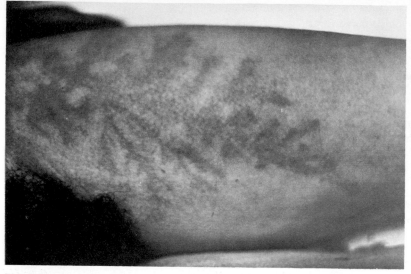

Fig. 9.7 Leaf- or fern-like pattern typical of some forms of lightning 'strike'.

continued artificial respiration. Burns lay on the ball of the right thumb and opposing aspect of the forefinger (between which the door-key was being held at the moment the lightning struck).

In another case seven persons were killed whilst sheltering under a corrugated steel-roofed park seat. A woman who was seated with a child of 5 on her knee fell dead with severe electric burns across the chest and down the front of the body, passing off the right knee. The child, surprisingly, escaped serious injury.

Lightning injuries aroused suspicion in the case of an Army motor-cyclist found dead near his wrecked machine on a deserted moor. The route of flash down the right side of head and (bent) leg from knee to foot and electrical charging of the machine made it clear that lightning was responsible.

Treatment consists almost entirely in endeavouring to restart the respirations which have become suspended, and in electrical defibrillation for those who are fibrillating. The former are revived surprisingly frequently by prolonged artificial respiration; those affected by fibrillation are almost certain to die.

In a series of 700 cases of injury by electricity which Maclachlan reported, there were 323 recoveries among 479 who had ceased to breathe. The Department of Trade recommends artificial respiration for as long as some hours; transfer to an intensive care unit is desirable.

Sometimes, in spite of 'recovery', residual cerebral confusion, blindness, deafness or palsies may ensue, the result of lightning injury or of anoxia from suspended respirations.

10

Disease, work stress and trauma

When death occurs suddenly or unexpectedly, especially when there has been no medical attention and the possibility of disease seems remote, it is only natural that thoughts of injury, some ill-effect of work conditions, even suspicion of poisoning or foul play, should pass through the minds of both relatives and the officials responsible for the certification of death, for registration and for burial. There is only one way of answering such doubts: an examination of the dead body must be made, if possible by an expert pathologist able to assess the relationship of any disease he may find with work stress, trauma or crime. Compensation—under private insurance agreements, by common law action or under the National Insurance (Industrial Injuries) Act—may depend upon the correct assessment of these relationships, of some criminal charge may follow upon proof of grave negligence or wilful injury.

It is vital that anyone who examines a body in order to determine these questions shall be familiar with the common natural causes of unexpected death.

Circulatory system

By far the most common cause of instantaneous death is coronary occlusion by atheroma, sometimes complicated by thrombosis or, if delayed for a few days (while infarction is developing), further complicated by rupture of the heart through the infarcted area. Specific intimal proliferation may also encroach upon the coronary orifices and occlude them. In either case an enlargement of—as for instance by hypertension—or weakening of the muscle—as for instance by senile or fatty change—must add to the likelihood of heart failure. Coronary embolism may effect the same sudden cessation of circulation through the heart, a portion of clot or vegetation derived from the left heart becoming impacted in one of the coronary orifices. Death is commonly instantaneous in such cases.

It is usual for death from simple coronary occlusion by atheroma to be precipitated by some exertion which has demanded more blood in the left heart than the diseased arteries can supply. Climbing stairs, sexual intercourse, working a hand-pump, digging over soil, lifting a weight, etc., may all precipitate such deaths, and where deceased was, at the time of collapse, engaged in some such work as part of employment, then a claim for compensation may be instituted.

The doctor may have to appear in civil proceedings and should readily admit the likelihood of precipitation of death by work stress, indeed by any exertion. If collapse during a period of exertion is followed by sudden death a few hours later, it is likely that autopsy will reveal a thrombosis developed in the coronary artery whose insufficiency was responsible for collapse; the stasis of circulatory collapse or sleep promotes thrombosis.

Myocardial degeneration—brown atrophy, fatty, fibrous or hypertensive changes—also causes sudden failure of the heart. Senility with its extreme brown atrophy is the commonest example of this. Recent years have also brought to light several types of cellular 'cardiomyopathy' which require microscopy for their identification. The first of these was fibroelastosis, but collagen and metabolic disorders, possibly some auto-immune states, may also cause sudden heart failure.

Rupture of an atheromatous aneurysm of the abdominal aorta is another common vascular cause of sudden, though hardly instantaneous, death. Dissection through the coats before final rupture into some large space takes some hours, during which pain or dyspnoea or a vague presentiment of trouble may have occurred. Hypertension, often with hyaline necrosis, atheroma and syphilis of the aorta naturally combine to encourage rupture, and here again the exertions of work may have precipitated the catastrophe, for such exertion will be bound to have increased the intra-aortic tension. In a famous test case (Clover Clayton & Co v. Hughes, 1910, AC 242) it was held that the mere tightening of a nut by a spanner could have provided this last straw, and compensation was awarded under the Workmen's Compensation Act provisions.

Neither cerebral haemorrhage nor cerebral thrombosis is likely to cause really sudden death. Collapse may be sudden, but death is more likely to be delayed some hours while the ultimate consequences of the cerebral lesions become developed: this takes time, usually hours, sometimes days.

This is not always true of the ruptures of 'congenital' cerebral aneurysms which become established, as life proceeds, at the site of developmental weakness at the stem of branches of the cerebral arteries. The initial leak from these is often small, causing pain in the neck or back of the head, and more extensive subarachnoid haemorrhage must follow before death results. Victims may die with inexplicable rapidity.

The arrival of negro immigrants into the UK introduced a previously unknown cause of sudden collapse and death—'sickle cell crisis'. The abnormal haemoglobin S and its sickle-shaped red cell predispose to cell 'sludging' in the capillaries and these cause microinfarctions that may very quickly become fatal.

Keith Mant describes a case in which a man surprised an intruder—a negro—coming downstairs in his house. The intruder attacked him with a screwdriver, but then suddenly collapsed, asked for a cup of water and died as he was drinking it. Sickle-cell sludging was widespread.

Pulmonary embolism is a very common cause of sudden death. Thrombosis of the leg veins is the likely source, and, although often a natural lesion, this may be encouraged by leg injury, especially a fractured femur, requiring an operative procedure and rest in bed. About 10-14 days after injury is a common interval before sudden collapse and death.

Nervous system

The vascular catastrophes of the brain have already been described. There are relatively few organic diseases of the brain which can cause sudden death. Blood or pus may rupture into the ventricles and any rapid swelling of the brain, as in the brain tumours, may initiate a medullary compression⇌intracranial-tension cycle of events which sometimes reaches a crisis quickly. A haemorrhage into the substance of a tumour may start the process.

Sudden functional inhibitions, the vagal reflex inhibitions, also provide a large variety of sudden, often apparently inexplicable, deaths. The principal sources of such vagal reflexes are:

1. Impaction of food or drink in the glottis; water, especially cold water, rushing into the nasopharynx or glottis may do the same, as in accidental drowning.
2. Intubation by anaesthetic or bronchoscopic apparatus through the glottis.
3. Sudden penetration of the pleura, rarely other serous sacs.
4. Sudden stretching or release of peritoneal sacs or abdominal organs—hernial sac stretching during operation, sudden emptying of a viscus, dilatation of sphincters (e.g. of anus).
5. Urethral dilatation.
6. Instrumental abortion.

Almost any sudden shock may have the same effect. The most famous case is that of the Scottish students' mock execution at which a college janitor, in terror of the lengths to which the ragging might be carried, had his neck fixed on a guillotine block and in mock solemnity was administered last rites, then suddenly flicked across the neck with a wet towel. He died instantly.

A taut emotional state is an important adjuvant factor.

A young man, in terror of needle exploration of the chest, said to his father, 'If they do it again I shall die.' He did collapse and die the moment the needle touched the pleura; it did not enter the sac.

The same nervous heightening of response is operating in many of the instrumental abortion deaths dying suddenly of reflex shock.

A woman was found dead with one leg in and one leg out of a bath, astride its edge, and leaning against the wall with a Higginson syringe still clutched in the hand by cadaveric spasm. She had died of shock whilst attempting an instrumental interference with a pregnancy.

Epileptic seizures, fixing the chest long enough, can precipitate death, the classic 'status epilepticus' seldom being present. The tongue is not always bitten.

Respiratory system

The suddenness of death in the event of impaction of food at the glottis has already been ascribed to vagal inhibition. Obstruction of the respiratory passages will more commonly cause asphyxia than precipitate a sudden death. Unexpected blocking of the air passages is most commonly the result of inhaled foreign bodies, including cold water, of acute oedema of the glottis (as in the acute allergies) or to fulminating membranous or sloughing infections. Asthmatic attacks can end fatally.

Something should be said, perhaps, of the remarkable swiftness of the course of classic influenzal pneumonia, if only because when the malaise, giddiness and vomiting which may accompany the onset of the disease is overlooked or regarded as migraine, and the subject goes to bed, quite unexplained death may follow within a few hours. Prostration, collapse, cyanosis, coma and death may all follow with such rapidity that no clinical illness is ever recognised. 'Cot deaths'—unexpected deaths of infants (sudden infant death syndrome SIDS)—may prove to be due to acute respiratory infections of microscopic proportions. As Boyd so aptly remarks: 'Life's little candle is easily extinguished.' Ancillary laboratory examinations are essential, but may be unrewarding.

Alimentary system

The only natural disease of the digestive system which may occasionally cause sudden death is perforation of a peptic ulcer. The sudden rush of irritating matter, including bile and blood, into the peritoneal sac may cause sudden grave collapse, even death. Some of these cases have compensation associations, as in the case of an engineer struck in the abdomen by a travelling gear, who collapsed and died immediately, autopsy showing a perforation of a chronic duodenal ulcer. Perforations of lower small and large intestines do not cause the intense shock of peptic perforations and never cause immediate death.

Pancreatic necrosis does not cause sudden death, though many persons not recognised to be seriously ill during a day or two's sickness are found dead from this cause.

There are many other diseases which will cause death after short and obscure illness, but these are not so likely to arouse suspicion as the conditions which cause death suddenly. Acute encephalitis or poliomyelitis, fulminating forms of meningococcal fever, acute adrenal insufficiency and the like are interesting diseases, but so much less likely to have forensic significance that they will not be discussed here.

'Status lymphaticus'

No one need doubt that there are variations in the degree to which the lymphatic tissues are developed, especially in children. There are constitutional variations in height and physique, and such things as obesity, flat feet and varicose veins, all of which are variations of build. But no excuse exists for using the names of such constitutional abnormalities as labels for causes of death. One might as well say that a man died of dwarfism or rotundity or flat feet—or, to carry the analogy further, of blue eyes and fair hair.

But persons who have constitutional defects may be rendered the more liable, by reason of them, to die of some cause which, in a 'normal' or more average person, might not be sufficient to precipitate death. Is this true of status lymphaticus?

The evidence is conflicting, and for this reason it must be laid before the student, who may judge for himself like the member of a jury presented with conflicting evidence. Where a problem excites strong protagonists and equally strong opposition its solution often lies between the extremes, containing the reliable elements of each.

What must be made clear beyond all doubt, however, is the fact that status lymphaticus can never be a *cause* of death. Is sudden death from trivial causes more common in persons with this constitutional build? The 'period' writing on this is historic.

Young and Turnbull (1931), in an analysis of 600 cases of sudden death in apparently healthy people of 15 years or over who had an abnormally large thymus, stated that they found no evidence that so-called status thymolymphaticus had any existence as a pathological entity, and a leading article in one of Britain's most critical medical journals, *The Lancet*, announced 'without sorrow, the end of the status' (1931).

Bratton (1925) emphasised the variation in size of the thymus under otherwise normal conditions, and Greenwood and Woods (1927) came to the conclusion after a strict analytical study of the subject that they could not assign 'the least importance to the recognition of these stigmata in the bodies of those whose deaths, apart from status lymphaticus, would in more pious, but not more superstitious, days, have been attributed to the visitation of God'. Cohen stated baldly that 'the term status lymphaticus used in the Coroner's Court is a meaningless expression'.

Yet Symmers, from the Bellevue Hospital, New York (1934), after equally extensive study, was convinced of its entity, finding it commonly in persons of unstable character, in suicides and associated with other glandular disorders such as Graves' disease or suprarenal insufficiency. In this respect Kemp (1937) agreed, suggesting that sudden deaths in lymphatism may depend chiefly on endocrine imbalance such as adrenal insufficiency and thyroid dysfunction—conditions which protagonists and opponents alike might accept as likely to cause death both suddenly and obscurely. Millar and Rose (1942) drew attention to another of the adverse conditions developed in lymphatism, aortic and general vascular hypoplasia.

Campbell, very reasonably, reconciled both views in the suggestion that there may well exist 'a condition of such lowered resistance and hyper-susceptibility that the patient so affected is in danger of sudden death from trivial causes'. Even those violently opposed to the use of the words status lymphaticus, like Greenwood and Woods (quoted above), admit that 'a nucleus of truth lies buried beneath a pile of intellectual rubbish, conjecture, bad observation, and rash generalisation'.

The only real danger seems to be the resort to a use of the term status lymphaticus to state the *cause* of death. Bad autopsy technique or sheer ignorance of some of the more trivial causes of death, such as vagal inhibition, allergy, air and fat embolisms, are likely to result in the pathologist finding 'nothing very much to account for death'. There always is a cause, and if it is not revealed by a careful autopsy it may safely be taken to be biochemical (as in acute adrenal insufficiency or hypoglycaemia) or functional (such as vagal inhibition).

> One of twins who had been healthy until the age of 18 years fell ill obscurely, lost weight, showed some proptosis and other evidence of thyrotoxicosis. At this stage the other died: the cause of her death remained obscure—in spite of analysis and bacteriology. Asthenia, anorexia, bouts of vomiting, melanosis and hypotension (85/40) ensued—and were thought to be due to adrenal crises upon admission of the second girl to a London teaching hospital. She suddenly collapsed under observation—urinary chloride being 346 mg/100 ml, and serum potassium variably high until death 48 hours later. Autopsy disclosed marked adrenal hypoplasia.

> A girl of 22, perfectly fit, 3 months pregnant, went to a sink and filled a glass with ordinary tap water. She 'tossed it back'—and fell back to the floor dead. Autopsy showed rather prominent lymphatic tissues but was otherwise negative, and the only possibility having any substance seemed to be vagal inhibition from the impact of cold water on the pharynx and glottis.

This problem deserves consideration at some length, for it frequently arises and is seldom given the balanced judgement which is necessary for a proper solution. The search for a precipitating cause of death must never be resigned because the subject shows some constitutional abnormality. This may have set the stage for death, but will seldom, if ever, have caused it.

Deaths during anaesthesia

There are two forensic aspects to this problem: (1) the addict's practice of taking anaesthetic drugs for self-indulgence or for sleep (also common among doctors and nurses), and (2) the problem of unexpected death during anaesthesia for some surgical procedure.

1. Habitual self-anaesthesia   The drinking of trichlorethylene, chloroform or ether or their inhalation for relief from overwork, depression or sleeplessness is not uncommon among hard-pressed senior students and 'inadequate' doctors or chemists.

A house surgeon of 24, taking his 'Final Fellowship' for the second time, overwrought by anxiety and 'too tired to sleep', found solace in chloroform inhalation at night. He was found dead in bed under the blankets, deeply anoxic, one morning, the bottle and a mask in his hands.

A ship's doctor was found dead in his surgery on board. He sat in a chair, slumped forwards, a syringe with needle fitted lying in the bend of the elbow, where a fresh venupuncture lay. A 1-g ampoule of Pentothal and distilled water were found nearby and analysis revealed about 0.5 g of this basal analgesic in the body. None had appeared in the urine, death having rapidly supervened—probably by accidental self-administration of the overdose: the margin of safety is very small.

Addicts' tolerance to many of these substances tends to increase: the dose has to be raised—and the danger is the greater as they press on to get the desired effect. Antidotes, if known, are seldom within reach, for familiarity breeds contempt. Irreversible circulatory or respiratory depression or both commonly develop, and deaths from these causes may ensue.

Self-indulgence in barbiturates, amphetamines, LSD, glues and spray vapours, toluene and carbon tetrachloride is currently in favour.

2. *Unexpected death during anaesthesia.* It is the practice to report to the coroner all deaths which occur 'before *full recovery*' from anaesthesia, and these provide a difficult forensic problem.

Deaths associated with anaesthesia and surgical operation

Fatalities during or soon after surgical intervention are often incorrectly referred to as 'anaesthetic deaths', although in fact deaths directly attributable to the anaesthetic agent or its administration form only a small proportion of failures to survive.

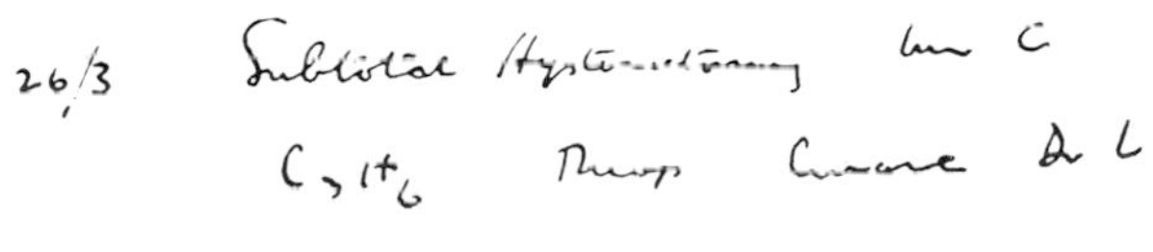

Fig. 10.1 The entire record of an operation and anaesthetic which was furnished to a coroner in the hospital records of an 'anaesthetic death'—a disgraceful dereliction of duty.

It is preferable to call such fatalities 'deaths associated with anaesthesia'. In England and Wales, all deaths during, or before full recovery from, an anaesthetic are reportable to the coroner; even after this period, any death which is considered by the doctor to be potentially related to the anaesthetic or surgical procedure must also be reported. For instance, a fatal pulmonary embolus some days after a gastrectomy should be reported, as it is unlikely that the fatal event would have occurred had the operation not been performed: it is no longer a 'natural causes' death.

Deaths associated with anaesthesia and surgical operations fall into the following major groups:

1. Those due to the injury or disease (often advanced) for which the procedure was carried out, the operation and anaesthetic playing no part in the death.

2. A moribund preoperative condition of the patient, due to the effects of age, disease or injury ... a 'last chance' procedure.

3. A postoperative event, such as pneumonia or a leg vein thrombosis and pulmonary embolism, which was due neither to the disease process nor to any defect in the operative procedure or anaesthetic.

4. A surgical mishap, unrelated to the anaesthetic, such as the inadvertent tearing or cutting of a major blood vessel, perhaps with air embolism.

5. A disease process, unrelated to that for which the operation was being carried out, either unforeseen or which had to be risked because of the urgency of the operation. An example would be a coronary thrombosis supervening in a patient operated upon for injuries.

6. An anaesthetic mishap or error—inadvertent overdosage, a mechanical error in the anaesthetic apparatus, etc.

The last category often presents great difficulty in investigation and cannot be left to the pathologist to evaluate. Often the autopsy findings are unrewarding, for the patient has been kept alive artificially, and the interpretation of the mishap rests largely upon the anaesthetist or the detailed recordings made during the operation. The pathologist must seek the close co-operation of both surgeon and anaesthetist at autopsy and in preparing his report for the coroner.

Anaesthetic deaths, proper, can be divided into several groups:

1. *Due to the anaesthetic agent itself.* These are uncommon but ventricular fibrillation and cardiac arrest sometimes take place from the direct action of the anaesthetic. Halothane has been the subject of considerable suspicion in recent years, especially where previous halothane anaesthesia has been given, even years earlier. 'Malignant' hyperpyrexia is an uncommon, but well-documented, genetic complication of certain muscle relaxants such as suxamethonium.

2. *Due to technique of administration of the anaesthetic.* Hypoxia (anoxia) is the most common error, often due to inexperience or inattention on the part of the anaesthetist, who may be relatively junior or insufficiently supervised. Obstruction of the airway, either within the patient's body or in the gas connections to the machine, is the most obvious. Where this leads either to death or to a decerebrate state from permanent cortical impairment, damages for negligence may be among the largest awarded for any type of medical malpractice ... provided the patient

survives, needing care and attention in what may be a 'vegetable existence'. Unfamiliarity with the machine and inexperience in the early detection of danger signs combine to make this a potent cause of avoidable
fatalities. A recent large survey of anaesthetic deaths in Britain emphasised this as the most common cause of fatalities.

3. *Due to malfunction of the anaesthetic equipment.* This is more common than might be thought, with crossed tubes, kinked pipes, faulty
valves and other mechanical errors often being compounded by the inexperience of the anaesthetist, who may be unable to recognise or deal
with the problems. Explosions, especially with ether and cyclopropane,
may rarely cause operating theatre tragedies.

Occasionally, when no organic cause for death is found at autopsy, it
may be necessary to discuss the possibility of some functional event such
as vagal inhibition. Vomit or tube impaction in the glottis, stretching of
the peritoneum as by emptying a viscus or tightening abdominal sutures,
intubation of the bronchus or urethra, needle puncture (especially of the
pleura) instrumental abortion, etc., may all induce such inhibitory reflexes, often with immediately fatal results. Even though the heart and
respiration may be restarted, their rhythm is unstable owing to the period
of collapse and anoxia, and failure may recur—without new reason.

Relationship of disease with work, trauma and crime

There are some pathological conditions such as coronary occlusion, the
relationship of which to exertion or work stress is so obvious that argument seldom occurs over compensation. Anything which demands a
quickening of the circulation and increases the strain on the heart may
be regarded as contributory to heart failure from coronary occlusion.
Exertions such as climbing ladders, lifting furniture, wielding tools or
holding tight against a strain may be sufficient, for the heart muscle may
be precariously short of blood already.

> A man of 47, engaged in the unloading of sides of beef from a ship, had to
> wheel them on a truck for some 25 metres up a slope and lift them off with
> the help of a loader on to a truck, swinging them up to a level of more than
> a metre on to a platform. After carrying and unloading two loads of sides he
> complained of pain in his chest and of being short of breath. He sat down for
> a few minutes and recovered. As he was wheeling the next load up the slope
> he collapsed, dead. Autopsy revealed moderately advanced coronary occlu-
> sion by atheroma, and compensation for acceleration by work stress was
> agreed without further litigation.

Many such cases arise in practice, involving innumerable variations of
the same principle.

The same arguments can be applied to the association of work stress
and the rupture of diseased and malformed (e.g. cerebral) arteries. Any
strain which demands an increasing flow of blood will raise the blood
pressure and be likely to precipitate the rupture of an artery. The aorta,

especially if already dilated and thinned by aneurysm, the elective vessels of cerebral haemorrhage (in the corpus striatum or pons) and the circle of Willis weakened by atheroma or developmental 'miliary' aneurysm defects, may all give way under the pressure of this increased arterial tension. As little exertion as that required to tighten a nut with a spanner was adjudged likely to have contributed towards rupture of an aneurysm in the famous Clover Clayton and Hughes case, and I (KS) have seen a very similar case where an aortic aneurysmal wall, stretched to paper thinness, gave way as a man was idly shovelling silt out of a tank at a battery works. He had only just taken on the job as a Sunday morning relief worker and collapsed at the second or third shovel stroke; acceleration by work stress was not denied.

> A man of 53, helping to load drums of electric cable, saw one rolling back down a slope and, putting his shoulder to it, held it by sheer strength till help came, perhaps some $1-1\frac{1}{2}$ minutes later. On releasing his hold he put his hand to his head and walked over to a packing-case, complaining of pain in the head. He became unconscious some 10 minutes later, and died $3\frac{1}{2}$ hours after, in hospital, autopsy revealing some cerebral atheroma and a massive cerebral haemorrhage. He was mildly hypertensive.

> A mechanic of 19, lying on his back tightening a sump drain plug under a lorry, was heard to cry out. Another man, hearing this call, turned to see a spanner topple out from under the vehicle. The mechanic was pulled out unconscious and died 7 hours later from a ruptured developmental aneurysm of the circle of Willis.

These are examples of natural disease the relationship of which to work stress occasions no argument. So long as it is admitted, as it must be, that the blood pressure is raised by exertion, so must the probability of acceleration by work stress be admitted.

The relationship of trauma to ruptures of blood vessels rests on simple principles. If it is of a kind that might suddenly jar or twist the vessel which burst, then trauma might well have precipitated rupture, and where the rupture is closely related in time to the injury the association is too likely to be denied. It must not be expected that the injury sustained will always be demonstrable.

> A bargee was prodded in the right upper chest by an oar; he complained of pain and started coughing, and after several coughs he spat up some blood. Small haemorrhages continued for some hours, and examination later showed he had right apical phthisis with cavitation. He died after a steady downhill course extending over some 9 weeks, and liability for acceleration by trauma was accepted. No mark of injury was ever demonstrated.

When criminal violence instead of simple trauma is involved the principle remains the same:

> An old bruiser of 72, long retired from the ring, was exchanging blows with his son of 46 in a heated argument when, after receiving a blow to the solar plexus and another on the point of the jaw, the son suddenly collapsed, falling unconscious. The old man tried to revive him by heating a flat-iron and applying it to the chest over the heart, but without avail. Death was due to

a ruptured developmental cerebral aneurysm, and medical evidence was given that, although the excitement of anger and the struggle, or the jarring blow to the head, might well have precipitated rupture, it was possible for the event to have occurred spontaneously. A charge of manslaughter that had been made was not pressed, and the magistrate discharged the old man. It was felt that he had suffered enough by the loss of his son under such circumstances.

The association between trauma and disease is not always as clear as this and it often has to be resolved into a balance of probabilities. A malignant growth or an abscess already present may clearly have its development accelerated by trauma which breaks down its natural barriers, but the relationship between trauma and the subsequent appearance of the disease is far more difficult to assess. Trauma is such a common event: anyone can remember some kind of recent injury to most parts of the body, and most patients with, say, acute ostiomyelitis or a brain tumour, when asked about trauma, can recollect some injury. When compensation may depend on the association, the memory tends to be encouraged—even in those with moral integrity; human nature has its weaknesses.

A butcher's boy of 17 was struck on the hip by a falling case of meat, sustaining some local bruising. Two days later he felt unwell and complained of acute pain in the same hip. By the fourth day frank osteomyelitis had become developed, and pyaemia and death followed.

Trauma can undoubtedly, by 'starting' a small juxtaepiphyseal haemorrhage, afford a nidus for bacterial infection, and when the relationship in time is very close, as in this case, it is reasonable to associate the disease with the injury.

In another case, a man of 47 sustained an injury to the left brow from a falling packing-case. Headaches commenced and continued intermittently for 14 months, when he suddenly collapsed with a paraplegia, dying 10 days later from hypostatic pneumonia. Autopsy revealed a malignant glioma of the right parietal subcortex ... in an area liable to contre-coup from the head injury sustained.

An association between trauma and the development of a brain tumour rests on less secure ground. The organisation of areas of brain trauma requires time and the interval between injury and the development of symptoms may be long. Even if these processes become malignant, this change also requires time. That it can happen is undoubted, for reparative processes are themselves new growths capable of all shades of activity, and of becoming irrepressible like keloids or frankly malignant like sarcomata of bone or muscle fasciae.

Some tumours, such as the aniline workers' bladder epithelioma, the English cotton mule-spinners' skin epithelioma (due to lubricating oil), tar-distillers' skin cancer, asbestosis and radioactive luminous paint-workers' sarcoma, are well established in their association with chemical carcinogenic irritants, and it is likely that trauma can be added as a factor in the localisation of pipe-smoker's lip and the chimney-sweep's scrotal cancers of former years.

Where trauma stands in some relation to a growth it is seldom a matter for proof. It is a matter of reasonable probabilities. Ewing formulated certain 'postulates' which should apply before a tumour is related to previous injury.

1. Previous integrity of the part.
2. Substantial—i.e. adequate—injury to the part.
3. A reasonable interval for the type of growth.
4. Tumour development at the site of injury.
5. Proof by microscopy of its nature.

Assessment of the first two factors depends so much on the veracity of witnesses who know that the success of the claim depends on their stories that they must always be tested with great care. The case of the brain tumour described above rests for proof on the exact site of the head injury, its character and the truth of the symptoms linking the trauma with the arrival of growth as much as on the more scientific generalisations set out above. Though it would not be unreasonable to associate the trauma with the growth, it is not a certainty. It is only a possibility, and such are the final assessments of most cases of the kind. Harvey Cushing felt, after a critical survey of his personal experience of glioma, that trauma of an authentic character could be associated in some 15 per cent of cases, and Parker and Kernahan, in over 400 cases, recorded a figure of 13.4 per cent associated with injury. To add a word of caution, they also found authentic trauma to the head in 10.4 per cent of a group of non-tumour-bearing patients, and 35.5 per cent of normal persons who could recall a significant head injury. Most of us can, and the problem clearly depends on the critical assessment of the Ewing postulates set out above. Courville concluded that in no case did a glioma prove to be of traumatic origin.

Injury that necessitates rest in bed, whether for surgical or other treatment, may also lead to two common complications—phlebothrombosis, which may end in fatal pulmonary embolism, and hypostatic pneumonia, seldom fatal since the coming of antibiotics.

Arguments in court over liability used to occupy days, and it is becoming increasingly clear that the 'no fault' system of acceptance (recommended by a Royal Commission in 1978 and which states that it usually takes two to cause an accident), already practised in some countries, will grow. Such agreement may, however, still leave room for argument on the contributory negligence of doctors and hospitals.

Workmen's diseases and injuries

National Insurance (Industrial Injuries) Acts

The Workmen's Compensation Act 1897 first established the responsibility of an employer to pay compensation for injuries incurred at work, so long as loss of earnings could be established. The Act was, after various amendments, finally replaced by the National Insurance (Indusrial Injuries) Act 1946 and its later amendments. From the appointed day, 5 July 1948, a special benefit became payable, as of right, on the sole basis of loss of faculty. All persons employed in Great Britain under a contract of service or apprenticeship are insured against incapacity, disablement or death due to an industrial accident in which the victim suffers *personal injury by accident arising out of and in the course of employment.*

The phrase 'injury by accident' includes any 'physiological injury or change for the worse' due to the work, and the word 'accident' means 'an unlooked-for mishap or an untoward event which is not expected or designed'. Certain industrial diseases, known as the prescribed diseases, are similarly covered by the Act; they should be distinguished from the 'notifiable' diseases of the Factories Act 1961, described at the end of the chapter.

Benefits may be payable even if an accident occurs when due to work-mates' misconduct, in emergencies, when travelling to or from work in an employer's vehicle, or when contravening or ignoring regulations or orders—provided the employee was at work and the act done for the purpose of and in connection with the employer's business. In civil courts the Law Reform (Contributory Negligence) Act 1945 allows damage to be apportioned according to fault.

Contributions are levied from employee and employer and these, together with an Exchequer supplement, are paid into the Industrial Injuries Fund administered by the Secretary of State for Social Services. In addition, 'supplementary schemes' can also be established from contributions to a special fund made by employees and employer: additional payments to all three forms of benefit may then be paid from the Fund. Only the National Coal Board has so far adopted the idea.

Payment of benefit is by means of a weekly sum except that a gratuity, and not a pension, is generally given for a disablement assessment of less than 20 per cent.

Three forms of benefit are provided:

1. *Injury benefit*, which may include allowances for dependants, is payable for up to 26 weeks' incapacity. It is never paid at the same time as disablement benefit in respect of the same accident.

2. *Disablement benefit*, which becomes payable whenever the victim remains disabled after injury benefit ends, from loss of physical or mental faculty (including disfigurement) due to an industrial accident or prescribed disease. The amount paid depends upon the assessment of disablement expressed as a percentage made by a medical board. Usually, of course, when a person returns to work after an injury, there is no remaining loss of faculty, and thus no disablement benefit.

Increased benefit in the form of a 'hardship allowance' may also be payable as an addition to disablement benefit if the claimant is incapable of returning to his regular job or of doing work of an equivalent standard. Increased benefit is also allowed for 'constant attendance' or hospital treatment.

3. *Death benefit,* which is payable to dependants if an insured person dies as a result of industrial accident or a prescribed disease. If a widow remarries, payment ceases but she is given a year's pension in the form of a gratuity.

Determination of claims

The onus of proof regarding an industrial accident or prescribed disease rests on the claimant. Claims are determined on a balance of probabilities, not by the Secretary of State but by an insurance officer and other independent authorities. The Secretary of State may not interfere with their decisions (see below).

An insured person is required:

1. to notify his employer of an accident 'as soon as is practicable', preferably entering particulars in the accident book;

2. to make claims in writing, accompanied by certificates and other supporting evidence, within 21 days for injury benefit, and within 3 months for disablement or death benefit claims;

3. to give notice of any change of circumstances, e.g. divorce, absence abroad, imprisonment, prolonged hospitalisation; and

4. to submit to medical examination, treatment, vocational training or industrial rehabilitation as may be required.

The employer on his part is required to take reasonable steps to investigate accidents, to furnish information for determining claims and to maintain an accident book.

Procedure upon claim

Industrial accidents   All claims are considered initially by an *insurance officer* appointed from the Department of Health and Social Security. He is a civil servant, and there is at least one at each National Insurance office. He decides, if necessary with medical advice, whether an industrial accident did indeed occur and whether *injury benefit* should be paid.

An initial right of appeal lies to a *local tribunal.* This has a solicitor as chairman, one member representing insured persons and another the employers. A medical practitioner may be asked to assist as an assessor.

The final right of appeal is to a *National Insurance commissioner.* The Chief Commissioner and the eight commissioners are appointed by the Crown on the advice of the Lord Chancellor, and must be barristers (or advocates) of at least 10 years' standing. A medical assessor, usually of consultant status, may be invited by the commissioner to assist him. No further appeal lies against a commissioner's decision, but it may be quashed by a divisional court of the Queen's Bench.

Disablement benefit questions of a difficult nature are reserved for determination by independent medical authorities. *Medical boards* determine whether an industrial accident has resulted in a loss of faculty and assess the appropriate degree and duration of disablement. The board is usually composed of two doctors from general practice. Appeal lies to a *medical appeal tribunal* composed of a barrister (or advocate) as chairman, and two consultants as members. On a point of law only is there further right of appeal to the commissioner.

Prescribed diseases   (listed below) may require the opinion of an *examining medical practitioner*, usually a local family doctor interested in industrial medicine. The insurance officer may then decide the claim himself; or refer the question to a medical board. Right of appeal from the insurance officer's decision is also to a board, and thence to a medical appeal tribunal. The commissioner can allow an appeal on a point of law.

Industrial lung disease and mesothelioma   Claims for the 'farmer's lung' and mesothelioma diseases, together with pneumoconiosis and byssinosis, are subject to special provisions.

Pneumoconiosis medical panels have been established to assist the insurance officer when a claim is received, and the *pneumoconiosis Medical Board*, drawing its membership from a panel, has a parallel role to that of an ordinary medical board. In special circumstances, an appeal on pneumoconiosis diagnosis is now allowed to an exceptionally experienced *central pneumoconiosis medical board* which conducts its proceedings on the same lines as a medical appeal tribunal.

Appeals against the decisions of an insurance officer go to a pneumoconiosis medical board, and if against a medical board (on the assessment of a pneumoconiosis) to the usual medical appeal tribunal, as with other prescribed diseases.

Persons engaged in certain occupations exposing them to the risk of pneumoconiosis have to submit to an initial examination before the end of the second month of employment, and periodically afterwards—giving a good basis for opinion of any changes found.

List of prescribed diseases

The prescribed diseases (other than pneumoconiosis and byssinosis) are set out in the first column of Table 10.1. Each disease is prescribed in relation to all insured persons who have been employed on or after 5 July 1948 in insurable employment in any occupation set against it in the second column.

Table 10.1 Prescribed diseases

Description of disease or injury	Nature of occupation
Poisoning by:	*Any occupation involving:*
1. Lead or a compound of lead	The use or handling of, or exposure to the fumes, dust or vapour of, lead or a compound of lead, or a substance containing lead
2. Manganese or a compound of manganese	The use or handling or, or exposure to the fumes, dust or vapour of, manganese or a compound of manganese, or a substance containing manganese

Table 10.1 (*contd*)

Description of disease or injury	Nature of occupation
3. Phosphorus or phosphine or poisoning due to the anticholinesterase action of organic phosphorus compounds	The use or handling of, or exposure to the fumes, dust or vapour of, phosphorus or a compound of phosphorus, or a substance containing phosphorus
4. Arsenic or a compound of arsenic	The use or handling of, or exposure to the fumes, dust or vapour of, arsenic or a compound of arsenic, or a substance containing arsenic
5. Mercury or a compound of mercury	The use or handling of, or exposure to the fumes, dust or vapour of, mercury or a compound of mercury, or a substance containing mercury
6. Carbon bisulphide	The use or handling of, or exposure to the fumes or vapour of, carbon bisulphide or a compound of carbon bisulphide, or a substance containing carbon bisulphide
7. Benzene or a homologue	The use or handling of, or exposure to the fumes of, or vapour containing, benzene or any of its homologues
8. A nitro- or amino- or chloro-derivative of benzene or of a homologue of benzene, or poisoning by nitrochlorbenzene	The use or handling of, or exposure to the fumes of, or vapour containing, a nitro- or amino- or chloro-derivative of benzene or a homologue of benzene or nitrochlorbenzene
9. Dinitrophenol or a homologue or substituted dinitrophenols or the salts of such substances	The use or handling of, or exposure to the fumes of, or vapour containing, dinitrophenol or a homologue or substituted dinitrophenols or the salts of such substances
10. Tetrachlorethane	The use or handling of, or exposure to the fumes of, or vapour containing, tetrachlorethane
11. Tricresyl phosphate	The use or handling of, or exposure to the fumes of, or vapour containing, tricresyl phosphate
12. Triphenyl phosphate	The use or handling of, or exposure to the fumes of, or vapour containing, triphenyl phosphate
13. Diethylene dioxide (dioxan)	The use or handling of, or exposure to the fumes of, or vapour containing, diethylene dioxide (dioxan)
14. Methyl bromide	The use or handling of, or exposure to the fumes of, or vapour containing, methyl bromide
15. Chlorinated naphthalene	The use or handling of, or exposure to the fumes of, or dust or vapour containing, chlorinated naphthalene
16. Nickel carbonyl	Exposure to nickel carbonyl gas
17. Nitrous fumes	The use of handling of nitric acid or exposure to nitrous fumes
18. *Gonioma kamassi* (African boxwood)	The manipulation of *Gonioma kamassi* or any process in or incidental to the manufacture of articles therefrom

Description of disease or injury	Nature of occupation
19. Anthrax	The handling of wool, hair, bristles, hides or skins or other animal products or residues thereof, or contact with, animals infected with anthrax
20. Glanders	Contact with equine animals or their carcases
21. (*a*) Infection by *Leptospira icterohaemorrhagiae*	Work in places which are, or are liable to be, infested by rats
(*b*) Infection by *Leptospira canicola*	Work at dogs kennels or the care or handling of dogs
22. Ankylostomiasis	Work in or about a mine
23. (*a*) Dystrophy of the cornea (including ulceration of the corneal surface) of the eye (*b*) Localised new growth of the skin, papillomatous or keratotic (*c*) Squamous cell carcinoma of the skin Due in any case to arsenic, tar, patch, bitumen, mineral oil (including paraffin), soot or any compound, product (including quinone or hydroquinone), or residue of any of these substances	The use or handling of, or exposure to, arsenic, tar, pitch, bitumen, mineral oil (including paraffin), soot or any compound, product (including quinone or hydroquinone), or residue of any of these substances
24. (Now covered by diseases 41 and 42)	
25. Inflammation, ulceration or malignant disease of the skin or subcutaneous tissues or of the bones, or blood dyscrasia, or cataract, due to electromagnetic radiations (other than radiant heat), or to ionising particles	Exposure to electromagnetic radiations other than radiant heat, or to ionising particles
26. Heat cataract	Frequent or prolonged exposure to rays from molten or red-hot material
27. Decompression sickness	Subjection to compressed or rarefied air
28. Cramp of the hand or forearm due to repetitive movements	Prolonged periods of handwriting, typing or other repetitive movements of the fingers, hand or arm
29. 30. } (Now covered by disease 28)	
31. Subcutaneous cellulitis of the hand (beat hand)	Manual labour causing severe or prolonged friction or pressure on the hand
32. Bursitis or subcutaneous cellulitis arising at or about the knee due to severe or prolonged external friction or pressure at or about the knee (beat knee)	Manual labour causing severe or prolonged external friction or pressure at or about the knee
33. Bursitis or subcutaneous cellulitis arising at or about the elbow due to severe or prolonged external friction or pressure at or about the elbow (beat elbow)	Manual labour causing severe or prolonged external friction or pressure at or about the elbow

Table 10.1 (*contd*)

Description of disease or injury	Nature of occupation
34. Traumatic inflammation of the tendons of the hand or forearm, or of the associated tendon sheaths	Manual labour, or frequent or repeated movements of the hand or wrist
35. Miner's nystagmus	Work in or about a mine
36. Poisoning by beryllium or a compound of beryllium	The use or handling of, or exposure to the fumes, dust or vapour of, beryllium or a compound of beryllium, or a substance containing beryllium
37. (*a*) Carcinoma of the mucous membrane of the nose or associated air sinuses (*b*) Primary carcinoma of a bronchus or of a lung	Work in a factory where nickel is produced by decomposition of a gaseous nickel compound which necessitates working in or about a building or buildings where that process or any other industrial process ancillary or incidental thereto is carried on
38. Tuberculosis	Close and frequent contact with a source or sources of tuberculous infection by reason of employment: (*a*) in the medical treatment or nursing of a person or persons suffering from tuberculosis, or in a service ancillary to such treatment or nursing; (*b*) in attendance upon a person or persons suffering from tuberculosis, where the need for such attendance arises by reason of physical or mental infirmity; (*c*) as a research worker engaged in research in connection with tuberculosis; (*d*) as a laboratory worker, pathologist or person taking part in or assisting at post-mortem examinations of human remains where the occupation involves working with material which is a source of tuberculous infection
39. Primary neoplasm of the epithelial lining of the urinary bladder (papilloma of the bladder), or of the epithelial lining of the renal pelvis or of the epithelial lining of the ureter	(*a*) Work in a building in which any of the following substances is produced for commercial purposes: (i) alpha-naphthylamine or beta-naphthylamine; (ii) diphenyl substituted by at least one nitro or primary amino group or by at least one nitro and primary amino group; (iii) any of the substances mentioned in subparagraph (ii) above if further ring substituted by halogeno, methyl or methoxy groups, but not by other groups; (iv) the salts of any of the substances mentioned in subparagraphs (i) to (iii) above

Description of disease or injury	Nature of occupation
	(v) auramine or magenta
	(b) The use or handling of any of the substances mentioned in subparagraphs (i)–(iv) of paragraph (a), or work in a process in which any such substance is used or handled or is liberated
	(c) The maintenance or cleaning of any plant or machinery used in any such process as is mentioned in paragraph (b), or the cleaning of clothing used in any such building as is mentioned in paragraph (a) if such clothing is cleaned within the works of which the building forms a part or in a laundry maintained and used solely in connection with such works
40. Poisoning by cadmium	Exposure to cadmium fumes
41. Inflammation or ulceration of the mucous membrane of the upper respiratory passages or mouth produced by dust, liquid or vapour	Exposure to dust, liquid or vapour
42. Non-infective dermatitis of external origin (including chrome ulceration of the skin but excluding dermatitis due to ionising particles or electromagnetic radiations other than radiant heat).	Exposure to dust, liquid or vapour, or any other external agent capable of irritating the skin (including friction or heat but excluding ionising particles or electromagnetic radiations other than radiant heat)
43. Pulmonary disease due to the inhalation of the dust of mouldy hay or of other mouldy vegetable produce, and giving rise to a defect in gas exchange (farmer's lung)	Exposure to the dust of mouldy hay or other mouldy vegetable produce by reason of employment: (a) in agriculture, horticulture or forestry; or (b) loading or unloading or handling in storage such hay or other vegetable produce; or (c) handling bagasse
44. Primary malignant neoplasm of the mesothelium (diffuse mesothelioma) of the pleura or of the peritoneum	(a) the working or handling of asbestos or any admixture of asbestos; (b) the manufacture or repair of asbestos textiles; (c) the cleaning of any machinery or plant used in any of the foregoing operations; (d) 'substantial exposure' to the dust arising from any of the foregoing operations
45. Nasal adenocarcinoma	Wood furniture manufacture
46. Brucellosis	Contact with bovine animals infected by *Brucella abortus*, their carcasses or parts thereof or their untreated products, or with laboratory specimens or vaccines

Table 10.1 (*contd*)

Description of disease or injury	Nature of occupation
	of or containing *Brucella abortus*, by reason of employment: (*a*) as a farm worker; (*b*) as a veterinary worker; (*c*) as a slaughterhouse worker; (*d*) as a laboratory worker; or (*e*) in any other work relating to the care, treatment, examination or handling of such animals, carcasses or parts thereof or products.
47. Poisoning by acrylamide monomer	Any occupation involving the use or handling of, or exposure to, acrylamide monomer.

In February 1976, viral hepatitis was added to the list under the Social Security Act 1975.

In 1977, angiosarcoma of the liver and osteolysis of the terminal phalanges of the fingers arising from exposure to vinyl chloride monomer were also added.

Additional diseases may be added from time to time on the advice of the Industrial Diseases Advisory Council.

The many medical questions which arise out of the legislation emphasise the vital importance of doctors keeping full and meticulously accurate records of all cases coming to them under the provisions of the Act. Reports are increasingly asked of doctors in the preparation of evidence, and they have a duty to give every assistance to ensure a full and proper hearing of cases. The Act imposes responsibilities which must not be discharged lightly. Patients rightly look to their doctors for the medical backing they need in litigation.

Factories Act 1961   By this Act every medical practitioner attending on, or called in to visit, a patient whom he believes to be suffering from lead, phosphorus, arsenic, mercury, beryllium, cadmium ... or their organic compounds, aniline, manganese, chronic benzene or carbon bisulphide, triphenyl or tricresyl phosphate poisoning; anticholinesterase action of phosphorous compounds; toxic anaemia or toxic jaundice; chrome ulceration; epitheliomatous ulceration; compressed air illness; anthrax; *if contracted in any factory*, shall forthwith send, addressed to the 'Chief Inspector of Factories, Department of Employment and Productivity, London', a notification stating the name and full postal address of the patient and the disease from which, in the opinion of the practitioner, the patient is suffering, and the name and address of the factory in which he is, or was last, employed, and shall be entitled in respect of every notice sent in pursuance of this section to the current fee. Failure to notify carries a liability to a fine. The foregoing will not apply if a letter, so worded, has been previously sent.

By the same Act (sect. 129) a practitioner must similarly notify any case of lead poisoning contracted in painting any building, unless it has been already notified; also of cadmium and beryllium.

The Factories Act 1961 also prohibits the employment of women or young persons in certain processes connected with lead manufacture, and in processes involving the use of lead compounds. All the notifiable lesions are compensatable under the National Health (Industrial Injuries) Act 1965.

Notification of infectious disease or food poisoning   The following diseases are notifiable:

Cholera*

Diphtheria*

Dysentery (amoebic or bacillary)*

Food poisoning or suspected food poisoning*

Lassa fever*

Marburg virus disease*

Meningitis (acute)*

Paratyphoid*

Poliomyelitis*

Rabies*

Smallpox*

Typhoid*

Viral haemorrhagic fever (ebola)*

Anthrax

Encephalitis (acute)

Infective jaundice

Leprosy

Leptospirosis

Malaria

Measles

Ophthalmia neonatorum

Plague

Relapsing fever

Scarlet fever

Tetanus

Tuberculosis

Typhus

Whooping cough

Yellow fever

All diseases marked with * should also be notified urgently by telephone to the medical officer of environmental health.

11

Suspicious neonatal and infant deaths

Perinatal and infant deaths are common, and their medico-legal aspects lie outside everyday obstetric and paediatric experience. Birth carries many hazards even when the infant is healthy and delivery is 'uncomplicated', and the first few days of life are like rough weather to a tender shoot, precarious unless handled with skill and care. Even after the immediate problems of the perinatal period are passed, there is the still unsolved menace of sudden unexpected death in infancy—'cot death'; and many children have also to survive the hazards of the 'battered baby'.

Doctors—and forensic pathologists—called to examine neonates and infants have to keep in view a broad spectrum of possibilities, and, whilst bearing in mind the ordinary risks (the current infant mortality is 16 per 1000) of birth and infant life, must always be alert to the possibility of 'accident' or crime.

Categories of infant death

1. *Stillbirth*—registrable if 'viable'—and *disposal* sometimes by *concealment of birth;* or
2. *Natural death*—from *prematurity, disease* or *birth hazards.*
3. *Want of attention* at birth—not criminal.
4. *Accidental happenings* at birth—e.g. into the toilet or under the bedclothes—not wilful.
5. *Wilful injury or omission* by the mother within 12 months—usually at birth; i.e. *infanticide.*
6. *Sudden infant death syndrome* (SIDS), often called *cot deaths.*
7. *Wilful injury* apart from the provisions of infanticide. *The battered baby* (manslaughter or murder).

The two further problems of 'cot death' and the 'battered baby' will be considered later (see pp. 170 and 172).

The law

A developing fetus is regarded by the law as able to have a separate existence if born at or after the twenty-eighth week of gestation: it is 'viable'. This is a legal term used in relation both to child destruction under the Infant Life Preservation Act 1929 and to the registration of stillbirths—required under the Births and Deaths Registration Act 1926 only for gestations of 28 weeks or more.

Child destruction is the rare offence of killing before birth of a viable child except as a proper therapeutic measure to preserve the life of the mother.

The law has, in the view of obstetricians, set a rather high standard for viability, for a glance at the statistics will show that something like 95 per cent of infants born at the twenty-eighth week fail to survive their first week of life. Its length—five times as long in centimetres as the number of months' gestation—is only 35.5 cm, and its weight a bare 1.15 kg: it is still very immature. But by the eighth month or so it achieves a weight of some 2.5 kg, and is regarded as obstetrically 'mature'. At this weight about 95 per cent will now survive their first week and thrive.

Doctors need not therefore be surprised if an infant of 28 weeks, though perhaps viable in the eyes of the law, fails to achieve a separate existence: it is so immature it is unlikely in the absence of skilled care to do so, and its death need occasion no suspicion. It is in connection with the death of the more mature infant that some more tangible cause must be sought: this usually necessitates autopsy.

Separate existence

A 'separate existence' is not quite synonymous with 'live birth' for a living fetus may be born in a living state but lie still and fail to breathe. The law says that an infant has achieved a separate existence when it has 'completely proceeded from the body of the mother and has breathed or shown some other sign' of being alive apart from its parent. It may be found to have a heart beat (or a 'pulse' in the umbilical cord), but mere movement (which might be due to gravity or some other factor) would not be enough. A post-mortem after a longer period of survival might reveal healing changes in the stump of the umbilical cord, or milk food in the stomach.

Autopsy will be necessary to reveal the expansion of the lungs that gives proof of breathing, and also the post-mortem findings may indicate the reasons for failure to survive. The colour of the skin is no help in this respect.

Offences under the law

In addition to the rare offence of *child destruction* already defined, the unborn child may (in Scotland only) have its existence 'concealed'. In the UK, the offence of *concealment of birth* is not often brought, since

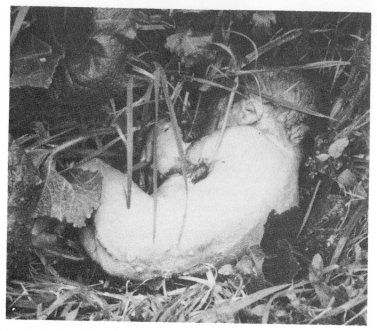

Fig. 11.1 Suspicious disposal of the newborn infant.

the infant has to be hidden in a place to which no member of the public has access: placing the newborn infant on the doorstep of a hospital, even discarded in a country ditch, is not 'concealment' in law.

Two gypsies who burned the body of a newborn infant in an Aylesbury encampment pleaded guilty to 'concealment of birth'; only a few bones could be identified in the ashes.

The Infanticide Act 1938

Like many similar statute laws in other countries, this was enacted in order to deal leniently with the mother of a newborn child who, often alone and unwilling to cell for help, causes its death by some omission or even a positive act of violence at a time of considerable emotional and physical strain. This is not some ordinary form of homicide like manslaughter by negligence or frank murder, for the woman's mind is likely to be too disturbed for her to have the guilt (*mens rea*) that the law needs to prove to convict of such serious crimes.

The Act sets out that 'where a woman by any wilful act or omission causes the death of her child, being a child under the age of 12 months, but at the time of the act or omission the balance of her mind was disturbed by reason of her not having fully recovered from the effects of giving birth to the child, or by reason of the effect of lactation consequent upon the birth of the child', then she shall be guilty of the crime of infanticide.

Any other person than the mother would face the ordinary charge of homicide: only the mother of the dead infant attracts such leniency.

The offence of infanticide has become comparatively rare since the Abortion Act 1967 has made it easier for a mother to rid herself of an unwanted child by a 'legal' abortion (see p. 176). This is not, of course, to say that a woman cannot be charged with criminal neglect, causing unnecessary suffering, or murdering her child, even if it is within the 12 months allowed by the Infanticide Act. For the latter, it still has to be said in evidence on her behalf that she had not fully recovered from the effects of childbirth. This has never proved to be a difficult obstacle, for sympathy runs high in her favour as a rule. The courts usually impose a 'binding over'—i.e. not to do it again within some prescribed period.

Medical examination in neonatal death

In practice the law takes the view that, until proof of a separate existence is forthcoming, the child shall be presumed born dead—or at least not to have achieved a life apart from the mother. This is of course the only fair way to handle cases where the child is badly decomposed or a near-skeleton, for it is possible for a mother (or someone else) to stuff a cloth into the mouth or tie the child up in wrappings after it has been born as a stillbirth or has succumbed to some cause such as inhaling birth secretions or blood, now no longer detectable because of the *post mortem* state. No charge of causing a newborn child's death can be properly founded until the infant has been shown to have had a separate existence. For how long this has lasted is of little importance except to help the police in their inquiries.

The condition of *maceration* —softening of the body of an infant that has lain dead several days or more in the watery amniotic fluid of the gestation sac—can answer the question whether an infant could have been born alive. If macerated, with wet peeling cuticle and softening body tissues—even the skeleton may collapse—it *must* have lain dead in the uterus. No macerated infant can be the basis for any criminal charge, for it must have been stillborn.

On attaining a separate existence, striking changes take place in the lungs of the newborn child, and these at autopsy may alone justify the opinion that an independent existence has been attained. No transient vagitus, a much overestimated phenomenon, can imitate the changes following upon breathing. The lung immediately begins to expand, a few minutes sufficing to aerate it in most parts. The birth mucus and debris of epithelium and amniotic fluid which lay in the principal airways is cleared, and air sacs rapidly fill out with air. The lung, previously airless, slate-grey or purple, solid and non-crepitant, covered by wrinkled slack pleural membranes, becomes distended with air, pink, spongy, finely crepitant and covered by a thin taut pleura. Whereas previously each lung weighed 30–35 g or about one-seventieth of the body weight, the new blood drawn into the expanding functioning lung increases its

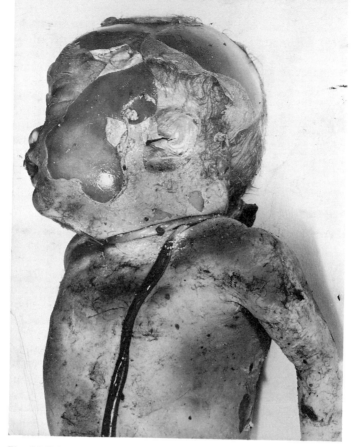

Fig. 11.2 Maceration precluding separate existence. The sodden peeling skin in a child freshly born, indicating death *in utero* several days prior to birth probably by cord strangulation *in utero*.

weight to some 60–65 g or one-thirtyfifth of the body weight (Fodéré's static test).

The lung may come to contain gases capable of causing it to float when decomposition has set in, and it is sound practice to refuse to give a positive opinion whenever any decomposition is present; the mother must be given the benefit of the difficulty, for the conditions prevent a sound opinion. It is often said, too, that artificial respiration may cause sufficient expansion of the lungs to obscure the issue. I (KS) have never seen it. On the contrary, manipulative artificial respiration tends gradually to collapse the lungs; only positive insufflation, as in mouth-to-mouth methods, expands them.

Where there is widespread fresh expansion in a reasonably well-preserved child a firm opinion should be expressed.

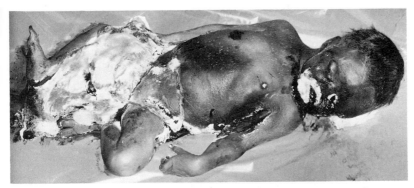

Fig. 11.3 Conditions of decomposition and mould formation likely to interfere seriously with the autopsy proof of separate existence. Newborn infant found after interval of 5 months in attic store-room.

Examples of the leniency of stating such a principle were seen in a case where a midwife, mother and grandmother all insisted that a newborn child had cried, but no expansion whatsoever could be found, and in another case where, after 7 hours of ineffectual breathing in hospital, conditions virtually indistinguishable from stillbirth were found at autopsy.

Such incidents should not deter one from a general view that a good degree of expansion in an undecomposed child must be seen to satisfy one that there has been a separate existence.

Air in the stomach is seen as often in stillbirths who gulp air in attempting to free their air passages of fluid obstructions as in live-births, who successfully attain a separate existence, and is of no practical value in confirming breathing. Breslau's belief that the distance to which air had entered the bowel could indicate the duration of a separate existence is quite unfounded.

Other evidence of separate existence

Drying of the cord commences rapidly after birth (and may continue after death). A ring of reddening appears around the attached end in some 36 hours, and in some 2 or 3 days the cord is hanging by a dry thread. In 5–6 days it sloughs off, and the ring scar is healed by the tenth day.

The foramen ovale and ductus arteriosus are open to a probe at birth, and for several weeks after, though functionally they are extinct. Three weeks or a month usually elapse before the ductus arteriosus is closed.

The umbilical veins and artery are quickly closed by thrombosis and the clot later becomes organised. Microscopy of these vessels may give help from about the sixth day to the third or fourth week, when little else but the length and weight are available.

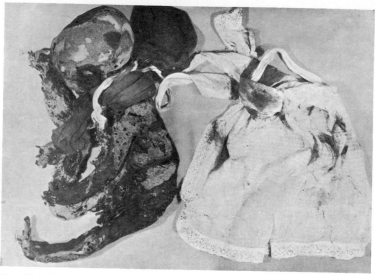

Fig. 11.4 Infanticide. Conditions of mummification (after 5 months) which preclude evidence of a separate existence. The ties (of a stocking and the strings of an apron) afford only presumptive evidence of a criminal act, for there is nothing to show the infant was alive or that asphyxia ensued.

The cause of death

The wording of the Infanticide Act demands that the child shall, having attained a separate existence, meet its death from some 'wilful act or omission'.

It must be remembered that many ordinary dangers lie in wait to snatch the newborn child from its new life. Although capable in law of living (viable), it may never attain a live birth owing to strangulation by entanglement with the cord, or to prolonged or unduly precipitate labour. When born alive it may immediately inhale birth fluids or fail to get into the stride of a strong respiratory cycle, atelectasis ensuing. Prematurity may limit the vigour with which it strives to overcome these obstacles. All of these events can be determined at autopsy, and any should at once dispose of suspicion of infanticide. They occur in spite of adequate care and attention at birth and do not reflect on the mother.

It is not without significance, however, that stillbirths are twice as frequent in illegitimate pregnancies as in legitimate ones. It is clear that many 'stillbirths' have to be labelled as such for lack of proof to the contrary. It is easy for a mother, not desiring a child, to see that it never gets a chance of drawing a breath through mouth and nostrils and exceedingly difficult to prove, when such an act is firm but gentle, that it was deliberate, or even to find evidence of it at all.

Many young girls experiencing labour for the first time, alone, in terror, shocked and faint from pain or loss of blood, may unknowingly commit some harmful act or omit some care which results in the death of the child. Many are genuinely taken by surprise when birth takes place. The mother may genuinely think that she is experiencing a difficult stool, and remain on the lavatory pan faint and helpless. In multipara, on the contrary, labour is very often brief and they may be little affected by it.

A housemaid delivered herself of a child weighing about 3.5 kg (7 lb 10 oz) into a lavatory pan during a period of some 30 minutes between doing her early morning 'chars' and serving breakfast. She did a normal morning's work, and walked 8 miles in the afternoon to dispose of the child's body. It was, she said, her first pregnancy.

Wilful omission rarely figures in charges of infanticide, many deaths being recorded, for lack of proof of wilfulness, as 'accidental' or 'due to lack of attention at birth', and so on.

The common wilful acts causing death are:

1. Suffocation or strangling.
2. Drowning.
3. Blunt injury, usually to the head.

Suffocation and strangling

The difficulty of proving that certain acts are, in fact, wilful acts demanded by the Infanticide Act has already been described.

A child found discarded in an attaché-case at London Bridge Station was found at autopsy to have died of suffocation, after the shortest possible separate existence. At autopsy there were intense asphyxial changes without mechanical cause. When traced the mother said she had given birth to the

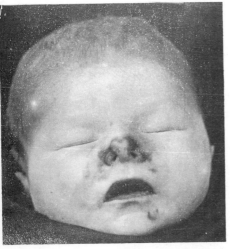
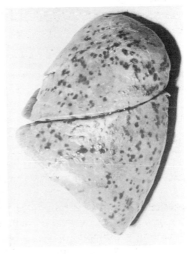

Fig. 11.6 Infanticide. Marks of the grasp of a right thumb and index fingers across the nostrils, of further fingers down the left side of the mouth, with a faint impression of the palm of the covering hand near the right angle of the mouth. The heart and lungs show many (Tardieu) petechial haemorrhages.

child under the bedclothes and did not hear it cry. She turned down the clothes to find the child blue and dead. No evidence was forthcoming to contradict her statement.

Sometimes, however (Fig. 11.5), clear evidence of a wilful act such as suffocation by the hand is provided by autopsy. Marks are usually present also in manual strangling, where finger-tip bruises or nail imprints may be found on the neck, the latter often crescentic in shape. Similar marks may result from attempts on the part of the mother at

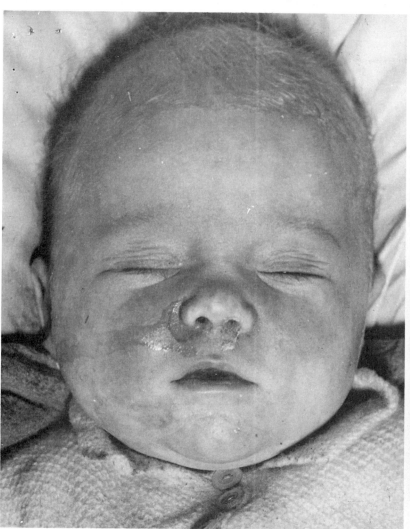

Fig. 11.6 White pressure marks around the mouth and nostrils of a dead child found face down, cannot be ascribed to suffocation, as identical appearances are seen as a purely post-mortem phenomenon. Blood-stained oedema fluid seen at the nostrils also commonly occurs in SIDS.

self-delivery, but these are usually widespread over the face and under the chin, sited wherever there is some purchase.

'Cot-deaths' are still a problem, for although petechiae are often present they are not asphyxial deaths (see p. 171).

Drowning

Precipitate deliveries commonly take place on the lavatory pan or chamber-pot, and the child may gulp a few breaths whilst drowning in the mixture of water and birth fluids (blood, vaginal mucus and meconium) in which it lies, dying from 'lack of attention at birth' (Fig. 11.7).

When a mixture of birth fluids is found in the air passages of a child who has breathed only to die of drowning, no medical grounds for suspicion of foul play could be maintained: only some mark of gripping by the hands could arouse suspicion. It is wise. if this is absent, to say

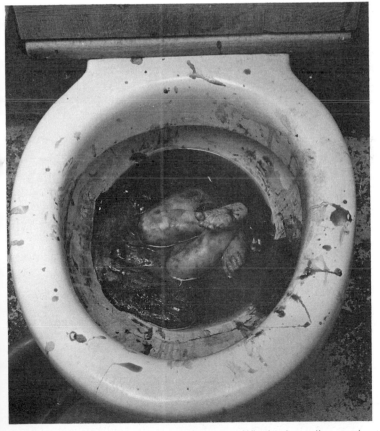

Fig. 11.7 Precipitate delivery into a lavatory pan. Whether born alive, starting to breathe (before immersion) or dying of some unexpected cause can be determined only by autopsy.

merely that death was due to asphyxia from inhalation of fluids. If there is no mark of injury to arouse suspicion of foul play this should be made quite clear.

Where, on the contrary, the fluid is foreign, death is likely to have been due to deliberate drowning.

> A hospital ward nurse, continuing to term with a pregnancy unknown to her ward sister, four nurses and two housemen, retired to the nurses' bathroom and there gave birth to and drowned a child weighing about 3 kg (6 lb 8 oz). Traces of carbolic soap (from the bath) were present in the faintly turbid fluid in the air passages, disproving her statement that birth took place unexpectedly on the bathroom floor.

The drowned infant is usually taken out of the fluid in which it met its death, wrapped loosely in some nondescript covering paper or cloth, and disposed of thus, or in a carrier bag or a small attaché-case, on dry ground. Drowning is a cause of death to bear constantly in mind wherever the body is found.

Blunt injury

The head may sustain injury from several causes during delivery. The caput must be distinguished, and the occasional fissure fractures of the vault plates which follow upon gross or rapid moulding must also be recognised as natural accompaniments of delivery. The absence of injury to the skin over such fissures will exclude local violence. Forceps injury and delivery fractures of arm and leg may also occur.

None of these bears comparison with the gross injuries inflicted by frenzied mothers upon their newborn children in infanticide.

> On one case where the external evidence of injury was limited to trivial bruises of the face, seventeen fractured ribs were found on autopsy; fragments of liver and spleen floated out through the incision made down the trunk for examination. The mother, who had at first denied violence, later admitted losing her temper and swinging the child by the legs against the bedrail.

Sudden infant death syndrome (SIDS)

The most common cause of infant mortality after the perinatal period in western countries, SIDS occurs in 1 of about every 500 live births. Also known as 'cot death' (or 'crib death' in North America), SIDS has a definite epidemiological pattern, although the causation and pathology are still in dispute.

SIDS shows the following features:

1. Occurs during sleep and usually in the small hours of the morning.
2. Has a higher incidence in premature and low-birth-weight babies, which partly accounts for the marked increase in incidence in twins, for whom the rate is two to five times that for singleton babies.
3. Shows a slight preponderance in male infants.

4. Has a marked seasonal variation, being more common in the northern hemisphere between October and April—the reverse being true in Australasia.

5. Has a definite social class incidence, being more common in socially less advantaged families as measured by father's occupation or the standard of housing.

6. Occurs mainly between 1 and 8 months of age, peaking at 3 months.

The common course of events is that a healthy child or one with minimal symptoms (usually of upper respiratory infection) is put to sleep at night and is found dead in its sleeping-place in the morning. Autopsy reveals little or no naked-eye changes, apart from some pulmonary congestion and oedema, and often petechial haemorrhage on the serosal surface of thoracic viscera. Unfortunately, the latter often suggested that some form of mechanical asphyxia or suffocation was the cause of death. This is now known to be quite untrue, and old theories of 'overlaying' or suffocation in soft bedding are unjustified.

Microscopically, few changes are seen; sometimes, minimal signs of a bronchiolitis may be found, but many deaths reveal no significant changes.

Theories as to the causation of SIDS abound, as in all syndromes of uncertain aetiology. Some of the more plausible include allergy to cow's milk protein, a subclinical virus bronchiolitis or some metabolic defect. Recently, most interest has been directed towards *prolonged sleep apnoea*, which although it may not be the basic aetiology, seems to be the final pathway to death. It seems probable that SIDS is a *multifactorial* condition, with varying factors in different instances, but all mediated via a terminal failure of the cardiorespiratory apparatus.

It is known that some infants, especially premature and immature babies, have an unstable respiratory drive. The SIDS rate in infants having such breathing difficulties soon after birth, or who have needed to be maintained in neonatal intensive care units, is much greater than in the general infant population. Is it postulated that a respiratory infection with its attendant hypoxia is such infants is likely to further depress respiration during sleep.

The hypoxia may further depress respiratory drive, lengthening the periods of apnoea during sleep, thus setting up a vicious circle of hypoxia–apnoea which may end in bradycardia and cardiac arrest. Some confirmation of this theory is given by the histological signs of chronic hypoxia reported by some researchers.

Whatever the basic causes of SIDS, the domestic consequences are considerable, as the mother almost always feels guilty. Unjustified talk about 'suffocation' or lack of care can greatly increase her self-recrimination and the family distress. The syndrome is now recognised by the World Health Organization's *Nomenclature of Disease* and can be certified as such. The risk of overlooking a deliberate suffocation may be remote, but it must not be forgotten although it is almost impossible to substantiate such suspicions on autopsy findings alone.

Overlaying and SIDS

Before it was recognised that the sudden infant death syndrome was a natural, if poorly understood, phenomenon, it was common to assume that where a child had died while in bed with an often-plump adult, the cause of the death was 'overlaying'—i.e. mechanical suffocation from the compression of the infant by the adult's body. Unfortunately, this assumption was reinforced by the frequent autopsy finding of intrathoracic petechial haemorrhages, now recognised to be non-specific and common in true SIDS where no possibility of suffocation could have arisen. To complicate the matter still further, in the relatively rare authenticated cases of true infant suffocation (usually accidental or homicidal), the so-called asphyxial stigmata of petechiae, etc., may be absent.

Where an infant is found dead in the maternal bed, the most rational view to take is that, as SIDS is so common (in western countries forming by far the greatest cause of postperinatal deaths), it should be considered to be the most likely explanation unless incontrovertible evidence to the contrary is available—and such evidence is more likely to be circumstantial than medical. Even if a mother finds herself lying upon her baby, SIDS may have anticipated her movement and there is absolutely no way in which an autopsy can distinguish true SIDS from the hypothetical, but unprovable, 'overlaying'.

These considerations warn every pathologist examining such infants to keep an open mind. The famous Boyd remarked that 'life's little candle is easily extinguished', and it would be tragic if false accusations against a mother were made on the grounds of dogmatic, but spurious, medical opinion.

Child abuse syndrome

Known also as the 'battered baby' syndrome or 'non-accidental injury in childhood', child abuse refers to deliberate, often repetitive, injuries inflicted upon an infant or child by the parent(s) or guardian(s). Although it was recorded in the medical literature of the nineteenth century, the modern syndrome was first described by an American radiologist, Caffey, whose publication of the association of subdural haemorrhage with long bone fractures released a flood of recognition during the 1950s and 1960s.

If no intervention takes place, there appears to be a 60 per cent recurrence rate; and there is a 10 per cent mortality rate in battered children. The most common cause of death is subdural haemorrhage, as described by Caffey, followed next by visceral injuries such as ruptured liver or intestines.

The following features are common in child abuse and should raise suspicion in the mind of a medical practitioner:

1. Multiple bruises, especially on the face, upper arms, around elbows, knees, wrists, neck and on the chest or abdomen. Typically, such bruises

are disc-shaped, often about 1 cm in diameter, due to the pressure of adult finger-pads gripping the child.

2. Bruising around the mouth and lips; laceration on the inside of the lips of children old enough to have teeth; and tearing of the frenulum inside the centre of the upper lip (Fig. 11.8). This is almost pathognomonic of either a slap across the mouth or forcible insertion of a feeding bottle.

3. Bruising of the ears or scalp and injuries to the eyes. Suspected victims of child abuse should be examined for vitreous haemorrhages, dislocated lens and detached retina; blindness may follow.

4. Skeletal fractures—either obvious or located radiographically. Where abuse is suspected, a full skeletal radiological survey is justified, in spite of the usual reluctance to expose to radiation. Particular fractures include skull, limb bones and ribs. Avulsion and chipping of epiphyses at the knee and elbow, and raised periosteum with subperiosteal calcification are particularly suspicious. In young infants, multiple rib fractures may occur, sometimes bilaterally, down the paravertebral gutter, where the ribs do not bend so easily, producing a 'string of beads' appearance radiologically when callus has formed. As with bruising, lesions of different ages are strongly suggestive of repeated violence.

5. More bizarre injuries, such as burns, scalds, cigarette burns, crushed fingers, etc., may be found.

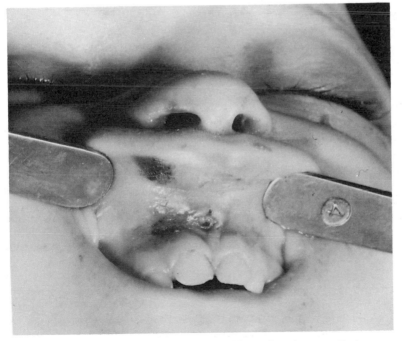

Fig. 11.8 A classic clue to battering ... bruised lips or frenulum, usually due to slapping across the mouth but sometimes due to ramming a feeding bottle into the mouth.

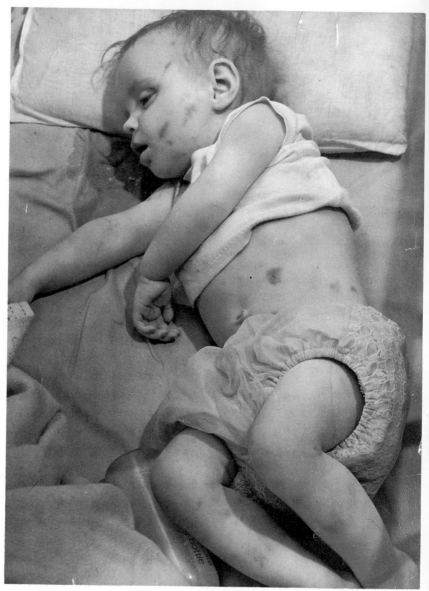

Fig. 11.9 A typical 'battered baby', found during a routine visit from a children's department visitor, crying and showing multiple bruises which the parents could not explain.

The major diagnostic problem is differentiation from true accidents, which undoubtedly do occur. Pointers which may be of assistance include the following.

1. A delay in seeking aid after injury—which is common.
2. A misleading story from the parent which is inconsistent with the clinical or pathological findings.
3. Variations in the story given on different occasions.
4. The child being taken to different doctors or hospitals at each episode of injury, in an attempt to avoid recognition.

Where doubt exists between battering or a genuine accident, the doctor should consult another, preferably a more senior or paediatric colleague. Although it is tragic to miss a case of true child abuse, the tendency to move to the other extreme and regard all child injuries as battering is unfortunate. Indeed, it has been reported that some parents fail to obtain medical care for their accidentally injured child because of the fear of being branded a child abuser. In fatal cases the diagnosis is often less difficult because of the gross nature of the injuries which have been sufficient to cause death.

The management of the battered child is a clinical and social problem of considerable magnitude, and the abundant literature should be consulted on this aspect. It is a grave mistake for a doctor merely to treat the current injury and discharge the child home to its abusing parent(s) without supervision. Removal to a place of safety may be necessary, if necessary by admission to hospital or by a legal order placing the child in the care of the proper authorities until the doctors and social agencies are satisfied that it is safe for the child to be returned home.

Most areas in Britain now maintain an 'At risk' register, in which suspected families are recorded, so that doctors can check rapidly—in total confidentiality—whether previous episodes of injury have occurred to the child in question.

12
Abortion

Abortion and miscarriage are synonymous terms for the premature termination of a pregnancy. The law is not interested in the stage of gestation at which this happens, though, in the Infant Life (Preservation) Act 1929, it recognised the right of the child to a separate existence after the twenty-eighth week. To 'destroy the life of a child capable of being born alive by any wilful act' constitutes 'child destruction', unless the act is performed 'in good faith and for the purpose only of preserving the life of the mother'. The charge is rarely brought, but the phrase 'in good faith' was for years an important test of a doctor's ethical right to terminate a pregnancy. A famous trial, R. *v.* Bourne, became a leading case in the interpretation of the words 'preserving the life of the mother', for the judge trying the case in London indicated his view that 'life depends on health'. This considerably widened the opportunities of terminating pregnancy on medical grounds, and the Abortion Act 1967 finally spelt out these grounds in clear terms.

The law

By the older Offences against the Person Act 1861 it is still an offence:

> Sect. 58. For any woman 'being with child, who, with intent to procure her own miscarriage, shall unlawfully administer to herself any poison or other noxious thing, or shall *unlawfully* use any instrument or any other means whatsoever with the like intent....'
> '... and whosoever, with intent to procure the miscarriage of any woman, whether she be or be not with child' ... shall do so.
> Sect. 59. Whosoever shall unlawfully supply or procure any poison or other noxious thing, or any instrument or thing whatsoever, knowing that the same is intended to be *unlawfully* used ... with intent to procure the miscarriage of any woman.

Both sections—the first for using some method of interference, and the second for providing the means of doing so—may involve the doctor. Before giving way to the temptation to indulge in some unethical (as well as unlawful) practice of this kind, the doctor would do well to pause and consider the ruin it may bring him. The privileges afforded to the doctor under the Abortion Act 1967 are set out below (see 'Therapeutic abortion').

Conviction carries a maximum penalty of 'life' for committing a criminal abortion, and of 5 years imprisonment for supplying or procuring some means of interfering with a pregnancy—or even a supposed pregnancy. Almost inevitably, also, the doctor's name will be erased from the Medical Register when his conviction is reported to the General Medical Council.

> In R. *v.* Pettigrew (Leeds Assizes) a doctor was charged with having provided a noxious thing—namely ergometrine—with the intent to procure abortion. The woman did abort, though possible not from this cause alone, and died. A criminal charge against the doctor failed.

When death follows, it is usually treated as 'manslaughter', because the evil intent, the *mens rea*, to kill was absent. The alternative is 'unlawfully using an instrument with intent to procure an abortion'. It is quite clear that, except where the woman herself attempts to disturb her own pregnancy, the law pays no regard to whether there was, in fact, a fetal sac—or whether abortion follows. It is the intent that matters.

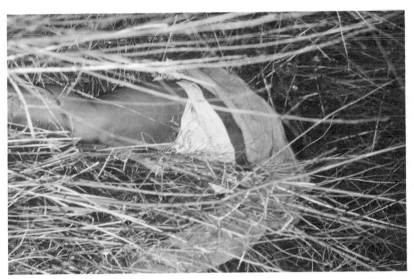

Fig. 12.1 Body of dead girl dumped on verge of road in Epping Forest—raising suspicion of either sex assault or abortion owing to the 'rolled-over' replacement of the panties.

Therapeutic abortion

Until the Abortion Act 1967 was passed, obstetricians performing abortions for good medical reasons had to rely on the permissive phrase 'in good faith and for the purpose only of preserving the life of the mother', derived from the Infant Life (Preservation) Act 1929, to make therapeutic abortions lawful.

By section 1 of the 1967 Act, it became lawful for a registered medical practitioner to terminate a pregnancy, provided that *two* registered medical practitioners were of the bona-fide opinion that either:

1. continuance of the pregnancy would involve risk to the life of the pregnant woman, or injury to her physical or mental health, or any existing children of her family (taking into account the pregnant woman's actual or reasonably foreseeable environment) *greater than if the pregnancy were terminated*; or

2. there is substantial risk that if the child were born, it would suffer from such physical or mental abnormalities as to be seriously handicapped.

Such abortions must be carried out in a National Health Service hospital or 'approved place'. The patient's consent should always be obtained. This does not prevent the emergency termination of a pregnancy to save the life or grave permanent injury to the physical or mental health of a woman—without two doctors' approval, and at home if necessary: consent is desirable, but not essential. The Abortion Regulations 1968 prescribe forms on which the reason for terminating the pregnancy is to be certified *before* the operation is carried out. Both certifying doctors must sign it if it is elective, or one if it is an emergency. Notification of details follows on another form to be signed by the practitioner who performs the operation, and these are to be sent within 7 days to the Chief Medical Officer, Department of Health and Social Security.* Provision is made in the 1967 Act to prohibit disclosure of detail. Doctors are also allowed to express a conscientious objection to taking part in elective abortion: it is usually on religious grounds.

In the first 9 months of the Act, 22 256 medical abortions were performed. In 1969 the total was 54 156, and by 1970 it had risen to 83 851. The 1975 total was some 140 000. About 60 per cent of these were performed in 'approved places' (i.e. outside NHS hospitals), but the disturbingly higher proportion of these in one London area (90 per cent in the NW Metropolitan district) raised anxiety as to the 'good faith' of some nursing-home operators. The reason given in nearly 80 per cent of cases was 'risk of injury to the physical or mental health of the woman'. Only 0.2 per cent were emergencies to save life.

Illegal abortion

It was estimated before the Abortion Act of 1967 that about 20 per cent of all pregnancies ended prematurely and that in some 40 per cent of these—probably more—there had been criminal interference. It was difficult to get at the truth in many cases, especially where abortion had been self-induced.

In making such assessments, it must not be forgotten that abortion

* In Scotland, to the CMO, Scottish Home and Health Department.

from natural causes is quite common. Many miscarriages result from serious illness in the mother—nephritis, grave heart disease, rhesus incompatibilities, placental or cord lesions that result in death of the fetus *in utero*. The passing of a macerated fetus is usually a natural event, and may never be reported in statistics.

Two factors have reduced the total numbers of abortions in the UK. The principal factor is undoubtedly the increasing practice of using the contraceptive 'pill', for only this could have decimated the number of unwanted pregnancies that caused so many young girls and women to seek abortion. The other factor is the introduction of the Abortion Act 1967 which spells out helpfully to doctors the conditions under which a pregnancy may be terminated lawfully.

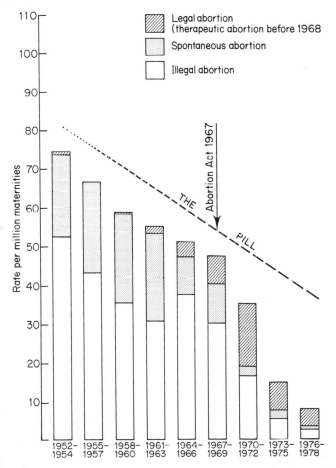

Fig. 12.2 Deaths per million maternities from abortion for the period 1952–1978, showing the effects of (1) increasing use of the contraceptive 'pill', and (2) the Abortion Act 1967 (see text). (Reproduced from *Report into Maternal Deaths*, HMSO No. 26, 1982, by permission of the Controller, Her Majesty's Stationery Office.)

Doctors are permitted, provided that the termination is undertaken in approved, registered, premises by registered medical practitioners who report the details as required by law, to terminate:

'... if continuance of the pregnancy would involve risk to the life of the pregnant woman, or injury to her physical or mental health, or any existing children of her family (taking into account the pregnant woman's actual or reasonably foreseeable environment) *greater than if the pregnancy were terminated ...*'

as well as if there is a substantial risk that the child might suffer some serious handicap—physical or mental—when born.

Those who set out the wording of the Act given in italic above can hardly have overlooked the fact that the risk of continuing a pregnancy to term and facing the risks of giving birth at that stage had always been—and still are—greater than those of medical termination. There are about 600 000 births in the UK per annum (about 12 per 1000 population, and the maternal mortality has gradually fallen to 0.10 per 1000 births. But the mortality of medical terminations is only 0.017 per 1000: *it has always been safer to terminate*. The risk of giving birth to a deformed or mentally handicapped child merely adds another freedom to terminate.

It must be said that the medical profession has—with very few exceptions in the early days of the Act—observed the terms of the Act with admirable professional honesty; and the early days of spurious 'nursing homes' which deliberately misused the permissive wording of the 1967 Act have been eliminated by refusal, as the occasion has arisen, to re-register them.

If this textbook were read only in the context of practice in the UK, it would be out of date to expand, as has been done in the past, on the picture of illegal or criminal abortion, often self-induced or in unskilled hands, which causes so much hurt, infection and illness to the victims. But this text is in use in many countries where religious attitudes and practices—and legal sanctions—are widely different (for example, in India and China and the Spanish-reading peoples of South America for whom it has been translated), and it would not reflect world experience to limit an account of abortion practices and their consequences to their state in the UK.

The time of interference   Nearly all criminal abortions take place at about the second or third month, when the woman has become certain of the cessation of her periods and morning sickness has confirmed pregnancy. Where means less certain to effect the desired abortion than instrumentation—pills or repeated vaginal douching—have failed, she may have reached the third or fourth month.

.After the seventh month the law further protects the fetus, now viable, by the Infant Life (Preservation) Act of 1929, which makes it an offence (child destruction) to commit any act causing the death of a child capable of having a serparate existence, except as a proper therapeutic procedure 'performed in good faith and for the purpose only of preserving the life of the mother'.

The duration of gestation is an important part of the medical examination in abortion, and tables which will act as a guide to maturity will be found in the section on identification (p. 27). The gestation period should be judged by the size of the ovum at 2, 3 and 4 months, remembering also that the placenta is formed at about the commencement of the third month. From the fifth month, the length of the fetus from vertex to heel should be used as a basis for measurement and certain ossification centres committed to memory. From the fifth month, the length in centimetres is approximately five times the number of months' gestation—at 5 months 25 cm, at 6 months 30 cm, and so on.

Means of procuring abortion   The common reaction of a woman to an unwanted pregnancy has always been first to try some simple method of disturbing it which she can practise herself. Drinking gin, repeated hot baths or vaginal douchings, or an enthusiasm for skipping, cycle- or horse-riding not previously practised might all be designed for such an end.

When these are unsuccessful a woman may perform some more deliberate act, often with the assistance of other persons. The more common means adopted are:

1. Local or more general violence.
2. Abortifacient drugs.
3. Instruments.

Violence   The tenacity of the ovum in a healthy subject has already been remarked upon, and general violence such as deliberate falls are more likely to cause grave injury than abortion.

> A woman of 24 had leapt to the ground of a concrete yard from the second floor of her home, a fall of approx. 7.5 metres (25 feet), sustaining injuries which proved fatal the following day, but failed to disturb a 2½ months' pregnancy.

> A woman of 37 had permitted her husband to deal her, with fist or boot or both, some five or six most violent blows over the breasts, the loins, over the lower abdomen, and to the perineum, without dislodging the pregnancy. She died 5 days later of uraemia from traumatic renal vein thromboses resulting from her loin injuries.

Drugs   In former years drugs were commonly used with the intention of causing abortion, but most of these had little or no effect upon a pregnancy. The increase in contraception and legalised termination of pregnancy have resulted in most of these drugs becoming of little more than historical interest in westernised countries, although they—or local variants—may still be encountered in less sophisticated communities.

In general, these drugs were intended to work in one of two ways:

1. By a specific effect upon the uterus or products of conception.
2. By causing such general disorder in the mother that abortion might follow.

The first group were intended to have a contractile effect upon the uterine muscle, and were formerly rather spuriously divided into 'ecbolics' and 'emmenagogues'. A host of vegetable compounds such as pennyroyal, savin (juniper), rue and apiol were in vogue; in tropical countries, unripe pineapple is also said to have a similar effect. These substances had little or no pharmacological action upon the uterus, a fact which was summed up by an official enquiry committee's view that 'the primary evils arising from their sale are the fraudulent exploitation of the mental distress of the women who buy them in the anticipation that they will cause abortion'. Other drugs had a better theoretical chance of success, although this was rarely borne out in practice. Ergot, lead, pituitary extract, quinine and prostaglandins all have a contractile effect on the uterus and, indeed, pituitary extract is used legitimately for this purpose in obstetrics. However, most illegal abortions are attempted in very early pregnancy, when such specific action is virtually absent, being applied to the small, undistended womb.

The second group causes general ill-effects upon the mother, usually in the form of purging from strong laxatives such as colocynth, croton oil, jalap, etc. This is highly unlikely to cause a miscarriage; indeed, as has been said of some of the allegedly more specific drugs such as lead, 'anything which kills the fetus is as likely to kill the mother'.

In summary, there is little or no evidence to show that any drug or other substance is efficacious in procuring abortion in the first two trimesters, although some medically used drugs such as oestrogens, ergot, pituitary and prostaglandin may well precipitate uterine contractions late in pregnancy.

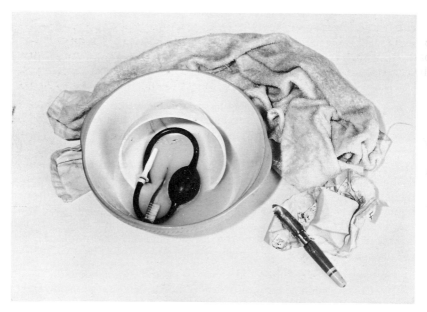

Fig. 12.3 Domestic preparations for an instrumental injection of soapy fluid into the uterus. A potato peeler shredded the soap and the bowl held the solution and a Higginson syringe.

Instruments (Fig. 12.4) This was, above all, the method of interference most resorted to among habitual illegal abortionists as, although beset with dangers, it is the most successful. Vacuum extraction is, of course, standard medical practice.

Among unskilled women using an instrument upon themselves, the commonest was the Higginson syringe.

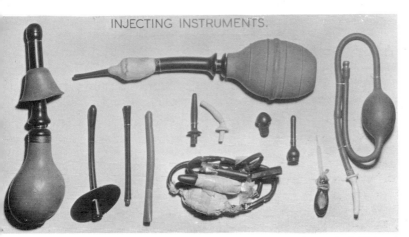

Fig. 12.4 Injecting instruments recovered from various abortion cases, including an adapted nozzle on a douching bulb, several shaped nozzles, a rotting irrigation tube and a fountain-pen filler.

The use of knitting needles, skewers, scent-spray nozzles, and similar probing instruments—nails, pencils, and cut lengths of 'slippery' elm bark (this also sometimes being left to swell and act as a 'tent' within the cervix)—was also more or less restricted to self-induced interference.

The semi-skilled abortionist, often an untrained woman who has ac-

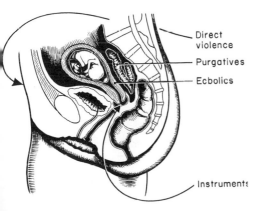

Direct violence

Purgatives

Ecbolics

Instruments

Fig. 12.5 Diagram of midline section of pelvic organs to illustrate the site of action of the forms of interference designed to abort. The fingers may guide an instrument safely into the cervix.

quired skill by experience, will usually confine herself to a fluid injection with a Higginson syringe. She is usually, though not always, wise enough to perform the operation outside her own home for fear of a death from shock (or air embolism) leaving her with a dead body on her hands.

A typical 'outfit', packed in a handbag, contained elm bark cut into 'tent' form for insertion into the cervix. The Higginson syringe had the flange-disc removed to enable it to be passed the requisite 12–15 cm up through the vagina and into the cervix, and a tablet of carbolic soap, popularly supposed to avert much of the risk of infection, was included to form the warm soapy fluid for injection.

The skilled professional abortionist, often a registered medical practitioner or nurse, is difficult to detect, for they usually use a catheter introduced, after adequate antiseptic measures, cleanly and without injury. The abortion takes place a few hours later, and if there is trouble and the woman is not already in a 'nursing-home', she has been told to

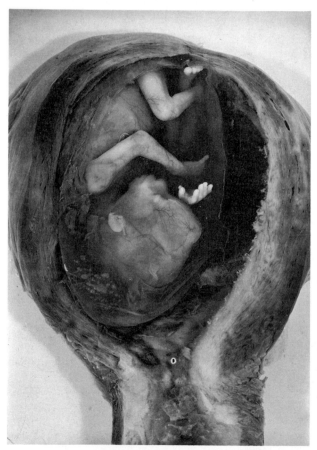

Fig. 12.6 Fetal sac displaced by an injection of soap and water (which has dribbled out upon dissection), leaving only a blood-tinged residue of soap solution.

present herself to a local doctor as a natural abortion or a 'flooding' of unknown origin.

The design of all instrumental interferences is to dilate the cervix (elm-bark tents), perforate the sac (any probe-like instrument), or introduce fluid to separate the sac from the interior of the womb (Higginson syringe injections).

The dangers of instrumental interference are as follows.

Shock Sudden collapse from reflex vagal inhibition may follow upon the mere touching of the cervix with an instrument, the impact of too hot, too cold or corrosive fluid, or the injection of fluid through the canal of the cervix. When death occurs, it is virtually instantaneous, and the few seconds which intervene allow only for the development of some congestion and cyanosis. These are the cases which may result in arrest and successful prosecution of abortionists, for the persons present at the time—and who often first tell a story of having the deceased visit them and collapse quite unexpectedly—are the persons who know what was going on at the time: they are almost certain to be responsible. The medical evidence as to the time lapse of a few seconds only in these cases is vital to the police inquiry, and, if death is due to shock, can be relied upon implicitly. Persons admitting themselves to be present at death in such cases are almost certain to have been parties to the interference.

Air embolism follows unexpectedly upon the introduction of a Higginson syringe nozzle and the squirting into the cavity of the womb of a mixture of fluid and air (Fig. 12.7). The latter is sucked inadvertently

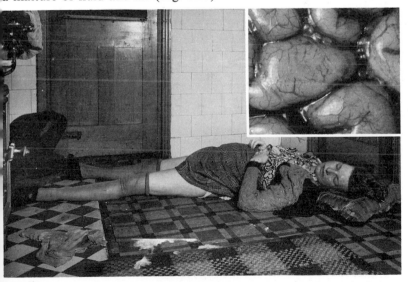

Fig. 12.7 A typical abortion case. An obviously pregnant woman found dead, the head resting on a pillow, the skirt half up, panties on the floor nearby—but no instruments. These were found in the kitchen, together with a note making an appointment with a woman suspected of making a living in abortion services.

Insert Air bubbles in the pial vessels in a case dying some few minutes after a Higginson syringe injection into the uterus.

into the syringe as the fluid level in the bowl or jug in use drops and so uncovers the sucking valve of the syringe. Some few minutes pass before sudden collapse with cyanosis and dyspnoea takes place; death then ensues almost immediately. Autopsy will reveal air bubbles in the interior of the uterus and its wall, in the uterine and ovarian veins, inferior vena cava and right heart, pulmonary arteries, left heart and systemic arteries. Cerebral and coronary air embolism are responsible for death. Rarely there may be some delay before uterine contraction drives the air into the mural veins—collapse and death then ensuing with the usual alarming rapidity.

Instrumental injury   Perforation of the lower vagina is uncommon except in clumsy, bungling self-instrumentation. The commonly expressed textbook view that the fornices are often perforated seems likely to be perpetuation of a view once expressed and little tested by experience. In a series of 100 successive instrumental injuries, the site of injury was:

Vagina	Fornix	Cervix	Endouterine	Fundus
15	4	48	12	21

The vaginal and cervix penetrations are more commonly due to sharp instrumental or elm-bark scratching and puncturing, and the deep uterine and fundus lesions to long rigid probes or to desperate pushing with a Higginson nozzle until 'something gives'. What is intended by this lay instruction is no doubt a perforation of the sac, but what in practice follows is a perforation of the fundus of the uterus (Fig. 12.8). Death may follow from shock and haemorrhage, but is more likely to result from subsequent infection.

Sepsis,   with or without injury, must always give rise to suspicion, though, of course, it may occur in spite of every professional care. Injury and the use of corrosives, even carbolic soap, may tend to the development of infection, and if the abortion is incomplete the probability of sepsis at once becomes greater (and suspicion the less). The development of chemotherapy has caused a striking reduction in the incidence of sepsis. Fatalities have almost disappeared.

Septic endometritis, infection of the uterine wall, broad ligaments and pelvic connective tissues may follow upon interference without damage, for the surroundings in these cases are often squalid and dirty, and the instruments unclean. The bacteriology is commonly mixed, including *Escherichia coli, Clostridium welchii*, haemolytic streptococci (about 45 per cent group A), and anaerobic streptococci. *Cl. welchii* may cause fulminating septicaemia (with a curious bronzed colour) in as little as 18–24 hours. It is surprising that the mortality of about 0.01 per cent is not far higher.

At trial, counsel for defence will often try to persuade the medical witness to say that the instrumental interference *could* have been self-inflicted. The proper answer is, without doubt, that '*It is possible* that even a clean, apparently skilled introduction of an instrument into the neck of the womb *might* be effected by a woman herself, unaided; but

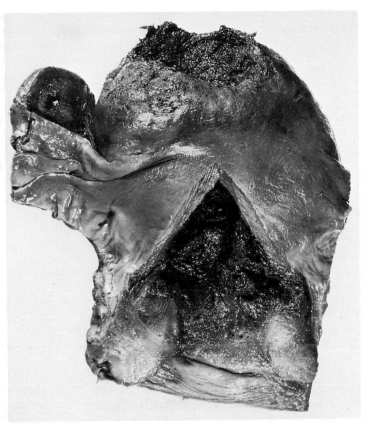

Fig. 12.8 A uterus opened in front, showing a complete instrumental perforation of the fundus. A sloughing infection spreading into this has caused it to swell and open out.

only remotely possible. The less the damage the more likely it is that help was given; the more gross the injury the more probable that it was the clumsy unaided effort of the woman herself.' Such reason will gain the approval of the jury, and usually also disarm counsel.

Doctor's duty in abortion

Decisions on problems of abortion need not cause the practitioner any anxiety provided he acts 'in good faith', as the law asks.

A well-informed Abortion Committee estimated in 1939 that some 120 000–150 000 abortions occurred each year in England and Wales, and that some 40 per cent of them were criminal. Yet the number of offences known to the police was usually around 250 and prosecutions seldom exceeded 50 each year. The provisions of the Abortion Act confirmed the committee's conclusions. Medical abortions now number about 150 000 per annum, and the number of inexpert criminal abortions has plainly fallen—since the necessity for back-street interference has gone: in 1981 there was not a single illegal abortion death.

Table 12.1 Deaths from abortion in England and Wales, 1981

Total abortions (England and Wales)	162 480
Performed by vacuum aspiration	142 000
Largest age group (20–24 years)	45 000
Deaths following abortion	1
Deaths in previous years: 1980, 3; 1979, 2; 1978, 6; 1977, 8	

Though the morbidity of terminations may be high, the mortality is remarkably low—under 0.01 per cent.

The doctor is, however, torn between preserving professional secrecy and his public duty as a citizen when attending cases of abortion, and has only his conscience to guide him. The view of the law, embodied in advice from Mr Justice Avory to a jury in 1914 and never altered, is that: '... the desire to preserve that confidence must be subordinated to the duty which is cast upon every good citizen to asist in the investigations of a serious crime. ...'

Long ago, the British medical profession, as represented by the BMA and the Royal College of Physicians, resolved that a medical practitioner should not under any circumstances disclose voluntarily, without the patient's consent, information obtained from that patient in the exercise of his professional duties.

The phrase 'without the patient's consent' enables the doctor to satisfy his conscience in both directions. He should endeavour to obtain her consent when her illness is due to the bungling of a dangerous habitual criminal abortionist taking fees. Such persons are a menace to society and the doctor should not hesitate to assist, with his patient's consent, in securing their prosecution. When, on the contrary, his patient has, after great anxiety and distress, induced herself by some more homely method described, the doctor may rest assured the police would be pleased to be spared such inquiries, incapable as they are of leading to any good result. Only the death of the patient necessitates reporting the case.

If death seems imminent the doctor would do well to obtain a dying declaration from his patient, provided he has reason to believe that some outside criminal abortionist is responsible. It will be admissible only after death.

The procedure of taking a dying declaration is described more fully elsewhere (p. 205), but it may be helpful to state here that the only absolute essentials in an abortion case are:

1. The death of the person making it must be the subject of the charge made.

2. The charge must be one of 'murder' or 'manslaughter', not merely of 'unlawfully using an instrument with intent to procure the miscarriage'.

3. The patient must be convinced that she has no hope whatsoever of recovery.

The conviction that death is both inevitable and imminent should form the preamble to the declaration, and the statement should follow, preferably in writing, witnessed after signature, though these latter matters are not absolutely essential to admission of the document.

In the event of death in any case of abortion arousing either suspicion or doubt in the doctor's mind, he should without delay report the circumstances to the coroner. Not to do so might suggest connivance in the affair.

Sterilisation

It is only a few decades since sterlisation of both male and female became legally acceptable, as hitherto it was considered a maiming procedure. Now it is performed both for medical reasons and for purposes of birth control.

The legal position mainly concerns *consent* to sterilisation. Where a surgical or, more often, a gynaecological operation coincidentally sterlises the patient (for example, a hysterectomy), then this fact must be included in the prior explanation necessary to obtain valid informed consent from the patient. In these cases, no consent need be obtained from the spouse nor where an elective sterilisation is to be performed for purely medical reasons, such as a woman with heart disease whose condition might deteriorate in a subsequent pregnancy. However, it is plainly both courteous and good medical practice to discuss the matter with the patient and the spouse, if the former agrees.

Where sterilisation is carried out for birth control purposes only (i.e. tubal ligation or vasectomy), strict law demands only informed consent from the patient, but it is customary to seek the agreement of the husband or wife. Where the patient is unmarried or separated, then the need for this precaution is less or even absent.

If the spouse refuses to agree, then the doctor must consider the best interests of his patient. Usually, he can proceed on the strength of the patient's own consent, but possible deleterious effects upon the union may need consideration.

In obtaining consent, the doctor must explain that absolute success can never be guaranteed, for legal actions are increasingly being brought by aggrieved pregnant women.

The position is more difficult where young persons are concerned, usually those under 16 years of age. Above this age, the position is as for adults, but it appears from a judicial ruling in 1976 that sterilisation of a minor for eugenic reasons such as the presence of hereditary disease, is unlawful. Where sterility will be the inevitable outcome of a surgical operation vital to the life or health of the young person, then the consent of the parents or guardian is all that is necessary.

13
Sexual offences

Two principal types of sexual offence come to the notice of the doctor. In the first the outstanding feature is a clear mental disturbance of which the crime is only a manifestation. Such cases afford scope for the psychiatrist but little for the student of forensic medicine, and the doctor's appearances in court in this kind of offence are chiefly to emphasise the disordered state of mind. Repeated *indecent exposure, indecent assaults* upon children, and the more sexual kinds of *sadism* or *masochism* fall naturally into this group of cases.

The second group of sexual offences involve no such aberration of the mind. The commonest are *indecent assaults* on females, *rape, incest and buggery*, and in country districts *bestiality* must be borne in mind, though it is comparatively rare.

Rape and indecent assault

In England and Wales rape had for long been defined as 'unlawful carnal knowledge of a woman by force and against her will'. The 1956 Sexual Offences Act rephrased this as 'unlawful sexual intercourse without her consent, by force, fear or fraud', but following the Report of the Advisory Group on the Law of Rape (the Heilbron Committee), the Sexual Offences (Amendment) Act 1976 defined rape as 'unlawful sexual intercourse by a man with a woman who *at the time* does not consent to it and, *at the time, he knows that she does not consent or is reckless as to whether she consents*'.

In addition to this offence, Scottish law has special provision for taking advantage of a woman who is drunk or asleep, defining it as 'clandestine injury on a woman', not rape. In one other comparatively unimportant respect also is there a difference of view, for whereas in England a boy is held to be physically incapable of rape before the age of fourteen years, there is no such limitation in Scotland.

The definition of rape as:

Unlawful ...
sexual intercourse ...

with a woman ...
by force, fear or fraud ...

provides convenient headings for a discussion of the subject.

'*Unlawful*' implies that there is such an act as a lawful sexual intercourse with a woman against her will. No man may be charged with the offence in relation to his wife, and should he find that his marriage is, unknown to him, invalid because his wife was under 16 at the time, any 'martial' intercourse he may have had is excused.

'*Sexual intercourse*' is held to mean 'the slightest degree of penetration of the vulva by the penis'. Penetration proper through the hymen is not necessary to the act, and in this respect the condition of the hymen will be of no value as medical evidence unless it is freshly injured. When it is already deflorate, ruptured by previous sexual intercourse, by masturbation or injury, it may be difficult to provide medical evidence to confirm a woman's allegations of rape. A great deal may depend upon her character and bearing, the substance of her story, the condition of her clothing, and the presence of even trivial injury to any part of the body. The doctor must on no account be satisfied with a mere examination of the vulva and hymen region. A painstaking investigation is demanded by a charge of this gravity and the routine which is desirable will be described in some detail below.

It is important for the doctor to attain familiarity with the various forms of intact hymen in their natural rather than their diagrammatic state. The doctor will rarely be in doubt about his findings, for evidence of a forceful assault freshly committed will be clear—or absent. There will be bruising, scratching or tearing of the vulva or hymen (Fig. 13.3), which may still be bleeding—or none.

Where the vaginal orifice is unusually large or the hymen vestigial or atrophied, it is less likely that injury will occur. It is possible that the only proof of penetration will come from the detection of seminal fluid in the vagina. A swab or smears should always be taken for this reason. In law the emission of seminal fluid is not essential to the proof of sexual intercourse, which is in fact no more or less than what it implies, but its demonstration may provide irrefutable proof of the act.

In practice it is more common to find seminal fluid on the clothing and injury, with or without bleeding, within the vulva. If no penetration is proved the accused may be convicted of an indecent assault under the Sexual Offences Act 1956.

The mere fact that menstruation is in progress at the time does not bar sexual intercourse, rape or some indecent assault. The doctor must remember, too, that the act may bring on a menstrual flow if it was about to start.

The development of gonorrhoea in a woman after alleged rape may sometimes be used as corrobative evidence, and culture as well as microscopy of a swab should be made if possible.

'*With a woman*' The Sexual Offences Act 1956 defines two degrees of sex assault upon a female—(1) sexual intercourse, and (2) an indecent

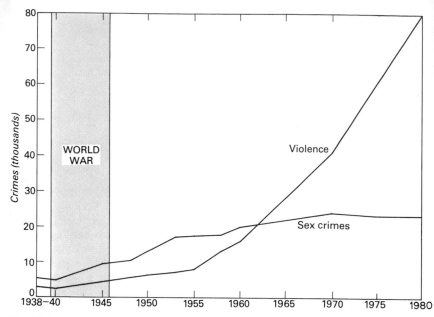

Fig. 13.1 Chart showing rise in sex crime during the period 1938–80. The rise has continued steadily since.

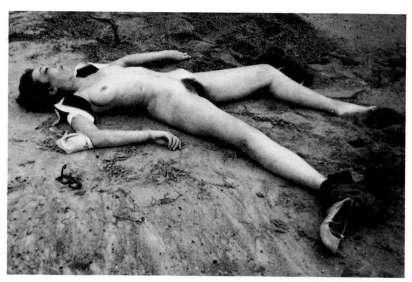

Fig. 13.2 Girl found dead on beach, stripped after being disabled by a head injury, rolled over, marking the sand, and raped: the dug-in toe marks can be seen between the ankles.

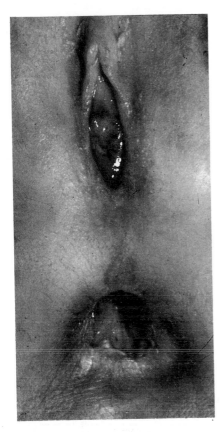

Fig. 13.3 Bruising at the vulva, and both dilatation and chafing at the anal orifice in an assaulted child of 5 years.

assault—and has laid down certain *qualifications with regard to age* in connection with these offences:

1. *Sexual intercourse* with a girl not yet 13 years old is rape—a grave crime, subject to severe punishment. Intercourse with a girl of over 13 but under 16 is 'an offence', dealt with less severely owing to the girl's age. The Act does not recognise 'consent' until the age of 16.

2. *An indecent* (i.e. sexual) *assault*, something short of actual intercourse, is 'an offence' if the girl is still under 16, irrespective of consent: she cannot give it by law. It is, of course, 'an offence' on any woman if without her approval, or if she is mentally handicapped.

It is clear that to have sexual intercourse by force, without consent, *at any age* is, thus, rape. It is only with respect to the question of punishment that the above amendments have been formulated. Under the age of 16 it is reasonable for the law to regard sexual intercourse as undesirable, and to make it an offence, though, of course, not the serious offence that intercourse with a girl not yet 13 must be.

Not infrequently it is said by the defendant that he had 'reasonable cause to believe that the girl was of the age of sixteen or over' and able to give her consent. If her physique, her manner of dressing, and her general conduct are such as to make this likely, the accused receives a lesser penalty, provided that he is not yet 24 years of age (Sexual Offences Act 1956). This applies only to the first such incident.

The Sexual Offences Act 1956 also states that it is an offence 'to have unlawful sexual intercourse with a woman he knows to be a mental defective, or with a woman who is under care or treatment in an institution, certified house or approved home within the meaning of the Mental Health Act 1959 or placed out on licence therefore or under guardianship under the Act'. It is made quite clear that sexual intercourse with a mental defective will be rape if it is without consent and an offence even though she consents. Her position with regard to consent is the same as that of a girl of not yet 16. The gravity of the offence is mitigated by consent though, in fact, the woman is not entitled in law to give it. It is an offence under the Mental Health Act for a person on the staff of a mental hospital or similar institution to take such advantage of any patient.

The Sexual Offences Act also makes it an offence to abduct an unmarried girl of under 18 from her parent or guardian, if with the intention that she shall 'have unlawful sexual intercourse with men—or a particular man.'

'*By force*' The essence of the offence is that it should take place against the wishes of the woman. If intercourse is had, unlawfully, whether:

1. by force, fear or fraud—e.g. threats of any kind;
2. by false pretences, as, for instance, under the pretence that an examination or operation is being performed;
3. by impersonation of her husband, as might happen after a drunken party;
4. when she is asleep or unconscious, or under the effect of drink or some drug that has stupefied her so as to make her unable to appreciate the real nature of the act;

then it is sexual intercourse without consent—i.e. rape.

In 1957 a man stood in Welling (Kent) Police Court accused of placing a chloroform-saturated cloth over the mouth of a girl with intent to commit a criminal assault. He had broken into the house, and, when arrested, said: 'I love that girl and will do anything I can to get her to marry me.'

The allegation that there was no consent must be examined with great care, for a woman sometimes concocts such a story only after her arrival home, when she is faced with giving some explanation to account for injury, blood-stains on her clothing, or a subsequent pregnancy.

In one such case with torn and blood-stained clothing (Fig. 13.4) the girl had met, quite casually, a soldier with whom she had walked a half a mile out of town and up a quarter-mile drive to a house which she knew was deserted; they had entered through a window and, she alleged, he had connection with her although she had struggled ('it was no good screaming, we

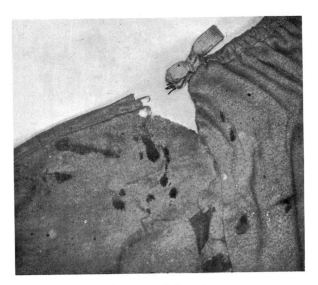

Fig. 13.4 Panties from a case of alleged rape.

were too far from anywhere'), pinning her against a sink in the scullery. The judge at trial directed the jury to stop the case if it were considered that she had, by going so far with the accused, given him reasonable cause to believe she was acquiescing in anything which might happen in that isolated deserted house. Torn and blood-stained clothing afforded no proper evidence in such circumstances to support what was otherwise an uncorroborated story of rape. The girl did not run away: she had sustained minor injury only to her private parts such as might naturally follow upon somewhat clumsy or over-eager connection.

In another case of belated allegation (Fig. 13.5) the police already had their suspicions that the story was fabricated before making further inquiries. The

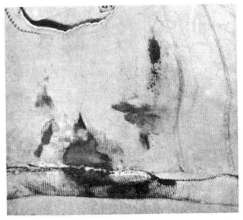

Fig. 13.5 Alleged rape. Pear-shaped blood-stain in two complementary parts of a slip evidently caused *before* tearing, throwing doubt on the girl's story that she struggled to prevent rape (see below).

girl, who produced a blood-stained slip, undoubtedly had a freshly torn hymen: but the pear-shaped stain on the slip was in two complementary parts through which a tear had (clearly subsequently) taken place. In a struggle to get possession of a girl the clothing would first be torn, if at all, the bleeding following as some forceful penetration is made. This complementary piece of staining proved, as was suspected, to be a deliberate act, effected to bring some pressure to bear on her fiancé who would not marry her. She had herself damaged the hymen, stained her slip, and subsequently torn it.

Inconsistencies in the story as compared with the doctor's observations are also important.

The question of consent is without doubt the most difficult of all features of a prosecution for rape. Pretence that there never was any encouragement, consent 'withdrawn' afterwards for fear of parents, fabricated tears and blood-stains, and entirely imaginary tales provide the principal difficulties. The whole evidence has to be weighed carefully against the character and background of the woman making the allegations.

When she is young and inexperienced, physically frail or nervous, she is the more likely to have been taken by surprise and overcome than when experienced in such matters, strong and able to give as good as she gets. It is doubtful indeed whether a woman can be raped by a man of anything like, or less than, her physique unless under threat of a knifing or some other such violence.

But she may be affected by drink or drugs, and so rendered incapable of proper resistance. The Sexual Offences Act 1956 makes it an offence to administer 'any drug, matter or thing to a woman with intent to stupefy or overpower so as thereby to enable any person to have unlawful sexual intercourse with her'. Although a significant proportion of allegations of rape eventually prove unfounded, it must be appreciated that many women who are genuine victims of sexual assaults never complain to the police or a doctor because of their well-founded fears of interrogation, medical examination and the publicity of a court case.

The male doctor or the dental surgeon may sometimes find themselves accused, to their astonishment, of indecent assault, even rape, as a result of dream or hallucinatory impressions occurring during anaesthesia, narcosis, etc. Such a possibility will be avoided by always having some other person present when a woman is being placed under the effect of a narcotic or anaesthetic drug for some medical procedure. Rarely does it happen, happily, that a doctor deliberately takes advantage of the opportunities afforded by examination or a narcosis to assault his patient; allegations of this kind are almost always found to be false. But they will be most damaging to the doctor and he would do well to foresee their possibility.

Medical examination in sexual assaults

The victim

The doctor should be certain that he has permission before undertaking an examination of a woman in cases of indecent assault or rape. Such permission should be written and witnessed, and a female chaperone present during the examination. The shorter the lapse of time between the alleged assault and examination the better; any delay should have a proper explanation.

A full examination by the doctor will have as its principal features:

1. Name, date, time of arrival and by whom examination is requested.
2. Observations on the woman's behaviour.
3. A full story in her own words.
4. Remarks on disorder of hair, clothing, tights, footwear.
5. Examination of body, general and local.
6. Taking of vaginal smears or a swab.
7. Writing a full report of this at once and keeping a copy of it.

This outline may seem unduly comprehensive, but when it is remembered that the sentence, in the event of conviction, may be imprisonment for a long period, the doctor will have no doubt of the responsibility he has undertaken. Some remarks will be justified about each of the principal parts of his examination.

The preliminary data are not merely perfunctory: the exact date and time of the examination and a note as to who requested it are essential pieces of evidence.

Behaviour It may be necessary for the doctor to say if, when he saw her soon after an alleged offence, she might be taken for a girl of 16 or over, capable of giving her consent, for this may be a proper defence for a first offence by a young man not yet 24.

The story in the girl's own words, must be written down at the time, for it will contain conversation the exact wording of which may be vital, and the doctor may be asked to recount it in court. No false modesty over detail or language should be allowed to interfere with this being a full record. It will gain by being graphic and tend to appear in its true light—authentic or false. It will be wise to ask her what her experience of sexual intercourse is at the end whether she is married or not: the doctor would be wise to bear this in mind in relation to the state of the hymen and the swab findings.

Disorder of hair, clothing, etc. Although the clothing may eventually be the responsibility of the police, for examination of it will be conducted by a laboratory expert, the doctor should include some remarks on the conditions as he saw them, for he has an advantage in time over the laboratory expert. Tangled, disordered hair and dirt-stained face or hands may not be recorded elsewhere. He may notice whether the condition of the clothing bears comparison with the story told, and should record tears and blood-stains in their broad outline; details will come from the laboratory expert.

Examination of body   With some reliable person present to assist, the clothing should be removed in the doctor's presence, and a careful examination made of every part of the body. The sexual offences examination kit provided by the Home Office forensic laboratories contains a sheet of brown paper upon which the woman stands to undress: any foreign material such as hairs, fibres or vegetation falls upon the paper and can be retained for scientific examination. Stories of being forced against something, pinned down, bitten, gripped by the arms, kicked or punched may gain corroboration from the finding of some comparable injury in the part described. This should include a search for 'love bites'.

Next, the local parts should be examined with the greatest care, using, whenever possible, the sex offence kits provided by the police:

1. Foreign hairs (Fig. 13.6)—to be placed in clean envelopes, sealed and labelled;

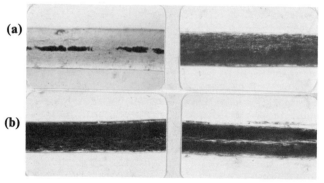

(a)

(b)

Fig. 13.6 Dark hairs identical with an accused's pubic hair sample found clinging to the vaginal entrance hairs of an auburn-haired woman raped and strangled in her home: (*a*) Auburn hair, and (*b*) near-black hair from deceased's body at post-mortem.

2. Seminal stains—to be smeared on swabs or slides;
3. Bruises, scratches or tears adjacent to the vulva and within it, as well as to the neighbourhood of the hymen;
4. The state of the hymen.

The significance of the last has been mentioned already. The orifice may be dilated or torn by many things besides the penis. It is common to overestimate the contribution of the hymen to the evidence—to regard it as the decisive thing in the case. No greater mistake could be made. It is the whole evidence considered together which tells in the end. Even if the hymen is freshly torn it is not decisive evidence with regard to consent.

Smears and swabs   Matted seminal-stained public hairs may be cut away. Dried thigh stains should be moistened with clean saline and smeared on glass slides. Lastly, vaginal swabs (vulval, mid- and high-vaginal) should *always* be taken. It has now become clear that spermatozoa can remain intact for a very long time in the vagina as well as in stains that have become dry. It is never too late to take a swab.

Report-making   Let the doctor make this out, without delay and with the possibility of court procedure in mind. Arranged in sections in something like the order outlined above, it cannot fail to be satisfactory. Many reports have been confined to a few lines, and were hopelessly inadequate. The occasion is a serious one and demands the doctor's most conscientious attentions.

The accused

It is less common for the doctor to have the opportunity of examining the man accused of a sexual assault: permission must be obtained and its voluntary nature made clear before commencing. The clothing may, on the contrary, be confiscated for examination as soon as lawful arrest has been made.

In our experience it has been common for such examinations to have been of secondary interest, murder having been committed during rape, and examination of the man following upon arrest for the major crime. Nevertheless it may be equally important to show that rape did in fact occur; the burden of proof of 'wilful murder' rests with the prosecution, not with the doctor.

The same routine cannot be followed as in the case of a woman presenting herself for examination, for the man must be officially cautioned before making any statement, and this will be the duty of a police officer, not a doctor. The medical examination will be likely to be limited to clothing and the private parts and the face and hands. The doctor will be on the look-out principally for foreign hairs on the clothing, adherent to the body or pinned under the prepuce, and stains such as that seen in Fig. 13.7. Injury to the penis is uncommon, but scratches

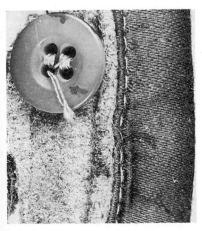

Fig. 13.7 Fresh stains noticed on the trouser 'fly' button and adjacent cloth of a man admitted to hospital for a lacerated arm shortly after report to the police of the assault and attempted rape of a girl by a window-cleaner who escaped by clambering over a glass-topped wall. The blood group was similar to the girl's, dissimilar to the man's group.

to the man's face or hands occur frequently in genuine rape. The presence, particularly in the neck region, of 'love bites' consisting of lip or teeth marks together with suction petechiae may help to corroborate sexual activity.

Laboratory tests for seminal fluid

Under ultraviolet light   seminal stains are markedly fluorescent; urinary and some faecal stains are only faintly so, if at all. A preliminary sorting of whitish or partly stiffened stains (Fig. 13.8) likely to be seminal may be effected by direct examination in this way.

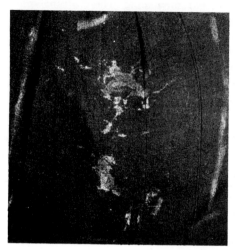

Fig. 13.8 Area of seminal stains on the frock of a girl alleging rape, seen by filtered (ultraviolet) light and outlined by chalk line. Marked fluorescence is shown. A specimen has been cut out for chemical test and microscopy.

Florence test   A portion of the stained cloth is cut out and teased gently in water or saline acidified by one drop of strong HCl to 30 ml. It is allowed to soak for several hours under cover and smear preparations are then made. When nearly dry they are treated, under a cover-slip, with a drop of Florence's solution: potassium iodide 1.5 g, iodine 2.5 g, in 30 ml water, when, if seminal fluid is present, a shower of dark-brown crystals, like haemin crystals in shape, but somewhat larger, will develop.

It is often said that this is not a certain test for seminal fluid, but if it is positive a painstaking search for spermatozoa is worth while. Electrophoretic tests can support colour tests in confirmation.

Microscopy for spermatozoa   Dried smears are fixed in a gentle flame and stained with haemalum or methylene blue for 20 minutes, washed, counterstained with eosin or neutral red, and examined under high power or oil immersion. Spermatozoa are about 0.055 mm long, consisting of head, neck and tail, the head one-tenth the length of the rest. The length is about the equivalent of eight red blood corpuscles. Although sperms may be demonstrated, still intact, in stains many months old, there can be no question but that drying tends to desiccate them, and that the chances of finding any intact sperms becomes much reduced. Absolute proof that the stain is seminal rests with identification of the sperm. The doctor may, under pressure in cross-examination, remind the lawyer that vasectomy could affect the findings.

Acid phosphatase test It has been found that the acid phosphatase content per millilitre of semen is so much greater in man (average 2500) than in animals (up to 12), that is a useful means of distinguishing human seminal fluid.

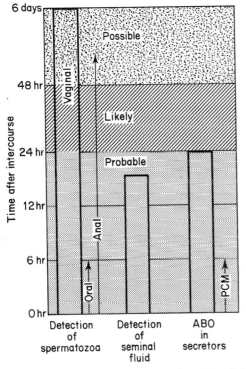

Fig. 13.9 Swab potentials in the living. (After R. L. Williams, 1978, *Police Journal*).

Incest

Sexual intercourse between a man and his granddaughter, daughter, sister or mother—or the corresponding relationship on the part of the female—is incest under the Sexual Offences Act 1956. The accused party must be aware of the prohibited relationship, or must accept the onus of disproving it, and the relationship need not be traced through lawful wedlock. Most cases concern father and daughter or brother and sister, and medical examination is concerned more frequently with demonstrating evidence of habitual intercourse than of fresh defloration.

Homosexual offences

Under the Sexual Offences Act 1967, the act of (or attempt to commit) anal intercourse (sodomy or buggery) is permitted between consenting adults, *if indulged in privately*. Members of the armed forces and merchant seamen are specifically excluded in the Act. The age of consent for the purposes of this Act is put at 21. It is, of course, still unlawful if practised upon anyone without consent.

A boy under 14 is regarded as sexually immature: he cannot be charged with the offence of rape or of buggery—merely of commiting an indecent assault.

Proof of penetration into the anus is necessary to the charge of buggery, but not emission of semen. Homosexual 'play' might be indecent or 'gross indecency'.

Examination in the case of an offence on a boy will usually disclose great tenderness around the sphincter, bruising or lacerations and stretching of the anal sphincter. In the older subject or in habitual partners the anus becomes dilated, loses its natural puckered orifice and develops a thickened keratinised skin. In either case seminal stains may be present on the passive participant and faecal soiling on the active. Traces of lubricant may also remain.

Before the coming into force of the Indecency with Children Act 1960, there was a gap in the law relating to indecency with children. If a

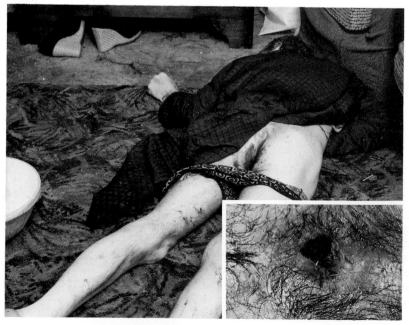

Fig. 13.10 Elderly victim of homosexual incident. The panties are drawn down: platform shoes lie nearby.
   Insert   Dilated and keratinised anal orifice in a habitual homosexual.

person, without any force, successfully invited a child to handle him indecently no offence was committed, as there was no assault. Now it is an offence for any person to commit an act of gross indecency with or towards a child under the age of 14, or to incite a child under that age to such an act with him or another.

Difficulties in the Medical Investigation of Sexual Offences

In recent years, there has been considerable criticism of the way in which doctors deal with allegations of rape and other sexual offences. Such complaints have come from women's action groups, the general public and the medical profession itself.

Firstly, there is the vexed question of the proportion of allegations of sexual interference which are true and those which are spurious. Some doctors claim that the majority of complaints are unfounded, whereas some feminist organisations insist that all are true. The latter claim is patently unrealistic, but in trying to assess the number of false allegations, it must be remembered that many women who have genuinely been sexually assaulted do not make a complaint either to the police or a doctor. The reasons may include personal repugnance to recounting the experience or the fear of a long and traumatic investigation by the police and of insinuations about their moral character by defence lawyers in eventual court proceedings. Thus perhaps a large block of the genuine cases are excluded from the cohort which contains less well-founded allegations, more commonly seen amongst younger girls who from reasons of fear of pregnancy or veneral contamination or spite against their boy friend, may retrospectively withdraw their consent to what was originally voluntary intercourse. It has been traditionally claimed that the longer the interval between the time of the alleged assault and the time when the complaint is made, the more likely is the allegation to be spurious, but this has recently been denied by some experienced physicians.

Doctors have also been condemned for their investigative role during the medical examination, it being claimed that questions by the doctor about past sexual activity are an invasion of privacy. However, it is clearly obvious that the doctor *must* inquire about the menstrual and pregnancy history and especially about recent sexual intercourse, if he or she is to make any sense of physical findings, including the presence of semen, in a victim of an alleged sexual assault.

More seriously, doctors acting for the police have in past years been condemned for their lack of expertise, lack of sympathy, brusque manner and reluctance to offer counselling to victims, being seen merely as technical tools of the prosecution.

In Britain, the activities of the Association of Police Surgeons have led to a marked improvement in standards, but increasing pressure is being brought to introduce facilities similar to those already established in parts of Australia and New Zealand, where 'Rape Centres' have been set up to provide optimum care and support for the victims of sexual assaults. Such centres have specially-trained women police officers, doctors and social counsellors on a 24-hour basis, where any women complaining of a sexual attack can be seen and cared for, irrespective of the possibility of a criminal investigation. Follow-up medical care and advice is offered about the possibility of veneral disease or pregnancy and physical and psychiatric after-care is provided. It is usually claimed that the doctor involved in the examination of sexual offences should be a woman and no doubt the majority of victims would prefer to be seen by a physician of their own sex. However, this preference is by no means universal and male doctors should not automatically be excluded from future participation in this most onerous of medico-legal duties.

14

Legal procedure

Dying declarations

The law of evidence is complex and the doctor need trouble himself but little about it. He may take it as a general rule that hearsay is not admissible as evidence, although there are some important exceptions to this rule. The doctor's principal duty in court is to answer the questions put to him: he may leave it to the authority of the court to decide what is admissible or otherwise.

One important exception to the general rule is the dying declaration which, if taken in accordance with the rules set out by law, may be admitted in evidence through hearsay. The services of a doctor are commonly required at the time such a declaration is made, for the subject is, in fact, dying or believed to be, and the initiative in securing such evidence before it is too late often lies with the medical man. The comparative infrequency of such evidence tends to reflect the comparative forgetfulness of doctors in the matter.

The essentials of the dying declaration are:

1. That the patient should, in fact, be dying—and from the injuries from which his grave condition has resulted. He must realise that death is inevitable. The statement should contain a preamble to this effect. The exact words are not fixed, but they must make it clear that no hope whatsoever of recovery was entertained at the time the declaration was made. 'Being without hope of recovery, I, John Smith, do say ...' would make a safe formula. Any words which could suggest that the declarant had some faint hope of recovery—such as '... no hope of recovery *at present* ...'—would undoubtedly invalidate the whole statement.

2. Death must follow; otherwise the statement becomes invalid.

3. Both the physical condition and the state of mind must be sufficiently sound to enable the declarant to formulate facts and to reason clearly. The doctor must be prepared to answer to this. It is assumed that a person who is dying will tell the truth, and that the statement has the integrity of evidence which might otherwise have been given on oath in a court of law.

4. The facts set out in the statement must be as full as possible. They must concern the criminal act responsible for the death of the patient and for which some person will be charged with murder or manslaughter; no other charge would permit of the declaration being used in evidence. The declarant may have been the only witness of the crime, and exclusion of his evidence might prevent a just charge being proved.

5. The doctor can himself take down the declaration in writing in the exact words of the patient, but it is preferable for him to leave the taking of it to a magistrate or a senior police officer. In a crisis the statement, which would then be likely to be very brief, might merely be committed to memory and later given in evidence. Questions may be included to clarify the statement and their answers appended.

6. The patient should sign the declaration, but this is not essential— merely desirable.

When death has taken place the declaration should be placed in the hands of the police without delay, for it may be the first intimation they have of some criminal act.

The death certificate

A doctor who has been in attendance during the last illness of a patient has a statutory duty under the Births and Deaths Registration Act 1953 to issue a certificate. No fee should be charged, though there is no regulation that specifically forbids this.

The registrar of births and deaths will not accept a certificate if the doctor has not seen the deceased person as a patient during the 14 days immediately preceding death. Although legally an alternative would be for the doctor to examine the body after death, most registrars are unwilling to accept this. It might be noted that Great Britain and the Republic of Ireland are the only countries in Europe which do not insist on a doctor's seeing the body before issuing a death certificate.

In England and Wales the certificate on the official printed form must be sent 'forthwith' to the registrar; in Scotland the doctor has 7 days' grace. It is usual practice for the relatives to take the certificate direct to the registrar, to expedite the matter. The postal services introduce un- desirable delay.

Although the strict letter of the law appears to make it mandatory for the doctor to issue a certificate where he was the attending physician, in practice it is usual for him to refrain from so doing if he is going to refer the case to the coroner or fiscal.

The registrar will always inform the coroner whenever he receives a certificate which is unacceptable, but it saves valuable time (especially at week-ends and holidays) if the doctor communicates direct with the coroner's office by telephone as soon as he decides that a death is re- portable. He should do this whether or not he has signed a certificate

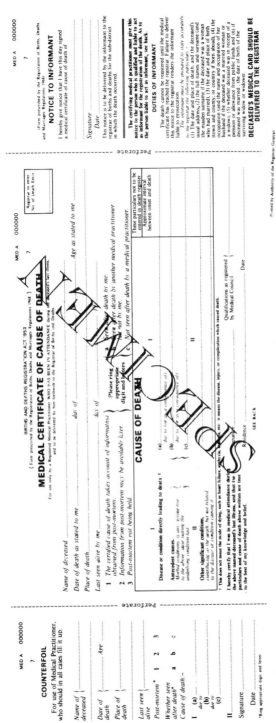

Fig. 14.1 Medical Certificate of Death.

PERSONS QUALIFIED AND LIABLE TO ACT AS INFORMANTS

The following persons are designated by the Births and Deaths Registration Act 1953 as qualified to give information concerning a death:—

DEATHS IN HOUSES AND PUBLIC INSTITUTIONS

(1) A relative of the deceased, present at the death.

(2) A relative of the deceased, in attendance during the last illness.

(3) A relative of the deceased, residing or being in the sub-district where the death occurred.

(4) A person present at the death.

(5) The occupier* if he knew of the happening of the death.

(6) Any inmate if he knew of the happening of the death.

(7) The person causing the disposal of the body.

DEATHS NOT IN HOUSES OR DEAD BODIES FOUND

(1) Any relative of the deceased having knowledge of any of the particulars required to be registered.

(2) Any person present at the death.

(3) Any person who found the body.

(4) Any person in charge of the body.

(5) The person causing the disposal of the body.

* " Occupier " in relation to a public institution includes the governor, keeper, master, matron, superintendent, or other chief resident officer.

Fill up where applicable

A

I have reported this case to the Coroner.

Initials of
Certifying Medical
Practitioner   } ....

Fill up where applicable

B

I may be in a position later to give, on application by the Registrar General, additional information as to the cause of death for the purpose of more precise statistical classification.

Initials of
Certifying Medical
Practitioner   } ....

NOTE.—The Practitioner, on signing the certificate, should fill up, sign and date the Notice to the Informant, which should be detached and handed to the Informant. The Practitioner should then, without delay, deliver the certificate itself to the Registrar of Births and Deaths for the sub-district in which the death occurred. Envelopes for enclosing the certificates are supplied by the Registrar.

A. Reported to Coroner ?

....

B. Further information offered ?

....

N.B.—If either Statement A or Statement B has been filled up, the fact should be noted in the appropriate place above.

Fig. 14.2 Reverse of certificate.

whenever the circumstances suggest that the coroner might have an interest in the death.

Reporting is usually to the coroner'as officer, an experienced police officer or civilian who conducts most of the administrative duties of the coroner. Once the doctor has given details of the death, he should take no further action—in particular, he should not attempt to sign a cremation certificate or seek an autopsy, as these are by then the coroner's prerogative.

Under the various provisions of the Coroners Acts of 1887 to 1926, 'where a Coroner is informed that the dead body of a person is lying within his jurisdiction, and there is reasonable cause to suspect that such person has died either a violent or unnatural death, or has died a sudden death of which the cause is unknown ...' the coroner assumes the responsibility of issuing the appropriate certificate after due inquiry.

The list of deaths which must be reported to the coroner, according to the Coroner's Rules 1953–1980 (Consolidated) are:

1. Where no doctor has treated the deceased in his or her last illness.
2. Where the doctor attending the patient did not see him or her within 14 days before the death, or after death.
3. Where the death occurred during an operation or before recovery from an anaesthetic.
4. Where the death was sudden and unexplained, or attended by suspicious circumstances.
5. Where the death might be due to an industrial injury or disease or to accident, violence, neglect or abortion, or to any kind of poisoning.

Although this list does not mention a number of other specific instances, these should also be reported; they include deaths in police or prison custody, where there is any allegation of medical or other negligence, and deaths of the recipients of war disability pensions.

A coroner cannot, in law, 'require' a practitioner to report a death to him, for he cannot act until he has been informed; in law that duty rests with the registrar. A doctor has, however, a duty to assist the law and should himself see that the coroner is informed without delay when the circumstances demand. Should he deliberately obstruct the coroner, he commits an offence for which he may be punished.

> In a case seen in a fashionable district of London a doctor had assured the relatives, who wished to 'avoid trouble of any kind', that they could rely on him. 'Leave this to me,' he said; 'you'll hear nothing more of this.' It was a case of death accelerated by a fall causing fractured femur, and the undertakers, noticing the shortening and eversion of the leg and the hip bruising, spoke of it to the registrar, who referred the certificate to the coroner. An unusually spirited inquiry followed.

> In 1950 a man was sentenced at Maidstone Assizes to 1 years' imprisonment for obstructing the coroner by concealing (by burial) the death of a foster child in his care. He had been found 'not guilty' of murder by suffocating the child.

The doctor must never deliberately omit some vital matter in his certificate 'in order to avoid trouble'—or for any other reason. The certificates in use in the UK are legal documents, deserving all the care a doctor would give to any other legal document.

The first essential is that the doctor should have been in attendance professionally, during the last illness, usually within the 14 days preceding death. It is not enough that the partner or locum tenens attended and left word or notes about the illness, or that the doctor 'had seen deceased about in the house getting more tottery and senile' and was 'quite satisfied' at the cause of death. The certificate makes the strictly personal and professional character of the visits quite clear, for it says at the top, 'For use only by a Registered Medical Practitioner who has been in attendance during the deceased's last illness', and again at the bottom where the doctor appends his signature, 'I hereby certify that I was in medical attendance during the above-named deceased's last illness'.

It is not even enough that he should receive information that a patient of his whom he had treated for hypertension has collapsed and died, for without professional attendance in that last illness he cannot be quite satisfied as to the cause of death. Every day provides autopsy findings of entirely unsuspected natural causes, and of injuries such as fractured skull, contused brain, or broken neck from collapse and fall from supposed 'strokes' or 'Heart failures'.

> In one such case a doctor who had attended a woman of 54 six months previously for angina pectoris issued a certificate upon 'hearing that his patient, still complaining of bouts of anginal pain', had been found dead in bed. The registrar stopped the certificate on the grounds that the doctor had not seen the woman recently. Autopsy on the coroner's instructions showed corrosive HCl burns of lips and mouth and some 20 ml (7 oz) of concentrated HCl in the stomach. The woman had committed suicide, unable to stand the torture of her angina–.

In most districts the registrar will refer a certificate to the coroner if the last professional visit took place more than 14 days prior to death, as shown under the heading 'last seen alive by me'. No period, however short, can ensure the exclusion of some extraneous factor such as violence precipitating death. Relatives who could benefit by the death might be tempted to hasten the event by some other means when natural diseases seems to dally overlong.

Dangerous as it may seem, all the law requires with regard to seeing the body after death is that the doctor shall 'ring' the appropriate words on the certificate. The importance of seeing the body when death has been reported cannot be over-estimated; in truth how can the doctor know without a visit that there is a dead body at all?

> A doctor gave a death certificate for an 'old lady' reported to him as dead the day after he had visited the house. The girl who came to the surgery for it forgot to explain that the 'old lady' now dead was in fact the mother of the one the doctor had seen, and carried away a death certificate for the 'old lady' who was still alive.

A doctor attending a child for bronchitis had last seen it 3 days previously. The mother said that she had fed it at 9 a.m. and put it into a cot. It had cried a lot, so she tried 'to settle it down' at 11 a.m. When she returned at 12.30 p.m. it was dead. This doctor noticed several small bruises over the face, and the mother said that it might have 'banged its little face against the cot' in its fits of crying. The doctor reported the case to the coroner, and at autopsy the bruises proved to be the marks of fingers gripping each side of the head; opposing thumb marks were found behind the neck. Seventeen ribs were fractured, and chest and abdomen were heavily crushed. Charged with murder, the mother admitted having lost her temper at 11 a.m., of having picked it up by the head and 'bashed it on the edge of the door'. If the doctor had not made a practice of visiting the dead body before issuing a death certificate this crime would have escaped detection.

When, however, the doctor:

1. is registered as a qualified medical practitioner,
2. has been in attendance during the last illness (within 14 days),
3. knows the cause of death,
4. is satisfied that the case does not demand the attentions of the coroner,

it is compulsory upon him to issue a certificate and hand the informant the 'notice' of the death for the registrar. The registrar will issue a disposal order for burial to the undertaker.

The vast majority of deaths are disposed of by these simple formalities. The doctor's only remaining difficulty is to fill in the precise entries relating to the 'cause of death'.

There are two sections. The first, headed I, asks for (a) the immediate cause and (b) the morbid conditions, if any, giving rise to the immediate cause. It would be sufficient, for instance, to write 'Acute general peritonitis' under I (a) and 'perforated gastric ulcer' under I (b). The second section, headed II, asks for 'Other significant conditions contributing to death, but not related to the disease or condition causing it.' There would be none in the example just given, but if uraemia and suppurative pyelonephritis were the I (a) and I (b) entries respectively, we might properly place 'carcinoma of the prostate' or 'diabetes mellitus' under II where the conditions warranted. All that is asked for is that a precise cause of death should be set out starting from the immediate cause and working back to the underlying disease responsible. There is a footnote asking that the terms which merely describe a mode of dying such as heart failure, coma, asthenia, etc., should be avoided. If the precise cause of death is not known the doctor should not take the responsibility of guessing at it nor start an autopsy to find out. The coroner is at hand to take the responsibility off his shoulders.

Preciseness is a laudable quality. The doctor who wrote:

'I (a) Heart failure.
    (b) Arteriosclerosis.

II Senile arterial degeneration over a long time. Dec. 1959, hemiplegia and aphasia; Sept. 1957, another cerebral haemorrhage; July 1958, another cerebral haemorrhage; Aug. 1958, heart attack—'

was informative to an absurd degree. 'Morbus cordis' is at the other extreme, being dangerously uninformative.

Avoid ambiguities such as 'Birth injuries', 'Cerebrovascular accident', or 'Termination of pregnancy', qualification of which must be given to make it clear that they were natural and not accidental or criminal occurrences. 'Fibrosis of the lung', possibly an industrial disease, will be certain to cause the registrar to refer the certificate. Indeed, vagueness of any kind is sure to result in the indignity of having the certificate refused by the registrar.

Under no circumstances should a doctor sign blank or partly blank death cerficates. He should also refer requests for copies to the registrar.

Scottish certification

In Scotland the coroner's counterpart is the procurator fiscal, and the relationship with doctor and registrar is virtually the same as that set out above. No provision is made on the reverse aspect of the Scottish certificate for intimating to the registrar that the case has been reported to the fiscal. The fiscal has to obtain a warrant from the sheriff in the event of his wanting more than a report on the clinical facts or a mere external examination; Scots law, curiously, permits any other doctor to certify.

Certification of live-births and stillbirths

A live-birth must be notified to the medical officer of health (under the Notification of Births Acts of 1907 and 1915), on stamped forms provided on request, and within 36 hours, by the father or some person in attendance at the birth, usually the midwife. Registration (in England and Wales under the Births and Deaths Registration Act 1874) must be made to the district registrar within 42 days, by anyone present or in charge of the child, and in Scotland (under the Registration of Births, Deaths, and Marriages Act 1854) within 21 days, by parents, nurse or person in charge of the child.

A stillbirth applies to any child 'which has issued forth from the mother after the twenty-eighth week of pregnancy and which did not at any time, after being completely expelled from the mother, breathe or show any other sign of life'. Certification in writing is then required from the doctor or certified midwife who was in attendance or examined the body after birth to the effect that the child was not born alive. The Acts providing for this are the Births and Deaths Registration Act 1953 in England and Wales, and Registration of Births, Deaths and Marriages (Scotland) Act 1965 in Scotland. The certificate is shown in Fig. 14.3.

It is still not fully appreciated that a doctor cannot possibly say, merely by looking at a newborn child, whether or not it has had a separate existence. Only autopsy can determine the facts, and the doctor would

SB 087860

COUNTERFOIL

For use of Medical Attendant or Midwife, who should in all cases fill it up.

Surname of Father (or Mother) ....

Date of Still-birth ....

Place of Still-birth ....

....

Cause of death

I (*a*) ....

(*b*) ....

(*c*) ....

II ....

Date of certification ....

Post-mortem*   1   2   3

Certificate issued to

(name) ....

of (address) ....

....

* Ring appropriate digit.

Fig. 14.3.

★ **CERTIFICATE OF STILL-BIRTH**   **SB 087860**

(Births and Deaths Registration Act, 1953, Section 11, as amended by Section 2 of the Population (Statistics) Act, 1960)

To be given only in respect of a child which has issued forth from its mother after the 28th week of pregnancy and which did not at any time after being completely expelled from its mother breathe or show any other signs of life.

| Registered at |
| Entry No. |

*I was present at the still-birth of a *male *female child born

on the .... day of .... 19...... to .... (NAME OF MOTHER)

at .... (PLACE OF BIRTH)

*I have examined the body of a *male *female child which I am informed and believe was born

I hereby certify that (i) the child was not born alive, and
(ii) to the best of my knowledge and belief the cause of death and the estimated duration of pregnancy of the mother were as stated below.

CAUSE OF DEATH

| | | Estimated duration of pregnancy |

DIRECT CAUSE
State foetal or maternal condition directly } (*a*)   I
causing death.   due to

.... weeks

ANTECEDENT CAUSES
State foetal and/or maternal conditions, if } (*b*) ....
any, giving rise to the above cause, stating } due to
the underlying cause last.   (*c*) ....

                 II

Weight of foetus (if known)

.... lbs.
.... oz.

OTHER SIGNIFICANT CONDITIONS
of foetus or mother which may have contributed to but, in so far as is known, were
not related to direct cause of death.

†{ 1   The certified cause of death has been confirmed by post-mortem.
    2   Post-mortem information may be available later.
    3   Post-mortem not being held.

Signature ....   Date ....

Qualification as registered by General Medical Council, or }
Registered No. as Certified Midwife.

Residence ....

* Strike out the words which do not apply.
† Ring appropriate digit.
* To be filled in by the obstetrician, midwife, or pathologist

THIS IS NOT AN AUTHORITY FOR BURIAL OR CREMATION

[SEE OVER

be wise when he has not been in attendance at the birth to report the case rather than presume the fact of stillbirth. The one exception is a state of maceration which gives clear evidence that the child died *in utero*.

If no qualified person is present, a declaration stating this and that the child was not born alive must be given by some person present at birth to the registrar, who may report the facts to the coroner.

Cremation certificates

The law dealing with this subject applies to England, Wales and Scotland, and is detailed in the Cremation Act of 1902, with amendments up to 1965.

A death certificate must first be issued, and the death must be registered in the ordinary manner. An application is then made by the relatives or executor to a cremation company or an undertaker for a cremation form. There are three parts to the document, each of which contains a number of detailed questions.

Form A is filled in by the applicant and must be signed before a person listed on the form as competent to verify the facts.

Form B is a medical certificate to be filled in by the doctor in attendance during the last illness. He will already have issued the ordinary death certificate. He *must* see the body.

Form C is a further, confirmatory, medical certificate filled in by a doctor not of less than 5 years' standing, and who must not be related either to deceased or to the doctor who filled in form B, nor be partner to the latter. He *must* see the body. As from April 1985, Form C is dispensed with, if there has been an autopsy.

These forms are then submitted to the medical referee of the cremation company who, if satisfied, grants authority (F) to cremate.

A coroner (or procurator fiscal) may give a certificate (form E), replacing forms B and C, in cases passing through his hands for autopsy. The medical referee may order an approved pathologist to perform an autopsy—or do one himself—thereby acquiring the information (form D) which would have appeared in forms B and C.

Only registered stillbirths for which the practitioner present at birth, or a pathologist examining the body, can both certify stillbirth and exclude suspicion may be cremated in the same manner.

If any circumstances demanding investigation by the coroner or procurator fiscal should come to the notice of the medical referee he must inform that authority and await written permission before authorising the cremation.

In the Waddingham case of 1936, the medical referee to a crematorium received, among the documents relating to the death of a wealthy woman who had died in a nursing home, a letter supposed to be in the lady's handwriting asking for cremation and adding 'and my last wish is my relatives shall not know of my death'. He stopped the cremation, and in due course it was proved that the matron of the nursing home had murdered her by morphine. A doctor had certified death as due to cerebral haemorrhage.

Where the person has not been identified, where the cause of death is still not clear, or where some further inquiry or examination may be necessary, the referee must withhold his authority for cremation. He must also do so when the deceased has left written instructions to the contrary. His most frequent cause for doing so is an unsatisfactorily worded medical certificate.

Procedure in deaths referable to the coroner or procurator fiscal

The coroner (England and Wales)

The ancient office of coroner, first mentioned in Saxon times but officially established by the Articles of Eyre in the reign of Richard I in 1194, derives its name from *custos placitorum coronas*—Keeper of the Pleas of the Crown. Originally concerned with many fiscal and administrative tasks, the coroner formerly investigated sudden and violent deaths, treasure trove, wrecks, catches of royal fish and even fires in the City of London. However, his present-day duties are concerned with enquiries into:

1. Violent, suspicious, unexplained or unnatural deaths.
2. Deaths in custody.
3. Removal of dead bodies out of England or Wales.
4. Ownership of treasure trove.

Under the various provisions of the Coroners Act 1887, as amended by the Coroners (Amendment) Act of 1926, 'Where a Coroner is informed that the dead body of a person is lying within his jurisdiction, and there is reasonable cause to suspect that such person has died either a violent or unnatural death, or has died a sudden death of which the cause is unknown, or that such person has died in prison, or in such place or under such circumstances as require an inquest in pursuance of any Act ...' the coroner must inquire into the death, may hold an inquest, and must file proper records of his inquiry and any inquest proceedings. He will issue a death certificate after due inquiry and this is sent to the registrar of births and deaths. He may also issue a cremation form E (dispensing with the medical and confirmatory cremation forms B and C) when a request for it is made.

In pursuance of his inquiries, which are usually conducted through his officer, he may ask for a report from a doctor, issue an order to a duly qualified person (preferably a pathologist) to perform an autopsy and furnish a report, and he may summon medical and other witnesses to an inquest should he consider one necessary.

Under the Coroners (Amendment) Act he can dispense with an inquest in cases of sudden death, the cause of which is unknown, if a post-mortem examination satisfies him that an inquest is unnecessary, and in these cases he sends his certificate (known as form B) stating the cause of death to the registrar.

In certain cases where the doctor has been in attendance but has had some cause to consult the coroner, inquiry may satisfy the coroner that the doctor's cause of death is acceptable without autopsy, and he may issue a certificate (known as form A) authorising the registrar to register the cause of death stated in it.

Where death was due to some simple accident or injury or to the ultimate consequence of some such thing, or to suicide—indeed *to any unnatural event*— the coroner may hold an inquest, and ... if it is suspected that death:

1. was due to murder, manslaughter or infanticide, or
2. occurred in prison or in such place or in such circumstances as require an inquest under any Act other than the Coroners Act 1887, or
3. was caused by an accident, poisoning or disease, notice of which is required under any Act to be given to a government department, such as a railway accident, or
4. was caused by an accident arising out of the use of a vehicle in a street or public highway (Road Traffic Act 1972), or
5. occurred in circumstances the continuance or possible recurrence of which is prejudicial to the health or safety of the public ...

an inquest must be held.

The coroner seldom now sits, as he did for so long, with a jury. The Criminal Law Act of 1977 abolished the requirement in cases where questions of criminal liability might arise—as after assaults, or the newer offence of 'killing by reckless driving', and also dispensed with the need for a jury in road traffic accidents.

A verdict returned at an inquest may no longer charge an individual with causing the death. The coroner has no power to issue a warrant for the arrest of such a person. Should criminal proceedings against some person be instituted, he must adjourn his inquest (under section 20, Coroners (Amendment) Act 1926) until after the conclusion of the case. He may then take evidence from a police officer of the verdict of the Assize Court, or await an official intimation from the clerk of that court.

The coroner cannot 'require' a doctor to report a death to him, but the doctor will find it advantageous to co-operate with the coroner, consulting him freely when in difficulty over a death, and recognising also that he may be subject to penalties for obstructing the coroner in the execution of his duties. The coroner has power to order an autopsy in any case that is reported to him, and autopsy may not then be performed except as ordered by him. He also has power to authorise further examinations such as analyses, and to incur certain expenses in these respects to satisfy himself as to cause of death.

The procurator fiscal (Scotland)

The procurator fiscal has not only to conduct inquiries into deaths of the kind set out as demanding the jurisdiction of the coroner in England and Wales, but also to prepare the evidence of witnesses and the conduct of the prosecution on behalf of the Crown in the sheriff courts. His investigations are private and his 'precognition' of witnesses, taken down in writing but not given on oath, may be used to enable him to make out a certificate of death, or, by forwarding the papers to the Lord Advocate, to institute criminal proceedings.

Under the Fatal Accidents Enquiry (Scotland) Act 1895 and the Fatal Accidents and Sudden Deaths Enquiry (Scotland) Act 1906, a public inquiry before a sheriff and a jury of seven is held into all fatal accidents at employment, fatal street accidents, or deaths in prisons, etc., when it is to the public interest that a public inquiry should be held.

Summons to a coroner's court in England or Wales and to precognition at a procurator fiscal's office in Scotland must be obeyed on penalty, but a doctor who is placed in real difficulty by such a summons will seldom find either official to be unco-operative. If his professional reputation seems likely to come into question he should take early steps to inform his defence or protection society.

15

The medico-legal autopsy. Evidence at courts and fees

The discovery of a body suspected to have died of violence or under circumstances requiring explanation is a common test of the doctor's training in elementary forensic principles. His first steps in the examination at the scene, and his first opinions, may make the difference between muddle-headed indecisiveness and a clean, swift investigation. An error in opinion may set in motion the wheels of a machine for criminal inquiry which may waste time and money—or, worse, cause grave distress, even injustice, to innocent persons. No doctor can afford to shoulder lightly the responsibilities of his first visit to the scene of suspected crime.

This does not mean that he should also undertake the more onerous responsibility of the autopsy. The day when 'any registered medical practitioner' was considered competent in this very highly skilled speciality has receded into the 'bad old days' of coroners' jurisdiction. The practitioner, who would not think of performing a thoracotomy or a delicate piece of orthopaedic surgery, also should no more think of performing an autopsy, on the accuracy and evaluation of which the machinery of justice may move. The spectacle of two doctors battling for over an hour to remove the cranial vault with a joiner's saw, two tyre levers and a coal hammer—only to have the battered remains come away in fragments—was one of lamentably bad judgement: no sound opinion could arise out of such a mess. The medico-legal autopsy requires training and experience: the ordinary practitioner would do well when called to the scene of supposed crime to limit his activities to a preliminary examination which will help to guide the inquiry into the proper channels (see Chapter 1).

Examination at scene

A doctor is called to the scene to make certain decisions that only a medical man can make—to ascertain the fact of death; to say, if possible, when it occurred; and to decide whether there are grounds for suspicion of foul play (see Chapter 1). He is not called as a sleuth and should not interfere with the police in their search for evidence—in rifled desks, jemmy marks, finger-prints, even the more sensational colour that marks some crimes. He should not hesitate, however, to ask for any information that may be relevant to his medical findings. It does help to know whether an overturned wardrobe has been lifted off a body when deciding the nature of a blunt wound to the head. The doctor should always know of the circumstances.

> The depressed fracture of the skull shown in Fig. 8.4 (p. 110) was found at autopsy in a man last seen talking to a group of men outside a works entrance. The body was found by a passer-by 20 minutes later, and suspicion that the man had been assaulted, kicked on the head, and killed was natural. A visit to the scene showed an ornamental wall, the surface markings of which were identical with the head injury. Autopsy disclosed sufficient coronary atheroma to cause faintness—even fatal collapse. Suspicion evaporated.

During his examination of the body and its immediate surroundings the doctor must be careful to avoid disturbing things, and in handling smooth surfaces such as furniture, telephone, weapon handles and the like that may bear finger-prints. Always ask, before disturbing anything at all, whether the scene has been recorded by photography—if it is so desired. Make a detailed note of the exact position of the body and of the state of the clothing irrespective of photography being done. Loose hairs and fibres should be removed by forceps and placed in sealed labelled envelopes. Five black hairs on the thigh of an auburn-haired woman found murdered in Folkestone went a long way to proving the guilt of the accused; to have disturbed them incautiously or to have permitted the undertaker to remove the body might well have been to lose this vital evidence. Scrapings of finger-nails are better done in a good light at the mortuary than in the light of a torch in a field. When you have finished, give approval for removal of the body; then have another look at the place where it lay, for sometimes an important clue lies concealed by the body.

Preliminaries at the mortuary

Where choice is possible, autopsy should be undertaken only in a good light under comfortable conditions and with proper equipment. Have a selection of swabs, glass bottles, bowls or plastic bags ready within reach for specimens. Label them at the time they are sealed.

Always in a criminal case, and preferably in all cases, have the body identified before commencing your examination. See that no unauthorised persons are present, but do not shut out the police officers or doctors concerned with the case, for your collaboration with them will be to the greatest mutual advantage.

Take a sample of blood and of the head and pubic hair (with skin attached) in all cases of crime, so that if necessary they may be compared with stains or a suspect's blood or hair. Take more specimens than seem necessary at autopsy, for you can discard them if unwanted, but rarely obtain them later if you forget to do so at the time. Vaginal or rectal swabs and nail scrapings often provide vital evidence.

The autopsy proper

Conduct this, in principle, like any routine post-mortem, and with the technique acquired in conducting autopsies during hospital training. There is no one way of examining the body: so long as the examination is thorough it will not miss anything of importance. Notes should be made at once—during the autopsy if they include measurements of wounds or directions of stabs or tracks of bullets. They can be used as the basis of a full report and may be produced to assist evidence in court if desired.

First examine any clothing which is still on, removing it with care piece by piece for evidence of violence, stains, etc. In most routine coroner's cases there is no object in paying detailed attention to clothing, but in cases of crime, especially of stabbing and fire-arm wounds, the character of the clothing and stains it bears may play an important part in the interpretation of these wounds. Do not allow the impatient cutting-off of clothing so often seen, for there is not the hurry for its removal or the need to limit movement that may arise in a live injured subject.

Next examine the body externally, from top to toe, lifting the arms and legs, opening the hands, and then turning the body on its face. Sooner or later, if you neglect to do this, you will be faced with an undiscovered injury of scar or tumour, coming to your knowledge for the first time in court, when it is too late to acquaint yourself with the facts. Be fussy over details rather than easily satisfied.

It is important, if you have reason to suspect some injury to the back, to cut through the skin at points such as the sacral and iliac prominences, the spine and the shoulder-blades, for bruises here may be invisible through the thick skin of the back. The proper reconstruction of injuries may depend on the presence—or absence— of deep bruises to the back.

Open the body by one of the routine throat to pubis or ear-thyroid-ear to pubis incisions, noting the volume and character of fluid effusions lying in the chest and abdomen.

Avoid enlarging surgical or other wounds. Cut alongside or across them at some entirely different angle if necessary. If you have doubts about the original character of wounds repaired in hospital ask for the surgeon who did the repair. In one case I examined, a stab wound which appeared to have transfixed the arm and entered the chest proved to have passed into the arm only, surgical exposure of a cut brachial artery and a stab drain in the chest accounting for the further complications found. Consultation with the surgeon will avoid such errors.

In taking out organs endeavour to remove them in groups rather than singly, so as to preserve their interrelationship. For instance, the entire tongue, neck tissues, chest contents and abdominal organs (less the intestines previously removed) may be taken out in one piece so as to keep the continuity of aorta, oesophagus and stomach (as in poisoning). Tie off lower oesophagus and duodenojejunal junctions if the stomach is going to be separated in a case of poisoning. Take samples of urine or cerebrospinal fluid or blood by sterile syringe before the organs are disturbed. Label them.

Evolve an order of examination which is adhered to as a routine, and no organs will be overlooked. In suspected air embolism, as from wounds involving veins, from venous infusion deaths and from instrumental air injection in abortion, commence with a dissection of the system of veins suspected to have conveyed the air to the heart and arterial tree—without opening any.

Complete your examination, including the brain—and, if suspected to be involved, the spinal cord—before being drawn into any conclusion regarding the cause of death. Delay a full report for microscopy if this seems desirable.

If you are unable to establish a cause of death you may ask for expert assistance. If poisoning is suspected, or analysis desired for its proof, remove the stomach contents by tying off both ends of the organ, washing its exterior and then opening it over a bowl. Do not take chances with a small-necked jar or you may see vital poison or pills disappearing down the drain. Preserve also samples of blood, of urine and of cerebrospinal fluid, and seal in bottles the brain, the liver, one or both kidneys, and a large square of muscles at the site of any injected poison. Lastly, in suspected arsenical poisoning take samples of hair (or skin with hair attached) and of the nails. See that these are sealed in the presence of the coroner's officer or the detective officer in charge and handed into his care. The coroner will direct any analysis which takes place.

Special autopsy techniques

In addition to a routine autopsy technique, the medico-legal substance of which will depend upon the forensic interpretations of the findings, there are certain special examinations which will be found necessary when attention is directed to some special region of the body not exposed by a routine autopsy.

Whenever the possibility of criminal proceedings arises in a case where blood could have been shed it will be wise to take a sample of the blood and ascertain its group without delay. It may later be important to know whether blood-stains found on a suspect are of a different group from the suspect's and similar to the victim's. For similar reasons it is important to retain samples of head and pubic hair. It is important in examining the extent of wounds to preserve them as much as possible, making single cuts across them, never extending them. In the event of re-examination such artificialities cause difficulties which need not arise; any exploratory cuts should be carefully noted.

The care necessary in dealing with gastric or intestinal contents and of urine in cases suspected, even remotely, of poisoning has already been remarked upon. Early refrigeration is vital.

The following special procedures are also demanded on occasion:

1. *The sinuses of the skull* may be opened direct from the interior of the vault by chiselling off the roofs of the middle ears and sphenoid, frontal and ethmoidal sinuses. The maxillary spaces may be similarly explored under the cheeks, preferably by turning forward face flaps extending from the incisions behind each ear made for the reflection of the scalp. It may be necessary to carry these incisions forward under the angle of the jaw to facilitate mobility of the flaps.

Far better exposures are obtained if the face is stripped off from the original post-mortem incisions behind each ear forward towards a hinge left down the centre brow, nose and chin, and the skull is sawn—as extensively and frequently as desired—to expose the sinuses. A paramedian split and subsequent saw-cuts made from the split surface afford excellent views. No difficulty is experienced in tying the skull fragments together again (with drill holes or saw niches to hold the ties), and turning back the face flaps.

2. *The spine* may be examined from behind for its laminae and canal, or from in front for bodies and discs. The most important preliminary is to raise the part next to be explored on a block. Inclined saw-cuts through the laminae from behind and then removing the loosened arch and spine by chisel or cranial key, taking care not to go deep enough to injure the cord, will give a good exposure of spinal canal and cord. Flat saw-cuts at deepening levels through the bodies carried right up the spine from pelvic brim to high neck, removing ribs where necessary for elbow-room, will give an excellent and rapid exposure of bodies and discs for dislocations, fractures and infections.

3. *The urinary system* may be examined as an integral whole, and this is of great importance in cases of injury. The kidneys are taken out of their beds as usual and are then drawn strongly towards the pelvis. The renal vessels, now under tension, are cut, but the ureters are left intact and dissected to the bladder. The bladder is next freed from its surroundings by skirting round it and, after taking a small block out of the symphysis pubis, the bladder is drawn forward and the urethra dissected from its bed, the penis being shelled out of its skin in the male. As an alternative, blunt-nosed scissors may be run down from the meatus through a gap sawn in the symphysis, up into the bladder, and thence via the ureteric orifices into each ureter *without removing the organs.* Any procedure which obviates the removal of organs and yet gives a clear view has two outstanding advantages: it limits the injury which may be done in exposing the parts, and it also preserves their relationship with their surroundings, a point of great importance in establishing the precise routes of penetrating injury or infection.

4. *The female genital tract* The same procedure may be used with equal advantage in examining cases of suspected abortion. Here above all is it essential that no injury should be made to the parts in removing

them, for small penetrations and scratches may be of vital importance in establishing the fact of an instrumental interference. Far better to inspect the whole system *in situ*. A single midline incision carried up along the front midline (after exposure by removal of a block of symphysis and dissection of the bladder and urethra off the vagina) will give an excellent view. With the legs splayed wide apart the front wall of the vagina may be inspected in advance of the blunt (probe)-ended scissors which is run up towards, into, and through the cervix. It is wise to have containers ready to collect any fluid lying within the uterus, for it may include soap, lysol, glycerine, or other matter injected to procure abortion. It will run out as soon as the cervical canal is laid open and the blunt end of the scissors enters the cavity of the uterus.

In both forms of exposure of the pelvic organs—whether they are examined *in situ* or dissected out before examination—a block should be placed under the buttocks. In suspected abortion it is wise to commence the autopsy by examining this region and the placing of a high block under the buttocks will be found to clear the field internally also, the intestines and any peritoneal fluid dropping back into the mid and upper abdomen.

Reports upon post-mortem examinations

Deaths which will not involve criminal proceedings

These reports may be couched in moderately technical terms, for they will be submitted primarily to either the coroner or the procurator fiscal, both of whom will have experience in such matters. They should be made out in keeping with the other official papers in such cases and preferably on a printed post-mortem examination form so that some standard lay-out may be followed. Sometimes a form will be issued, to be filled out after examination. It matters not a great deal precisely how or in what order the observations are recorded, so long as the report contains (1) the place and date of the examination, (2) the name of the subject as identified at autopsy, (3) how long dead, (4) full details of external and internal examination findings, and (5) the cause of death. It must be signed, with the medical qualifications added, and should again be dated.

The Scottish report must include a certification 'upon soul and conscience' that it was by authority of the procurator fiscal that the examination was made.

Some space for an explanatory summary such as that used in the report form illustrated, under the heading 'Other remarks', is of the greatest value in placing on record, in the report of bare findings, an opinion. Many cases of sudden death from natural disease, such as coronary occlusion, occur while the subject is at work. The nature of this work may be such as could well have accelerated death from such causes, thus introducing an extraneous factor which might justify compensation under the National Insurance Act 1946. The autopsy itself will, of course, give no evidence of this, but bearing the possibility in mind, the examiner will do well to include in his report some such phrase as: 'There is nothing from autopsy *to distinguish this from* a death from natural causes.' Such a remark will afford an opportunity to qualify the interpretation of the autopsy findings in the light of subsequent evidence. When the doctor is informed or hears upon oath of the exact nature of extraneous factors alleged to have contributed to death, he can, if necessary, modify his opinion.

In the example of a routine autopsy report shown in Fig. 15.1:

> Alexander S., aged 66, who had been depressed by ill-health following duodenal ulceration and by domestic anxieties, failed to return home one evening. He was found dead in his office upon search, hanging by a thin rope which encircled the neck from a water pipe which ran close to the ceiling. An overturned chair lay nearby, but there was no other disturbance. He had left no note indicating his intention.

Deaths from crime

Where crime is suspected a pathologist should accept the coroner's routine instructions to conduct an examination of the body and furnish a report with reluctance. If the case seems likely to place weighty decisions on his shoulders and results in his appearing as a medico-legal expert in the witness-box at trial in a criminal court, then he should not hesitate to suggest to the coroner that an expert be called at the outset.

Usually the coroner and the police will already have come to the conclusion that the case is one for an expert pathologist and the doctor will merely be given the opportunity of attending the autopsy. He has no right in law to attend such a post-mortem examination unless given permission by the coroner, and will, of course, earn no fee by his attendance. It will, however, be foolish of him to neglect such an opportunity: mutual benefit is likely to follow from such a 'consultation': it is encouraged in the Coroners' Rules 1953.

As this account is not intended for experts in forensic medicine, nothing will be said of the form of report in such cases, except that it will be carefully prepared with the criminal proceedings in view—further need for the hand of the expert.

It may be that after a routine autopsy the doctor is unable to state the cause of death. He should then draw up his report as far as possible with his observations and indicate what conclusions, if any, he has been able to draw. The coroner will take steps to further the investigation, being authorised to ask for another autopsy, for analysis, or bacteriological or other special laboratory examination in order to satisfy himself as to the cause of death.

Occasionally the cause of death is literally 'unascertainable'. The coroner is entitled, after due inquiry, to return such a finding.

POST-MORTEM EXAMINATION.

Name Alexander SMITH   **Stated Age** 66 years

At London Mortuary   **Date** August 10th., 1980

EXTERNAL EXAMINATION

Nourishment ...   .

Marks of Violence,

Identification, etc. ...

Height 5ft 10in

Of a general physique in keeping with the age.
Old upper abdominal operation scar - and internal evidence of older gastro-enterostomy
DEEP IMPRESSION OF NOOSE encircling neck, lying at about upper thyroid level across the front of the throat and around the R side of the neck, rising to a suspension point behind the L.ear - a single line, most deeply imprinted under the R lower jaw.
Well marked vital asphyxial changes along the line of constriction, and in the head and neck above it.
No other mark of recent injury.

How long dead 24 hrs (approx)

INTERNAL EXAMINATION

Skull ...   ...

Normal

Brain Meninges ...

Deep engorgement and cyanosis, with occasional petechiae scattered in the white matter. No disease.

Mouth, Tongue, Oesophagus ...   ...

Larynx, Trachea, Lungs ...

Fresh fractures of the cornua of the R half of the hyoid and thyroid beneath the line of constriction.
Larynx otherwise uninjured.
No disease of the respiratory passages or in the lungs.
Well marked asphyxial changes in the latter, with deep engorgement and many scattered subpleural petechiae.

Pericardium, Heart and Blood Vessels ...   ...

No organic disease. Deep engorgement and cyanosis in all compartments. Dilatation principally R sided, but without anoxic petechiae. Mild coronary atheroma only.

Stomach and Contents ...

Old partial gastrectomy and gastro-enterostomy: no residual ulcer. No growth. No poison.
Stoma wide and apparently functioning well.

Peritoneum,

Intestines, Etc. ...   ...

Liver and Gall Bladder ...

Spleen ..   ..

Kidneys and Ureters...

Bladder, Etc. ...   .

Generative Organs ...   ...

Normal.
No disease. Terminal engorgement and cyanosis only.
Engorged and cyanosed only.
No organic disease.
Some terminal engorgement and cyanosis only. No urinary obstruction, though some benign prostatic enlargement present.
Normal.

Other Remarks ...   ...

The autopsy findings are consistent with deliberate self-suspension and give no cause for suspicion.
An older gastric operation appears from examination to have produced a good local condition.
No other painful or distressing disease was present.

Histology, Bacteriology. Toxicology

CAUSE OF DEATH 1a
(See International Form) b
    c
    2

Asphyxia, due to
Hanging.

Signed

M.D.,Lond(Pathologist)

Fig. 15.1 Example of an autopsy report.

Medical evidence

It is so often said that the ordinary medical witness was weak, or unintelligible, or made a poor impression for a 'skilled witness', that there are likely to be some grounds for this criticism. The reason is, of course, that he is expected to be good: he is well educated, a man of science, not ignorant of the art of both logic and argument, and capable of making reasonable deductions from an array of facts. He is, however, like all other witnesses, somewhat nervous in an atmosphere to which he is unused, and often obsessed with the feeling that he is in the box to be badgered. Let him remember that his sole duty is to present his medical observations, and to construct reasonable deductions from them. His aim is the truth: there should be no taking sides and no evasion. The doctor is called to help the court come to a correct decision.

Several simple rules will help to make the doctor the 'skilled witness' he is supposed to be by law:

1. Be familiar with the details of your evidence before entering the box: anticipate certain questions on it, and be prepared with the answers to them in advance.
2. Take all records, reports, details of observations and any other data to be quoted into the box. Do not attempt to memorise.
3. Stand up; do not lounge in the box.
4. Speak clearly: good diction is cultivated and requires effort.
5. Listen carefully to the questions. Answer only what is asked.
6. Do not evade a question. Say 'I do not know' if it is true ... no one can know everything.
7. Answer without heat: do not argue. Disagree firmly and repeatedly—but do not lose your temper.
8. Make only reasonable deductions. Be strictly fair.

Evidence which might be lucid and impressive is often made obscure by faulty diction or bad grammar, or its essentials lost among qualifications and asides. Evidence should be concise and clear, a simple description of the truth, so transparently honest in its deductions that its integrity is beyond doubt.

The array of evidence should be brought forward in a natural order, constructing a case in such a way that the conclusions become self-evident and do not require proof; cross-examination will be shortened in this way. In most courts an experienced coroner or skilled counsel will extract the details in a natural order suitable to the presentation of the case; answers such as 'Yes' and 'No' are civil, direct, sufficient, and do not provide further material for counsel's use. The habit of answering 'I did' or 'It was not' instead of 'Yes' and 'No' is stilted and tends to give the impression of testiness.

A coroner is addressed as 'Sir', a magistrate as 'Your Worship', a County Court judge as 'Your Honour', and a High Court (e.g. Crown Court) judge as 'My Lord'.

As to phraseology, court conditions demand some stock sentences which cannot be bettered. 'I formed the opinion [or view] that ...' is unequalled for implying a careful weighing of the evidence. The doctor must not feel hurt by opposing counsel saying: 'But that is only an opinion, doctor.' Since this was what the medical witness was asked for he will disarm counsel by saying so. Another stock phrase: 'the findings [or observations] were consistent with ...' is also sound, for it is not incapable of yielding ground. Other interpretations of the same facts may be admitted, but this one seems the most consistent. Phrases such as 'My conclusions, based on the observations stated, were as follows' sound pompous.

A sound knowledge of the evidence to be given, studied diction, plain English, and strict confinement to the facts or to reasonable deductions arising out of them—these are the hall-marks of a good medical witness. Avoidance of medical terms is desirable, though not always possible. And a final danger to avoid at all costs is stepping outside the field of one's own competence.

Attendances at court

Coroner's court

A coroner who directs a doctor to make an examination of a dead body and report to him in writing on his findings may subsequently hold an inquest on the case and can summon the doctor to attend and give evidence on his findings. The doctor must obey such a summons. Similarly, if a doctor has been in attendance on such a subject in life he may be summoned to give evidence. He should take his records of visits and any reports that he had filed in connection with the case and use them in giving his evidence from the box. Sometimes the coroner's officer will have asked him at an earlier stage for a statement of his professional attendances and findings, and it will smooth his subsequent passage through the witness-box if he complies. There is no compulsion about this preliminary service to the coroner, but the doctor should always co-operate so far as he can.

The coroner's court is a court of record. Its judicial acts, such as committing to trial, have now become obsolete under the Coroners (Amendment) Rules 1977. The doctor may expect to receive every courtesy, being allowed to sit in the court during the inquest and often, upon request, being called at as early a stage as possible and released after giving his evidence. The coroner will obtain from him the evidence he requires, and the doctor should use his own notes freely in giving his replies. Far too many doctors rely, to their disadvantage, on their memory; it is unwise and quite unnecessary. This court is not bound by the strict rules of evidence, except in cases of crime, and hearsay evidence may be given at the discretion of the coroner.

Criminal courts

The following are the forms of criminal courts: (1) Petty Sessions Magistrates' (or Police) Court, (2) Crown Courts, and (3) Courts of Appeal— which, under the Criminal Appeal Act 1968, consist of civil and criminal divisions. Further recourse lies to the House of Lords on points of law 'of general public importance'.

The Magistrates' Court is the lowest of the criminal courts, and is composed of justices of the peace (magistrates), or a police magistrate, or a stipendiary. It has jurisdiction over all kinds of offences against the criminal law which may be tried summarily. This court also makes the preliminary inquiry into all indictable offences, and when it is satisfied that a prima facie case has been made out by the prosecution the accused person is sent for trial on indictment before a jury. Relatively 'petty' offences, such as common assaults, matrimonial separation, road traffic offences, drunkenness, etc., are also tried in this court. The justices of the peace are advised on points of law and practice by their clerk, usually a solicitor. The stipendiary is always a barrister and sits alone.

Crown Courts fall into two classes, the *lower* being presided over by a lesser judge, nominated by the Lord Chancellor. In a borough a recorder, who is a senior barrister nominated by the Lord Chancellor, presides. The jurisdiction of this court is limited, but it hears all indictable offences which are not sent for hearing to a higher Crown Court. It also hears appeals from convictions from the Petty Sessional Courts. There is a jury except in appeal cases. An appeal lies from this court to the Divisional Court, and in certain cases to the Courts of Appeal.

Higher Crown Courts try the more serious criminal cases, such as treason, murder, manslaughter, rape, etc. They are presided over by a judge of the High Court. Judges used to travel on a circuit, of which there were seven in England and Wales, and the court sat at the 'assize' town in each county. The Central Criminal Court (the Old Bailey) is a Crown Court which sits in the City of London. Higher Crown Courts also try civil actions.

The Court of Appeal (*Criminal Division*) hears appeals from sentences at the Crown Courts. The Lord Chief Justice presides over this court and is assisted by other judges of the High Court, there being never less than three; always an odd number capable of a majority decision.

Under the Criminal Justice Act 1967, much evidence that used to be given verbally is submitted in the form of statements, signed by the witness. These are served to both sides and either can ask for the attendance of any witness to give evidence if it appears desirable.

The doctor who has to give evidence in a case in which one of the more serious criminal charges has been brought will appear at the Petty Sessional or Magistrates' Court, where his evidence on oath will be taken down in writing by the clerk of the court. He should give his evidence at dictation speed, watching the clerk, and, in the event of a counsel or solicitor representing the accused at this stage desiring to ask questions, should answer these also at dictation speed. His evidence will be read over to him by the clerk, and he should not hesitate to interrupt to correct errors, or to clarify anything which does not seem to him to represent exactly what he said. He will sign the papers and will be bound over before leaving the court to appear at the trial on a recognisance to which he will merely assent. The evidence thus taken forms the deposition of the witness: points from it may be raised again at trial.

At a later date, if a prima facie case has been made out and the accused is committed for trial, the doctor will attend either at one or other of the Crown Courts, according to the gravity of the case, and will there again give his evidence on oath. He should again take his notes with him into the witness-box and use them freely: anything he has said in evidence at the preliminary hearing before the magistrates, having been taken down in writing, will now be before the court, including counsel who appear to prosecute or to defend. The doctor will be examined by prosecuting counsel, and cross-examined by the defending counsel, who will not hesitate to point out any inconsistencies.

At the Crown Court the accused is on trial before a judge and a jury sworn to try 'and a true verdict give according to the evidence'. The trial is conducted in an atmosphere of established custom and dignity; for 'justice must also be seen to be done'. Doctors should always avoid taking sides. Truth is the real object, and impartiality will be likely to create an impression of fairmindedness on any judge or jury.

When the doctor is called to court the outline of his evidence will first be put to him in a series of questions, by counsel for the prosecution. He will then undergo a 'cross-examination' by defending counsel, to whom he should answer fairly and calmly, yielding points when it is reasonable to do so and resisting, denying, possibilities which are (to him) less reasonable. The doctor will never have a bad time if he is fair, impartial though firm, and refuses to be drawn into anger—even resentment. If counsel makes an obviously unfair suggestion which is intended to rouse the doctor, let him say, without heat, that he does not agree or even that the suggestion seems to him to be improper. The judge will uphold him if it is so.

After cross-examination the prosecuting counsel may once more get up to re-examine his witness, to strengthen any parts of the evidence which may have been shaken by cross-examination.

Lastly, the judge himself may put any pertinent matter which he thinks it necessary to clarify for the jury.

The doctor who has to orientate himself in this atmosphere would do well to locate the jury at an early stage, for it is primarily for them that his evidence must be made clear—to whom he may think it wise to demonstrate on his own body the position of some wound he is describing. This may seem to be unnecessary advice, but in older Crown Courts the jury is sometimes tucked so compactly into a corner that it requires a piece of deliberate searching to pick them out. Counsel will often indicate when he wishes the doctor specially to show something to the jury by saying: 'Now, doctor, will you show the jury . . .'

Lastly, the medical witness should never assume that when he comes down from the box his attendance at this court is no longer required. At the criminal courts it is common for a doctor to be recalled to answer some medical question which has subsequently arisen, and unless his release has been asked for in open court and the judge has asked defending counsel if he thinks he may desire to recall the doctor and the answer has been a clear negative, the doctor must stay. As a rule the judge or prosecuting counsel will suggest release from the court as soon as the medical witness has finished giving his evidence and has dealt with cross-examination and re-examination. The ordinary medical witness should collect his fee before leaving (see p. 231).

Civil courts

The County Court   is an inferior court of civil action, and the atmosphere is entirely different from that in the criminal court. This court was created by the County Courts Act 1846, and various subsequent Acts have extended its jurisdiction. Many civil proceedings are now within its range and actions commenced there are of the same nature as those in the High Court. It also has jurisdiction in equity, bankruptcy, and the winding-up of certain company matters.

In actions commenced in the County Court in contract and tort (which is a wrong independent of contract) the claim must not exceed a sum of £5000 unless the parties agree in writing. Claims commenced in the High Court can be remitted to the County Court, but are usually too substantial.

In actions heard in the civil courts the counsel who appear will endeavour to establish or dispute the claims of a plaintiff. The feeling of sides may be strong, and a doctor may sense that he is being pressed to take one or other side for which he has been called to give evidence: he must try to avoid bias.

A common type of case demanding a doctor's services would be a claim for compensation for some physical disablement alleged to have followed from a defect or piece of negligence for which the defendant was said to be responsible. Medical details of injury and of clinical observations on the course of an illness, or of the autopsy findings, will be the subject of argument by examination, cross-examination, re-examination, maybe further cross-examination by opposing counsel, as well as of pertinent questioning by the judge who presides over this court. There may be a jury, but the doctor's notes and records, which he should always have with him and use, and his expressions of opinion should be directed to the judge. The same desire for a lucid description of clinical detail and observations, and the same quiet fairness of opinions, should actuate the doctor as in other courts. Where opposing views are also tenable the doctor would do well to admit of both, giving each the value he himself thinks proper. He should avoid at all costs the apparent taking of sides.

In civil actions he must allow for delay and disappointment as affairs are often difficult to run on a fixed schedule. He may find that at the last minute as settlement has been arranged between the parties and his attendance is no longer required. He must accept these difficulties with as good grace as he can. He will already have received conduct money, and maybe also promise of a fee for his appearance in court, and he is entitled to both in compensation for the inconvenience caused him.

The High Court is the superior Court of Record and is divided into various sections, which have replaced the old Probate, Divorce and Admiralty Divisions. The new sections consist of Chancery, Family and Queen's Bench Divisions, the last having Commercial and Admiralty sections. In London, the High Court sits in the Royal Courts of Justice, in the Strand, whilst in the provinces and Wales they use the same courts (and often the same judges) as the Crown Courts, which have criminal jurisdiction. The procedure in court is much the same as in the County Court, and when the doctor appears as a witness in the High Court it will, as a rule, be for a plaintiff or defendant in claims of a value much in excess of those taking place in the County Court. He will give his evidence in the same manner as has been detailed in respect of other courts.

A Court of Appeal of the High Court sits as occasion demands to hear appeals from the courts below, but the doctor will not be likely to be called to give evidence in this court as appeals are almost always on points of law or procedure.

Fees

Whereas, in the past, fees set by Regulations in respect of the various services given by doctors and scientists in connection with coroners' or police investigations, and for attendances and expenses in connection with the giving of evidence at court remained in force for long enough to justify setting them out in a textbook, they now become revised at such short intervals that they are likely to be out of date before a text-book can get into circulation. They will not, therefore, be set out for standard services for police work, nor for the coroners' or magistrates' or criminal courts.

Doctors, scientists, pathologists and the like will, by and large, have to rely on the *Schedules for Payments* available on the day, but should not forget to make application and sign any necessary forms on completion of the service in question—and to keep their own records of service in detail until full settlement.

Experts are paid such allowances as the court considers reasonable. Application for such additional items as 'preparing to give evidence' (qualifying fee) may be made through Crown counsel. An office operates these payments, which may be collected before leaving court.

Legal aid in both civil and criminal cases assesses the remuneration of witnesses (for either side) upon the recommendation of the Law Society. The sums awarded follow, in general, those fixed by statute, and little room is left for even the expert to manœuvre.

Civil courts In the *County Court* and the *High Court* the expenses are subjected to the approval of a registrar and a taxing master respectively at the time the costs are 'taxed'.

The medical witness falls into one of two classes. If a witness of fact, of the details of clinical records and of recorded diagnoses and opinions, he owes a duty to the State to give evidence and must be content with statutory allowances. If an expert, called to express opinions on the facts already recorded, he is in a position to make a bargain with the legal adviser for the side for which he appears to pay him an agreed fee. Or he can waive his fee, as doctors often do in cases of undoubted poverty or for their fellow-practitioners.

'Conduct money', to cover expenses of travel to court and sustenance—usually £1 for courts in a nearby district or town—used to be paid at the time he was subpoenaed to appear as a witness by the party for whom the doctor is to appear, before he could be made to attend. Now a fee is paid for attending to give evidence, plus a 'qualifying' fee if claimed. Where a doctor is doubtful about getting his fee he may indicate so before giving his evidence. No witness is less helpful than an unwilling one, and the position seldom arises.

In the *High Court* the award of special sums for medical evidence may depend to some extent on the sum the successful litigant can obtain from the unsuccessful litigant who is ordered to pay the costs. These are in an ordinary case 'taxed' by the taxing master after the hearing when the costs are lodged with him, together with all receipts, for disbursements.

With regard to keeping conduct money or claiming fees when a case is settled out of court, the doctor is entitled to do so if he has done anything—lost appointments, made reports, or prepared case-notes, etc.—to justify a fee.

16
Medical ethics

It is important that the public shall be able to distinguish between a qualified medical practitioner and an unqualified person professing some skill in healing. Because of a deteriorating situation in this respect in the middle of the last century, a body was set up by the Medical Act of 1958, then called the 'General Council' and now known as the General Medical Council, this name being officially adopted in 1950.

The functions of the General Medical Council (GMC), which is responsible to the Privy Council, include:

1. The establishment of a Medical Register.
2. The supervision of medical education.
3. The setting and maintenance of ethical standards.
4. The exercise of disciplinary functions within the profession.
5. The determination of the fitness of sick doctors to practise.

By the terms of the various Medical Acts, the latest dated 1978, the unregistered practitioner is prevented from using any title or pretence of qualification, recovering fees at law, supplying poisons on prescription (Pharmacy and Poisons Act 1933), signing death certificates (Births and Deaths Registration Act 1874), attending maternity cases (Midwives and Maternity Homes Act 1936) or treating venereal disease (Venereal Diseases Act 1917). Further, he may not hold public service, insurance or Crown appointments.

A registrar makes the entries of both provisional and full registrations and erases where loss of contact, death or instructions, after inquiry, from the Council make it necessary. The restrictions imposed by provisional registration last for a year, subject to a satisfactory report, and consist mainly of excluding the new doctor from unsupervised practice and from signing certificates outside his hospital employment.

Since the radical reconstitution of the GMC in 1979, sweeping changes have been made, including the types of registration. The following categories now exist.

1. *Provisional registration* for those qualifying in the UK.
2. *Full registration* after satisfactorily completing a preregistration

233

year. In addition, reciprocal registration exists for the graduates of certain overseas universities within the Commonwealth, for nationals of EEC countries in certain circumstances, and for foreign graduates holding limited registration who are entitled to proceed to full registration.

3. *Limited registration* is offered to graduates of 84 countries who hold acceptable qualifications and who have a minimum of 1 year's acceptable experience. Limited registration cannot exceed an aggregate of 5 years and, before being granted, the applicant must satisfy the Professional and Linguistic Assessments Board (PLAB) test. Limited registration is granted only for specific medical appointments. Holders may proceed to full registration if the GMC consider that their ability and experience are suitable.

4. *Visiting overseas specialists* and EEC doctors may be granted temporary full registration for specific purposes.

The constitution of the GMC

Following the Medical Act of 1978, a Council of 95 members now has a majority (50) of members elected by postal vote by all medical practitioners. The other 43 comprise 21 members appointed by the university medical schools, 13 appointed by the royal colleges etc., 9 lay members and 2 from the Privy Council. A President is elected from amongst the members. The GMC premises are at 44 Hallam Street, London W1N 6AE.

Disciplinary functions of the GMC

The GMC is not concerned with civil disputes between doctors and patients concerning alleged medical negligence, unless the conduct of the doctor is sufficiently serious and repetitive as to constitute *serious professional misconduct*. This phrase is the only type of lapse which the GMC disciplines. It was formerly described as 'anything which would reasonably be regarded as disgraceful or dishonorable by his professional brethren of good repute and competency'.

A doctor's behaviour may come to the notice of the GMC either (1) by notification by the courts of any conviction of a doctor, or (2) by an accusation of 'serious professional misconduct'. The latter may come from an official body such as the health authorities or from a private individual. Until 1970, divorce courts were obliged to notify the GMC of any doctor cited in a divorce action as the co-respondent, but this is now done only if the injured party claims that the doctor was guilty of professional misconduct.

A conviction in the courts has to be accepted as proven by the GMC, who have only to decide whether the crime constituted serious professional misconduct. Other allegations of misconduct are examined in the GMC by the President or his 'preliminary screener', and unfounded or malicious complaints are rejected.

In the remainder the doctor may be asked to comment and to clarify the matter, and, in the light of his explanation, the complaint may either be dismissed or sent on to the Preliminary Proceedings Committee, whose function is similar to that of examining magistrates deciding whether or not to send a case for trial. They may warn the doctor or dismiss the matter, but serious cases are sent to a Professional Conduct Committee, which used to be called the Disciplinary Committee. Here, the doctor will be summoned to a hearing, which has similarities to a trial in court. Legal representatives attend on both sides and the usual rules of evidence are applied. At the conclusion of the hearing, the Committee can take one of several courses in disposing of the matter:

1. Dismiss the case.
2. Admonish the doctor.
3. Postpone judgment, and place the doctor on probation.
4. Make his registration conditional for a period of up to 3 years, as long as he complies with various directions of the Committee (e.g. restriction on prescribing dangerous drugs).
5. Suspend registration for a period of up to 1 year.
6. Direct that the doctor's name be erased from the Register.

Suspension and erasure mean that the doctor can no longer work as a registered medical practitioner, which effectively excludes him from most type of practice, including any NHS or government job.

A doctor whose name has been erased cannot apply for restoration to the Register until at least 10 months have elapsed. He has 28 days in which to appeal against the verdict to the Judicial Committee of the Privy Council.

In Scotland appeals are also made to the Privy Council. Those instigated by dentists (Dentists Act 1957) in appeal against erasure are also dealt with by the Privy Council.

The principal forms of professional misconduct are published in a 'Blue Booklet', which may be obtained on request from the GMC. Any kind of offence may, of course, come before them for consideration, but convictions in a court of law are reported to the Council as a routine by the police, and a doctor so convicted may 'expect to hear in due course' of the more serious ultimate effects of his conviction. Alleged offences may be reported by patients, relatives, a local Executive Council of the NHS, or other members of the public, and inquiry may—or may not—follow.

The more common offences are sometimes described as 'the 5 As':

Abuse of a doctor's privileges (mainly with drugs)
Association with unqualified persons
Advertising, as by canvassing, improper publicity, etc.
Adultery—arising out of professional relationships
Abortion—if not 'in good faith', or contrary to the regulation of the 1967 Abortion Act

to which one might add a caution on alcohol and addiction.

The types of cases considered by the Preliminary Proceedings Committee (and its predecessor, the Penal Cases Committee) over the years 1973–82 inclusive were:

Type of case (total number 1101)	%
1. Disregard of personal patient care	5
2. Abuse of alcohol	27
3. Abuse of drugs	13
4. Improper prescribing of drugs	4
5. Breach of professional confidence	1
6. Improper sexual and emotional relations with patients	4
7. Dishonesty	16
8. Violence	4
9. Indecency	5
10. Advertising and canvassing	5
11. False certification	3
12. Improper financial transactions	2
13. Others	11

In many cases, the Professional Conduct Committee merely admonishes the doctor or places him 'on probation' by postponing judgment.

Providing National Insurance (or indeed any certificates) without examining the patient, prescribing drugs irresponsibly or providing a known addict with heroin when not licensed to treat addicts, or sheer neglect of one's duties as a doctor are bound to come to light in the end—and to reach the ears of the GMC. They constitute a frank abuse of doctors' privileges.

In 1969, at the prosecution of a man called Thompson, it was stated at the London Sessions that a Dr Christopher Swann, given a 15 years' sentence for various offences, had prescribed 'the staggering total of 3500 purple hearts in just over 6 weeks'. Thompson, hardly surprisingly, had become an addict.

Association   with unqualified persons includes the employment of an unqualified or unregistered assistant or the mere countenancing of such practice, the assisting of an unqualified person as by giving anaesthesia for some procedure, or having relations with unqualified persons which enable them to practise midwifery (except under personal medical supervision). The providing of certificates, notifications or other kindred documents which enable such practices to occur (covering) also amounts to 'serious professional misconduct'.

Advertising   with a view to personal gain or sanctioning it in agents, particularly if deprecatory to other practitioners, is wrong, and so too is canvassing or even accepting employment in a firm which canvasses or advertises for patients—as distinct from advertising the efficacy of some remedy. Broadcasting and television appearances by doctors are now less frowned upon by the GMC. The practice of sending reprints of an article advocating some personal practice for which superior skill appears to be claimed might come close to canvassing if not restricted to personal acquaintances or those with kindred interests. Notification in the lay press of surgery hours or of a change in address is not permitted, though a practitioner may, of course, allow his name to be printed in the official Department of Health and Social Security (DHSS) list of doctors.

Adultery constitutes an offence when one of the parties is married and the affair arises out of the opportunities of a professional relationship, but a breach of professional behaviour may, of course, follow from a doctor taking an improper advantage of a professional relationship with a patient. There is, happily, nothing to stop a doctor choosing a life partner from among his single patients.

Abortion is perfectly legitimate if performed for a proper medical reason and in good faith. A practitioner engaging or assisting in—as by recommending knowingly—some contravention of the 1967 Abortion Act commits an offence, conviction for which will result in his name being forwarded to the GMC for disciplinary action.

Alcohol tempts men and women in all professions, and some are a prey to it. The doctor may, like any citizen, be found drunk and disorderly, drunk and incapable, or drunk in charge of a vehicle, and although the GMC may deal leniently with one, even two, such offences it cannot in the end overlook the menace of drunkenness to the proper skilled practice of medicine.

Discipline in the National Health Service General practitioners and dentists are responsible to Family Practitioner Committees under the disciplinary direction of Service Committees. The local authority provides clinic, welfare, nursing and other supportive services. Discipline in hospital service is obtained by larger Regional Health Authorities responsible for both professional services and maintenance, mainly through District Health Authorities. Teaching hospitals have, since April 1974, disbanded their boards of governors.

Doctors' duties are prescribed in the 'conditions of service', and failures to give the proper professional attentions to patients on the accepted 'list' are answerable in the first instance to the local Family Practitioner Committee; domestic affairs are best settled domestically, and patients with complaints like to feel that they have an 'ombudsman' within reach. Most go no further.

Regional Committees have, however, power to punish lapses by practitioners, and usually do so by withholding a stated sum commensurate with the offence from the next services cheque. An appeal to the Health Authority is seldom successful.

Professional responsibility

Further matters of conduct may conveniently be considered here, although they are not the concern of the General Medical Council.

Responsibility towards a patient is undertaken as soon as a doctor agrees to examine the case. *Consent*, implied by a nod of the head, verbal or, for operations, written, must always preface treatment.

The doctor should beware of casual examination of cases: no child or adult may be examined without permission, and an action for assault might follow in its absence. A visit for consultation implies a request to examine, but the 'health examination' of, say, officials or workpeople at the request of an employer carries no such assurance.

Negligence (or malpraxis) is the term used to describe a lack of reasonable care or skill as a result of which the health of the patient suffers. 'Damages' may be assessed in money where a patient has suffered, but there is no liability just because something goes wrong; there must have been lack of care. Degrees of skill vary, but everyone is capable of showing reasonable care and prudence, and the doctor is expected to add to this a degree of competence in keeping with his status in the profession. He may make mistakes in diagnosis with impunity provided he has displayed reasonable care and skill in making them! He cannot be expected to know of all the current trends in research and treatment, but he is expected to show *some* competence.

Actions for negligence are always civil (criminal lack of care results in a manslaughter charge in a Crown Court: such trials are rare), and a large proportion of these involve claims for damages alleged to have resulted from the failure to x-ray injuries or to ensure that due care is shown in giving treatment. It is a wise precaution to x-ray all potential bony injuries, even though it seems unnecessary at the time. Accusations of malpraxis should be referred without delay to the defence society or union which the doctor will have joined the day he registered.

Where liability for the negligence of others is involved, so far as it concerns doctors the position is broadly as follows: a principal is liable at law for the negligent acts of servants whether or not they require skill or special knowledge, and a hospital or local authority or doctor who employs nurses, radiographers and others under contract of service is likely to be held liable for their negligence. Dispensers and private nurses fall into the same category.

In the case of Gold *v*. Essex County Council (1942), long and considered judgments were given in the Appeal Court holding the County Council liable for the negligence of a radiographer in their employ, who burned the face of an infant plantiff during Grenz-ray treatment. A long-standing judgment (Hillyer *v*. St Bartholomew's Hospital (Governors), 1909) was criticised by the Lords Justices, who decided that this well-known and often quoted authority was not binding upon them. (The Hillyer case had made a distinction between the ministerial and the professional duties of nurses under contract of service to a hospital.)

Lord Justice Denning put the matter at its clearest when he said (of the supposed distinction between the Hillyer and Gold cases) 'I think it [liability] ... depends on this. Who employs the doctor or surgeon; is it the patient or the hospital authority? If the patient himself selects the surgeon or doctor as in Hillyer's case, the hospital authorities are, of course, not liable for the negligence ... but where the doctor or surgeon, be he consultant or not, is employed and paid not by the patient but by the hospital authorities, I am of the opinion that the hospital authorities are liable ...'

In Roe *v*. The Ministry of Health (1954) a part-time consultant anaesthetist who had injected a spinal anaesthetic which caused paraplegia and was later shown to contain traces of a phenol due to defects in the ampoules was found not negligent—but the Appeal Court took the view that had negligence been proved the hospital authority would have had to bear responsibility.

The term 'Consultant' is, in the words of Lord Justice Denning, 'merely a title denoting his place in the hierarchy of the hospital staff'. Every member of a staff appointed by the DHSS and paid by them is likely to be assumed to be carrying out the duties imposed by the Secretary of State. As the law puts it: '*respondeat superior*'.

Professional secrecy   Much of the close confidence between a doctor and his patient arises from the feeling that matters divulged or found on examination will not go further. Damages may be awarded, if, in casual or deliberate conversation, some harmful remark is made more public.

In the famous Kitson *v.* Playfair case £12 000 was awarded against a doctor who discussed with relatives an abortion in the case of his sister-in-law whom he was attending. Her husband was abroad and the doctor, regarding the pregnancy as illegitimate, sought to have her allowance stopped. He would have been wise to have confined his attentions to professional matters.

A doctor may be compelled, on pain of being penalised for contempt of court, to divulge such secrets if the judge so directs. He may do so with expressions of reluctance, but he can no longer refuse to divulge the information gained in a professional relationship if ordered to do so by the judge. He may write a particularly private matter on paper and pass it to the court for restricted circulation. The doctor has no option but to bow to any direction the court may give in such a matter; the occasion is privileged and he cannot be held liable for civil action for what he then divulges.

Privileged communications   may be a source of some anxiety to the doctor, and it is well that he should know how far the law will stand by him in divulging information he considers proper, for some ethical reason, to pass on to another person or to an authority.

A doctor has, of course, to give evidence about his knowledge of a patient's health when requested to do so in court, or in giving statutory notification of births or infectious diseases. The chief difficulties which arise concern examinations of those whose employers have a direct interest in their welfare and state of health. The best way of avoiding trouble is to press the employee to change his job to one in which his disability will not invoke risk to his employer or to the public, or to divulge the information himself. If he will not and the matter is vital to the well-being or safety of the employer or the public, the doctor has every right to communicate the facts to the employer himself, whether or not the patient agrees to such a proposal. A barmaid who develops a chancre or open tuberculosis is no fit person to be serving drinks to the public, and a bus driver whose blood-pressure is rising over 200 is unsafe to be in charge of a public vehicle. The swimming-bath should be prohibited to those with gonorrhoea, and no one will criticise the doctor who takes it upon himself to safeguard the public by divulging information which will eliminate risks of this kind, provided it is imparted to the proper authority. Communications such as these would be held to be privileged.

Relatives, even parents, are not entitled to know the results of examination of persons who are of age unless the patient consents, and naturally remarks or reports to persons not vitally concerned or responsible, say to the press, or to other users of a bus or taxi service, or of a swimming-bath in danger of pollution, would be liable to civil action.

With regard to knowledge of crime the doctor's position is less difficult. A 14-year-old girl who is pregnant has obviously been the victim of a crime, though the doctor may well consider that he has done enough when he sees that her parents know of her condition. When, however, a man attends for treatment of a finger freshly bitten off, and the doctor reads in the evening paper of a rape in the local park in which a girl screaming for help managed to bite the hand that was clapped across her face, he has a duty as a citizen to give information.

Suicide attempts are no longer subject to police action, since the Suicide Act 1961 eliminated this act from the list of offences at law, although aiding and abetting, counselling or procuring suicide are still offences. A dying declaration, which can only become valid after death, may help the doctor to record vital evidence without risking his reputation for tact and consideration among his patients.

Donation of organs and tissues

The donation of easily regenerated tissues such as blood and bone marrow given during life presents no ethical problems, except when the donor is a minor. The doctor must ensure that no harm can befall the donor, even when there is parental consent to the transplant from a minor.

No donation during life can be made if this leads to any mutilation or if there is a substantial risk to the donor, however willing the potential donor may be. Obviously, no unpaired vital organ can be removed, but in some countries the live donation of a kidney is more common than cadaveric transplants.

Where cadaveric organs or tissues are used, as in renal, cardiac, vascular or corneal transplantation, the position is regulated in the UK by the Human Tissue Act 1961.

However, before this Act comes into effect on the death of a donor, there are usually other ethical problems in relation to the definition of death. Where organ donation is concerned (but not corneal grafting), present surgical practice requires that the donor organ be removed with a beating heart supplying oxygenated blood, so that the chances of a successful transplant are maximal. This means that any such donation must come from a patient in an intensive care unit, who is on life-support equipment. As organs cannot be removed from a living donor, death must be certified on the grounds of brain stem death, while the heart is still beating but, by definition, no *spontaneous* respiration is present.

'Brain stem death' must be certified according to conditions published by the DHSS in a *Code of Practice* booklet, last revised in 1983. Two doctors, experienced in such matters, must fulfil the requirements of this code of practice, based mainly on tests of cranial nerve function. (In the UK, the use of electroencephalography is not essential to arrive at the diagnosis of brain stem death.) These doctors are part of the caring team and must not be identified with the surgical transplant unit.

Once the decision is made to terminate life support, this is communicated to the relatives, who then may be approached by the transplant team to request donation of organs or tissues.

The Human Tissue Act 1961   enacts that:

1. If the deceased has, during life, given permission for the use of his tissues after death, donation may be proceeded with. This usually takes the form of a signed 'kidney card' in the clothing or papers of the deceased. Although, legally, a relative cannot countermand this authority, no hospital would be likely to proceed with transplantation if there were family opposition.

2. If no such *ante mortem* permission exists, the person lawfully in charge of the body (normally the hospital authority) may give permission for removal of tissues if, having made such reasonable enquiries as may be practicable, he has no reason to believe that:

(a) the deceased has ever expressed any objection to donation;
(b) the surviving spouse or any surviving relative has made such objections.

The interpretation of these regulations is rather vague, especially concerning what degree of relationship need be canvassed and what are 'reasonable enquiries'. The matter is usually resolved by obtaining the permission of the nearest relatives who are about at the time of death.

As most donations will be taken from the bodies of the victims of head injuries sustained in traffic accidents, the coroner will have to agree to such donation, in case the procedure may interfere with the investigations of his pathologist. However, this is usually arranged by prior consultation about the principle of the matter, rather than discussed afresh in every instance. Where any criminal charge is likely, the body must be left untouched for the forensic pathologist's autopsy.

17

Medico-legal aspects of insanity

Testamentary capacity

The law defines the capacity to make a will as the possession of 'a sound disposing mind'. It is not concerned with whether the testator is suffering from some mental illness, but merely whether at the time he is about to make a will:

1. he knows of what property he is possessed and how he is able to dispose of it—i.e. what a will is;
2. he knows to whom he may reasonably give it, and the nature of the undertaking he is about to perform;
3. he has some good reason for his action—is not obsessed with some unreasonable dislike or affected by delusions which prevent a sense of right and wrong.

A patient may be unable to speak, but he may signify by a nod or a shake of his head his approval or otherwise of questions put to him, and is not prevented by this disability from making a will. He must appear to understand the purport of the questions dealing with the dispositions of his property, and if this is so he will be looked upon as possessing a sound testamentary capacity.

If the testator lacks the mental capacity to make a will, a judge can, by the Administration of Justice Act 1969, authorise another person to make a will on his behalf—rather as the Mental Health Act 1959 enables a judge or master or nominee of a Court of Protection to do so for an inmate of a mental hospital.

There must be no undue influence by any other person and, above all, by drugs or alcohol with the giving of which a doctor or nurse who may benefit by the will has been concerned. To establish undue influence, coercion or some kind of fraud has to be shown. The medical practitioner is often present at the time his patient is about to make his will, for many testators have a habit of postponing that act until almost the last, and may be seriously ill when the will is made and signed. A gift to the medical attendant may for this reason be looked upon with suspicion as

242

obtained by undue influence. A doctor is often called upon to attest the signing of a will, and he may be a valuable witness if, as not infrequently happens, a will is later contested by some dissatisfied relative who may try to establish that it was executed while the testator was of unsound mind or that undue influence was exercised upon him. Death may take place years after the will was made and the doctor who has attested the signature (thereby providing a record that a medical man was present) can be called upon to give evidence as to the capacity of the testator at the time his will was executed if the matter ever proceeds to court for trial.

The will should be signed at the end in the presence of two witnesses who will be present at the same time and in the presence of each other, and at the request and in the presence of the testator when he signs the will (Wills Act 1837). A mark by the testator is sufficient if he is too ill to write, and he may even direct some other person in his presence to sign for him. The will should always be read over just before it is signed.

A gift to an attesting witness is void, and so it is to the husband or wife of an attesting witness; a legacy given to a doctor or to his wife is not effective if either of them attests the will.

Criminal responsibility

No child under the age of 10 years can be guilty in law of any offence (Children and Young Persons Act 1963), for its is deemed incapable of forming sufficient malice aforethought to be guilty of a criminal act. A child of 2 years who deliberately suffocated a newly arrived brother of 4 months with a cushion came into this categogy.

With regard to children between the ages of 10 and 14 there is a presumption of innocence which is rebuttable except in respect of certain sexual crimes.

All persons over the age of 14 are subject to the criminal law, although a person found guilty of capital murder may not be sentenced to life imprisonment if still under 18 years.

It is an established presumpton of the law that every person is sane and responsible for his actions—even their ultimate effects—until the contrary is proved. The burden of proof to the contrary rests with the accused.

Mental illness may have no bearing on culpability for a crime for which full responsibility may have to be borne. It may, on the contrary, have such an influence on the mind as to excuse a man from punishment. He may, when brought before a jury for trial, be excused because he is:

1. *'Unfit to plead'* (whether guilty or not guilty) ... i.e. unfit to try.
2. Guilty of the act, but not wholly responsible in law owing to an 'abnormality of mind ... as substantially *impaired* his *mental responsibility* for his acts' (Homicide Act 1957).
3. Not guilty by reason of insanity (Criminal Procedure (Insanity) Act 1964).

Unfit to plead   has regard simply to the ability of the prisoner to plead *at the time of his trial*; he may or may not have been equally insane when the crime was committed, but this is no part of such a verdict. It is likely that the most gross and obvious insanity—idiocy, imbecility, dementia, general paralysis, or other grave psychoses—will be present, and that it will be plain to everyone that the prisoner is incapable of making an intelligent response to the charge. He is, in court, unfit to plead. He is found so after medical evidence from the prison doctor has been given in court and is ordered to be compulsorily detained in hospital without limitation of time. If he later recovers he may be required to stand trial.

In Scotland no jury is required, a judge at Sheriff Court having the power to detain a person who is found unfit to plead.

> Fritz Podola was said by his counsel to be unfit to plead because he had amnesia—he just couldn't remember the incident in which he had shot a PC resisting arrest. The jury—and most of the public who followed this unusual defence—thought Podola was 'spoofing' amnesia. He was tried, convicted and hanged for 'capital murder'.

Impaired responsibility   is a term which was introduced by the Homicide Act 1957. It reflects a more enlightened view of mental illness, as distinct from frank insanity, that might properly be said to have had a bearing upon an accused person's actions at the time of killing. Section 2 sets out that:

> 'Where a person kills or is a party to the killing of another, he shall not be convicted of murder if he was suffering from such abnormality of mind (whether arising from a condition of arrested or retarded development of mind or any inherent causes or induced by disease or injury) as substantially impaired his mental responsibility for his acts and omissions in doing or being a party to the killing ... but shall be liable instead to be convicted of manslaughter.'

This concept comes closer to the Scottish law that accepts 'diminished responsibility' because of mental weakness (short of insanity) as an extenuating circumstance. It virtually does away with the older legal views of insanity and criminal responsibility which were formulated in 1843 by a panel of judges after McNaghten had been found insane upon trial at the Old Bailey on a charge of murdering Mr Drummond, secretary to Sir Robert Peel. These were for long a yardstick by which juries were asked to assess criminal responsibility in cases of murder.

Not guilty by reason of insanity   is a verdict which demands evidence that at the time of committing the crime the accused was insane. This verdict may lead to detention in a 'special hospital' (the former 'criminal lunatic asylum') for life; consequently the plea is seldom put forward except to escape the death penalty—and with the abolition of hanging will be rarely heard.

The clear definition of this, the substance of a defence on the ground of insanity, has arisen from what are known as the McNaghten* Rules,

---

*Also spelled 'McNaughton', as on contemporary documents—the indictment and the death certificate.

and the student should know something of their substance. They are the replies to certain questions put to a panel of judges in 1843 after McNaghten was tried at the Central Criminal Court for the murder of Mr Drummond, and a verdict of insanity had been returned by the jury. Their substance is as follows:

1. Every person 'is presumed to be sane and to possess a sufficient degree of reason to be responsible for his crimes until the contrary is proved' to the satisfaction of a jury.
2. That 'to establish a defence on the ground of insanity, it must be clearly proved that, at the time of committing the act, the accused was labouring under such a defect of reason, from disease of the mind, as
   (a) not to know the nature and quality of the act he was doing, or if he did know it,
   (b) that he did not know that he was doing what was wrong.'
3. If the accused suffers from delusions it will depend upon the nature of these in relation to his crime as to what responsibility accused must bear. He will be in 'the same situation as to responsibility as if the facts with respect to which the delusions exist were real'.
4. A medical man, though not seeing the prisoner prior to trial 'but who was present during the whole trial and the examination of the witnesses' can, where the facts of the case are not in dispute and the question of accused's responsibility becomes a question 'substantially one of science only', give his opinion on the state of the prisoner's mind at the time of the crime.

Intoxication by alcohol or drugs does not excuse a crime unless it could be shown that such was the state to which accused had been reduced at the time of committing the act that he was 'incapable even of forming the intent to commit the act'.

A man of 42 returned to a friend's flat after a prolonged Christmas 'pub crawl' of gin and beer drinking. Both were hopelessly intoxicated. Accused awoke during the night to find a body lying on his bed. He took it to be a dummy put there as a joke and threw it to the floor, stabbing it with a bayonet. He fell asleep and only realised the real substance of his act in the morning upon waking. The blood alcohol of a sample from the dead man was 303 mg per cent, and it was assumed that that of accused was likely to be much the same—for the purpose of defence—at the time of the crime (see Figs. 5.16 and 5.17).

In the appeal Kirkwood v. HM Advocate in 1939, Lord Normand, the Lord Justice-General, said that mental weakness, short of insanity, was regarded by Scots criminal law as an extenuating circumstance having the effect of modifying the character of the crime or justifying a modification of sentence—or both. The electroencephalogram has been introduced in support of a defence of insanity in recent years, but its reception has been cool as it fails to decide more than that accused did not possess 'a normal personality'—a fact already quite clear. Ten per cent of 'normal persons' have abnormal EEGs.

The Home Secretary may order the state of a prisoner's mind to be inquired into after conviction. In the past the Home Secretary was empowered to order a prisoner's state of mind to be reassessed, but the Mental Health Act 1959 repealed these regulations. In those cases where the court has restricted discharge for the protection of the public, the patient may appeal to the Home Secretary after a year's interval. Mental Health Review Tribunals are available for this purpose.

Well as these 'McNaghten Rules' worked in most cases, there was no category for those with a degree of mental immaturity or some frank aberration of the mind which fell short of what was required by the strict McNaghten standards of 'knowing' the nature and quality of the act that had caused death, or 'knowing' that it was wrong. Juries faced with such extreme alternatives as 'guilty' or 'insane' must undoubtedly have felt strong urges towards verdicts that paid some attention to the punishment that would follow as well as to the evidence.

> In the case of R. *v.* Heath at the Old Bailey in 1946 the psychiatrist called for the defence was asked by Crown counsel whether he thought Heath had bound, gagged, beaten and killed his victim out of a feeling that he was right to satisfy a craving for sexual lust—something that he was unable to resist because he was a sex pervert. The doctor said he thought so, and that this should excuse him from criminal responsibility. By McNaghten standards it clearly did not. Heath was convicted.

The Homicide Act also allows of extenuation for provocation 'whether by things done or by things said or by both together' that may cause a person to lose his self-control. It leaves the assessment of this to the jury, and although not usually a matter in which any question of the mental state arises, this may nevertheless be another aspect of criminal law practice in which the doctor may find himself playing a part: an ill mind may plainly give way more easily to provocation than one that is content, and it may be left for the doctor to say so.

The forensic aspect of mental disease

Although a textbook of forensic medicine is no place for a classification of mental diseases, certain offences are so frequently related to diseases of the brain that an outline of their association is essential to a proper understanding of criminal responsibility, the law of which has been set out above.

Malingering

A person accused of a grave crime sometimes feigns insanity to avoid sentence of death or prolonged imprisonment; it is more comfortable to escape to a mental hospital on a verdict of not guilty by reason of insanity than to take the punishment which would be meted out to sane persons held fully responsible for their act. It is, however, seldom difficult for a psychiatrist to distinguish between an assumed form of insanity, the details of which the lay prisoner has had to arrange and the continuation of which, without relaxation, may be too great a strain for him, and real insanity. Insane persons may also feign symptoms, but they are likely to be standard malingerings recognised as reflections of their insane state.

Perhaps the most common form of malingering, not always entirely deliberate, is the plea of a 'black-out' or amnesia in relation to the circumstances. Hopwood and Snell, reviewing a hundred male inmates of Broadmoor criminal mental hospital, showed that, although a very frequent defence, amnesia as a mental state excusing crime is not frequently successful. It is too often dependent on the accused's words alone, and this seldom satisfies a jury made familiar with malingering by counsel or the judge's remarks on it during trial. Chronic alcoholism, a psychopathic personality or neuropathic hereditary traits are common backgrounds to a confused recollection of the facts. A sudden return of memory almost certainly indicates malingering.

Inebriety

Acute intoxication by alcohol, mere drunkenness, is no excuse for a crime until it is so developed as to prohibit the accused from forming any criminal intent (a *mens rea*). To be drunk at the time of committing a homicide or rape may in fact aggravate the offence. Only when the accused becomes so drunk as to be incapable of forming any specific intention, or knowing that what he is doing is likely to endanger life, may he escape the full consequences of his act. If, through not recognising the dangers of suffocation because of his drunkenness, a man places a hand over a girl's mouth to stop her screaming and she dies, a charge of manslaughter might be substituted for one of murder; drunkenness falling short of this, merely encouraging a man to give way to some violent passion, is no excuse in law (R. *v.* Beard, 1920).

Insanity due to alcohol, as distinct from loss of control due to inebriety, will be discussed in the section dealing with insane states which follows.

Drug addictions

These affect both mind and body, whether as mild as the current adolescent drift into cannabis (pot) or as serious as the moral and physical depravation of heroin and cocaine addiction. Veracity and a regard for discipline are not features of addicts' behaviour, and the fundamental defects of character that lead young people to 'go a bit further' with drugs often leads them into court.

Most young smokers need several doses to get a pleasurable 'high', and the inevitable drift into dejected apathy which follows makes aggressive behaviour rare. Occasionally, however, the amphetamine or LSD addict goes berserk, gets wild hallucinations, and may harm himself and others.

A young man known to be in possession of 'purple hearts', leaving a cellar session near London Bridge, was seen to start waving his arms, to clamber on to the stone parapet, and dance along, for a few yards, with hands in side pockets, waving his overcoat in flying gestures, then to 'fly' out into space— to drown. When recovered, the body had decomposed, but traces of amphetamine were recovered from the blood and urine.

Toxic confusional states ('the horrors') induced by heavy doses of amphetamines, LSD or cocaine are the most likely reasons for enforcement of restraints, in clinics or by temporary admission to hospital under the Mental Health Act. Too many cannabis offenders were sent to prison in the earlier days of 'pot' smoking.

Most addicts to drugs drift back to them after treatment, for they regard hospital as a sad interference with the 'free existence' and permissiveness of life outside.

Older addicts, mostly to heroin, deteriorate physically with frightening rapidity. The expectation of a 20-year-old who gets 'hooked' on 'hard stuff' is about 5 years. The physical aspects of the subject are dealt with in the sections on toxicology.

Mental impairment

Those classed by the Mental Health Act 1983 as suffering from arrested or incomplete development cannot be held responsible in the ordinary way for their impulses. The 'severely subnormal' and those whose subnormality requires supervision may be unrestrained morally, rape or rob with violence, or commit arson. Such acts require no critical intellect or judgement and cause no sense of wrong, and mental defectives, if not restrained, may repeat their unlawful acts, deriving great pleasure from, say, a series of bonfires in haystacks, or from a sexual satisfaction, with or without consent. Moral imbeciles display strong vicious instincts and a complete lack of moral sense, of fair play or ethical feelings, and incorrigible thieving, cruelty and wilful—even boastful—indulgence in crime are common consequences.

Dementia

Dementia, or deterioration of intellect, sometimes results in criminal acts, because the disorders of behaviour are encouraged by strong delusions. Long planning and very considerable cunning may precede the crime, so that it comes unexpectedly and may not provide evidence to indicate the person responsible.

Psychopathic disorder

This is defined in the Act as a 'persistent disorder or disability of mind which results in abnormally aggressive or seriously irresponsible conduct on the part of the patient, and requires or is susceptible to medical treatment'. Such patients may plan crime with great cunning.

Schizophrenia (dementia praecox)

This is the commonest of all psychoses to be associated with homicidal assaults, often based on delusions of a sexual character. The subject, usually in his 20s, has often been a 'bad mixer', sensitive and introspective, and sometimes emotionally cold. A total stranger or some plainly harmless person may be selected for the attack, and it may have an impulsive character.

> The dead body of a pantry boy was found naked in a gulley on the roof of a university college. A student aged 21—described as 'unsociable, secretive and religiously fanatical'—subsequently admitted killing the boy, telling with interest how he had attacked him with a hockey-stick as he entered the study, strangled him with a piece of string, stripped the body, inflicted numerous cuts of a frenzied sexual character, and thrust a walking-stick into the anus. Several efforts were made to dispose of the body, between which accused took his usual lunch with other students, apparently in a normal frame of mind, and afterwards enjoyed a short sleep in his chair.

The question of responsibility may be difficult to judge owing to the 'split' between the mind of emotion and thought: a criminal act may be committed—and skilfully covered up—while the emotional state is so disturbed as to be plainly psychotic, though knowing the act to be wrong. The subject of criminal responsibility is discussed elsewhere (p. 244).

Paranoia

Paranoia, a systemic delusional insanity, may have grave criminal associations. Subjects of the disease shade imperceptibly from those who can perceive the falsity of their frequent misrepresentations of the trivial happenings of the day to those who become obsessed by such delusions and develop persecutory mania. They may single out an individual for assault to redress their grievances, or address themselves in important phrases to prominent people, take action, and allege bribery and corruption among the judges who dismiss such actions. Everyone's hand is against the wretched victim, but his spirit is aggressive and his intellect otherwise sound, so he may secure adherents for his incurable 'righting of wrongs'.

Only when he indulges in bursts of violence to redress his grievances is serious harm likely to follow.

Manic–depressive insanity

This results in alternating moods of exalted well-being and abysmal gloom. At one period the subject is occupied in a restless buoyancy of mood, intolerant of restraint, subject of grandoise flights of ideas, and at other periods there exists the most absolute gloom and melancholia. Both conditions may be accompanied by hallucinations and either may drive the subject by 'irresistible impulse' to some criminal assault.

Melancholiacs are frequently suicidal, for they may be convinced of their irretrievable ruin, of their doom from a filling-up of the intestines, or of unpardonable sin whose only expiation is death.

Some maniacs tend to lose their self-respect, becoming dirty and careless of ordinary decencies of behaviour; indecency may ensue.

Confusional insanity

This includes various forms of confusion of the mind, from mere extremes of mental fatigue, or childbirth or other grave physical stresses, to toxic forms where exhausting bouts of acute fever encourage a wandering delirium.

In mild forms a state of exhaustion and mental apathy develops. Restlessness and insomnia tend to aggravate the bewildered, confused, tired state of the mind, and the wretched victim may wander heedlessly into danger, or merely forget his identity and whereabouts, having to be taken into the care of some hospital for sleep and food.

Acute confusional states are preceded by a period of restlessness which suddenly breaks out into the most violent mania, with uncontrollable excitement, wild delusions and exhausting shouting. Restraint is an urgent necessity, for personal danger is unrecognised and grave injury may follow leaps through windows or 'escapes' over electrified tracks, and the like.

A state of stupor follows upon exhaustion, the victim remaining in one heedless posture for hours at a stretch, taking no notice of his surroundings, desiring no food and showing no emotion or response to calls. The states of acute confusion and of stupor pass away to reveal a blank memory, entirely unaware of the events which took place during the 'attack'. Crimes of violence are rare, however, and loss of identity is likely to be the chief consequence of such a 'breakdown'.

Puerperal mania

This may take various forms, but commonly pursues a course like the confusional state described above. Delusions of unworthiness may cause suicide; and sometimes revulsion from a husband, and violent hatred for the newborn child may result in infanticide.

'Insanity' due to epilepsy

Many epileptic subjects drift into a moody irritable state before the fit commences, and may commit impulsive assaults whilst in the mood. By far the most common forensic aspect of epilepsy is, however, the grave psychic disturbance which may precede, or come immediately after, the motor fit. When the fit is imminent the moody irritability may reach a crescendo in which consciousness is confused. Acts of violence and grave criminal assaults may be committed without the victim being properly aware of even the facts, far less the forensic quality and significance of his actions.

During the postseizure stage the same confusion may exist, 'automatic' acts of indecency, dangerous handling of knives and firearms, theft, rape or murderous assault taking place without proper legal cognisance of the act. It is fair to say that recourse to epilepsy is more commonly a despairing grasp at some form of defence for a criminal act than a proper explanation of it.

Insanity due to alcoholism

Acute confusional states very similar to those from other causes may occur, pursuing much the same course, and one particularly striking form, *delirium tremens*, may be seen on withdrawal of alcohol. It has few forensic aspects, although visual and auditory hallucinations of such striking intensity may arise as to cause the victim to seek escape from his terrifying new world by suicide.

Korsakoff's syndrome, with its extreme dissociation of perception and thought and the loss of memory, is more likely to come to the medical specialist than the jurist.

All kinds of alcoholic insanity tend eventually, however, to end in *alcoholic dementia*, where the mind, becoming a little stupid and befuddled, suspects the more simple faults such as marital infidelity, grows jealous, loses critical faculties and memory, and suffers outbursts of violent recriminations without fair basis. Unfair accusations based on jealousies, themselves founded on delusion or hallucination, lead to violent quarrels and cruelty. Commonly the besotted husband makes the wife the subject of these outbursts, and he may eventually kill her or his whole family 'in revenge'.

No description of the *functional nervous disorders* such as hysteria or neurasthenia will be given. They have little forensic significance, and are almost wholly the province of the psychiatrist.

Care of the mentally ill

The Mental Health Act 1983, now in force, rejects the older terms 'mental subnormality' and 'mental handicap' in favour of 'mental impairment' as 'indicating a state of arrested or incomplete development of the mind' and 'associated with abnormally aggressive or seriously irresponsible conduct'. Such vulnerability might not be a basis for compulsory detention, it may be said, but the alternative might be imprisonment. The emphasis is on the need for special care and treatment rather than detention, and by October 1984 the older 'mental welfare officers' were replaced by 'social authorities officers'. 'Lunacy' and 'asylums for the criminal lunatic' are both things of the past, and the Crown Courts seek to impose suitable conditions of treatment rather than the rigours of punishment.

Application for emergency admission on just *one* doctor's recommendation has been rescinded, and replaced by a request from an approved social worker within 24 hours of the patient being seen. This is admission for assessment and lasts 28 days—it includes any necessary treatment. An appeal to a mental health tribunal may be made within 14 days, although in fact the management of the hospital has the power to discharge the patient.

Approved mental nurses, for the first time, have 'holding power' to detain a patient for 6 hours to that a doctor may sign an appropriate (section 30) Order. Patients compulsorily admitted have the right to appeal to tribunals at regular intervals—and to refuse treatment.

Compulsory detention has now to be renewed—first for two 6-month periods and then annually so long as a mental disorder exists or there is a risk to the health or safety of the patient.

The 1983 Act carries power to enable courts to remand anyone charged with a criminal offence to a psychiatric hospital—although not to any named hospital. Tribunals, the chairman of which must now be a senior judge, can order the discharge of restricted patients, and there are to be mental health commissioners whose duties will include visiting mental hospitals and making themselves available to patients wishing to see them. Consent to treatment will always be a difficult area, for many handicapped or psychotic patients are quite unable to understand the nature or purpose of the treatment proposed.

Criminal cases

A person charged with a crime but suffering from some 'mental disorder' may be committed to 28 days' hospital observation on the evidence of two doctors, who may or may not be asked to give evidence; an order cannot be interfered with by relatives.

Mental Health Tribunals are available to those who feel aggrieved, and under the new Act doctors may be employed by either the patient or the relatives in their interests.

It must not be forgotten that both the older McNaghten Rules (see p. 244) and the provisions of the Homicide Act 1957 (p. 49) still apply to those who make 'insanity' or 'impairment of responsibility' their defence when facing trail on a charge of unlawful killing. If already in custody in a prison, the 'hospital' to which the accused is committed will be the nearest available prison hospital: the prisoner can, of course, be seen there by his own lawyer and any doctor who is called in to help the defence.

The various certification forms issued under the provisions of the new Mental Health Act are to be obtained from HM Stationery Office; they will not be set out here, for the current trend in handling mental disorder is to put off the evil and outmoded day of certification as a 'lunatick' until no other course appears to be profitable. The Scottish procedure differs only in minor detail.

Aggressive psychopaths detained on a hospital order may represent a greater potential danger than the psychopath in custody. If there is no restriction order they may be discharged from hospital on purely medical grounds, only to commit another vicious crime.

A man with previous convictions for assault and attempted rape attacked an elderly woman not known to him, striking her violently in the face and knocking her over a stone wall. He had been released from hospital 2 months previously following detention under a hospital order alone.

A woman with a history of mental disorder attacked and killed a man with an axe. She was found unfit to plead and sent to Broadmoor. She had been discharged from hospital less than a year previously following detention on a hospital order after attacking a neighbour with an iron bar. No restriction order had been made and she was discharged from that hospital after only 4 months.

Mental hospitals are reluctant to admit the criminal psychopath, for he is likely to disturb the other patients, the staff and the orderly hospital routine.

Civil actions for wrongful certification or detention (as a result of certification) come before the courts from time to time, but are seldom difficult to defend, provided that certification was 'in good faith' and reasonable care had been shown in considering the circumstances before the order was made.

In 1960 the Court of Appeal gave leave to a man to bring an action for damages for false imprisonment against a Duly Authorised Officer who had, on a doctor's advice, forcibly removed the man's wife from her home into an ambulance. The doctor had, it seemed, said no more than that she needed observation and psychiatric treatment. He had not said she required certification. She had nevertheless been detained in a mental home against her will. It all arose out of her son's determination to marry a girl she thought unsuitable.

Junior doctors in hospital are sometimes faced with an alcoholic, drug or acute confusional insanity that presents an urgent problem they may have to shoulder themselves.

The correct way to handle this difficulty is undoubtedly under section 36 of the 1959 Act. Doctors are entitled to call a police constable to remove a person who appears to be suffering from a mental disorder from 'a place to which the public have access' to either a police station or another hospital where he may be detained for 72 hours pending examination by the mental welfare officer and another medical practitioner.

18

Laws regulating sale of poisons

In the UK the sale of poisons and the prescribing of medicines are controlled by statute law. The doctor in practice must abide by the rules set out in the three principal Acts.

Poisons Act 1972

The Poisons Act 1972 has replaced the Pharmacy and Poisons Act 1933, which controlled the storage and sale of all poisons, commercial or medicinal, and listed two major categories classed as:

1. Medicinal products—to be sold only by registered pharmaceutical chemists.
2. General, mainly commercial or domestic, poisons—to be sold by registered (shop) sellers.

A Poisons Board of experts was set up to prepare Poisons Rules, which are issued from time to time under the Poisons Act 1972.

Medicines Act 1968

The Medicines Act 1968 has replaced the Pharmacy and Medicines Act 1941 and the Therapeutic Substances Act 1956. This 1968 Act has little bearing on the general practice of medicine, being concerned mainly with the listing of medicinal substances into one of three categories:

1. General sale list (GSL) medicines.
2. Prescription only medicines (POM)—replacing the older Schedules I and IV known to doctors in the past;
3. Pharmacy medicines (P)—not listed as GSL or POM.

The student and practising doctor cannot possibly be asked to memorise the long lists of medicinal substances set out as 'GSL' or 'POM' substances, and even practising pharmaceutical chemists need an official guide to them. The Pharmaceutical Press has published a *Medicines and Poisons Guide* (3rd edition, 1982) to which those in practice are advised

---

Name and address
of patient.

Address of Doctor
prescribing.

Date

R   Name and quantity of ingredients,
including *dose* and *total amount* of product
to be supplied.*

To be repeated (if desired) X times
at N days interval.

(Date stamped
when dispensed.)

Signature (not initials) of
prescribing doctor.

---

*Except for recognised BP, BPC, or BNF preparations.

Fig. 18.1.

to turn. Such medicines have strict rules of storage, labelling and sale to which doctors in practice as well as chemists must adhere.

The form of *prescription* for scheduled drugs or medicines must be adhered to, and all POM prescriptions and records must be kept for 2 years unless they are NHS medicines. All such medicinal products must also now have set out as a part of the labelling the words 'Keep out of reach of children'. Containers have been devised to make their opening difficult for the young ... and have proved an even greater problem for the elderly with arthritic fingers. See below for details of prescription writing required by law in the case of POM preparations and the drugs even more strictly controlled by the third Act about which doctors must have a working knowledge.

Misuse of Drugs Act 1971

The Misuse of Drugs Act 1971 has effectively replaced the Dangerous Drugs Act 1967 and also the Drugs (Prevention of Misuse) Act 1964. It deals with the more danger-of-habit-forming drugs to which addiction was common, and uses the words 'controlled drugs' (CD). Regulations place such drugs into four categories (A, B, C and D) according to their potential (see p. 259) and in general control is the more strict from A to D. Moreover, special Regulations now apply to those who have become recognised to be addicts, and doctors who abuse the privilege of handling and prescribing controlled drugs may—by the Regulations and Orders under the Act—be deprived of such licence. The prescription form required for POM substances and that for controlled drugs are so nearly alike that they may be described as follows. *Prescriptions* (subject to the 2-year retention) must:

1. be written indelibly, in handwriting or type;
2. be dated and contain the name and address of the prescribing doctor, together with his qualifications;
3. state the name and address (and age if under 12 years) of the person for whose treatment it is intended, or, if a veterinary preparation, the name and address to which delivery is to be made;
4. indicate—for a repeat prescription—to repeat only according to directions. Single prescriptions must not be dispensed later than 6 months after issue;
5. where not stated 'repeat', be dispensed on not more than two occasions.

A doctor may order a medicine to be prescribed by telephone or by word if he covers it by the approved prescription within 72 hours, but this does not apply to a drug controlled by the Misuse of Drugs Act 1971 regulations.

Certified midwives are permitted, on a Midwives Supply Order, to possess and to give pethidine in the course of their practice. Although at one time this gave rise to anxiety as to the possibility of addiction among them, the regulations concerning the keeping of records for inspection have cleared this shadow.

Pharmacists may now also supply, in an emergecy, a repeat prescription for not more than 3 days' treatment—where the doctor happens not to be available, but this does not apply to a controlled drug (C or CD) under the Misuse of Drugs Act 1971 nor to a barbiturate other than one to be used to control epilepsy. Great thought has been given to public need whilst keeping some control in the effort to prevent accumulation of drugs, exchange of surplus pills or capsules among patients, and loose or careless use of medicinal substances. Sadly, pharmaceutical chemists' premises and doctors' surgeries are prone to 'breaking and entering' for theft, and the indiscriminate sale of drugs in clubs and public-houses is still a menace.

The control of addiction

An 'addict' is so defined for the purposes of Regulations if he has as a result of repeated administration of a drug 'become so dependent upon that drug that he has an overpowering desire for the administration of it to be continued'. Early 'Dangerous Drugs' Acts and Rules were mainly concerned with opium, morphine, cocaine and synthetics such as pethidine and heroin. Then it became apparent that drugs such as the amphetamines, mescaline and lysergic acid needed stricter control, and, after some years' trial of a Drugs (Prevention of Misuse) Act of 1964, the Misuse of Drugs Act 1971 was passed. The older Acts concerned with the drugs of 'addiction' or 'misuse'—the Dangerous Drugs Acts— were all repealed. The notification of addicts was reconfirmed in Misuse of Drugs (Notification of and Supply to Addicts) Regulations 1973, under the provisions of the 1971 Act.

The Misuse of Drugs Act 1971 and Regulations 1973

1. *Set up an Advisory Council* on the misuse of drugs, to keep the Secretary of State informed of trends in the use of drugs thought likely to 'constitute a social problem', and to advise on regulations.

2. *Regulates the production, possession and supply* of such drugs as it lists in *class A, B or C* as liable to misuse. *Class A* contains the more dangerous addictive drugs, such as cocaine, morphine, pethidine and heroin; *class B*, the middle range, oral amphetamines, cannabis and codeine; and the *class C* range such drugs as methaqualone and chlorphentermine, which have more nuisance value than danger. Barbiturates are not mentioned.

3. *Permits the possession and supply* by doctors', dentists' or veterinary surgeons' prescriptions of the special drugs listed, unless the Secretary of State decides that a *special licence* has become necessary—and makes a specific order to that effect:

> ... whilst retaining a right to enforce the **furnishing by the doctor of particulars** of the supply of such drugs to anyone he considers (or has reasonable grounds to suspect) is an addict, and also, ... **the right to prohibit any doctor** from giving such drugs to addicts unless licensed to do so.

Misuse of Drugs (Notification of and Supply to Addicts) Regulations 1973

These require a doctor, whether in charge of a treatment centre or not, to notify an addict under his care.

There is nothing, of course, to prevent a doctor who has morphine or some other listed drug in his possession from giving an injection to a person involved in an accident or some other emergency in order to relieve pain—even if the victim is a known addict.

Where a doctor has been convicted of an offence in connection with the use of any of the specified drugs, he becomes liable, by the 1971 Act, to be prohibited altogether from having such drugs in his possession.

The 1971 Act also makes it an offence for occupiers of ordinary premises to allow the production, supply or smoking of controlled drugs, preparing opium for smoking, or smoking cannabis. It is also an offence to frequent such a place.

The various penalties for such offences are no concern of the practising doctor. As always, they seem to be too trivial to hurt either the pocket or the person, and all too likely therefore to be ineffectual.

The full list of 'controlled' drugs set out in Schedule 2 of the Misuse of Drugs Act 1971 is as follows.*

---

* Modified by the Misuse of Drugs (Modification) Regulations 1973, 1975 and 1977.

Controlled Drugs*

Class A drugs [Part I]

1. The following substances and products, namely:

(*a*) Acetorphine.
Allylprodine.
Alphacetylmeythadol.
Alphameprodine.
Alphamethadol.
Alphaprodine.
Anileridine.
Benzethidine.
Benzylmorphine (3-benzyl-morphine).
Betacetylmethadol.
Betameprodine.
Betamethadol.
Betaprodine.
Bezitramide.
Bufotenine.
Cannabinol, except where contained in cannabis or cannabis resin
Cannabinol derivatives.
Clonitazene.
Coca leaf.
Cocaine.
Desomorphine.
Dextromoramide.
Diamorphine.
Diampromide.
Diethylthiambutene.
Difenoxin.
Dihydrocodeinone *O*-carboxymethyloxime.
Dihydromorphine.
Dimenoxadole.
Dimepheptanol.
Dimethylthiambutene.
Dioxaphetyl butyrate.
Diphenoxylate.
Dipipanone.
Drotebanol.
Ecgonine, and any derivative of ecgonine which is convertible to ecgonine or to cocaine.
Ethylmethylthiambutene.
Etonitazene.
Etorphine.

Etoxeridine.
Fentanyl.
Furethidine.
Heroin (see diamorphine).
Hydrocodone.
Hydromorphinol.
Hydromorphone.
Hydroxypethidine.
Isomethadone.
Ketobemidone.
Levomethorphan.
Levomoramide.
Levophenacylmorphan.
Levorphanol.
Lysergamide.
Lysergide and other *N*-alkyl derivatives of lysergamide.
Mescaline.
Metazocine.
Methadone.
Methadyl acetate.
Methyldesorphine.
Methyldihydromorphine (6-methyldihydtromorphine).
Metopon.
Morpheridine.
Morphine.
Morphine methobromide, morphine *N*-oxide and other pentavalent nitrogen morphine derivatives.
Myrophine.
Nicomorphine (3,6-dinicotinoylmorphine).
Noracymethadol.
Norlevorphanol.
Normethadone.
Normorphine.
Norpipanone.
Opium, whether raw, prepared or medicinal.
Oxycodone.
Oxymorphone.
Pethidine.
Phenadoxone.
Phenampromide.

* Brand (trade) names prefixed in official documents by the code 'cd' contain 'controlled' drugs.

Phenazocine.
Phenomorphan.
Phenoperidine.
Piminodine.
Piritramide.
Poppy-straw and concentrate of
poppy-straw.
Proheptazine.
Properidine
(1-methyl-4-phenyl-piperidine-4-
carboxylic acid isopropyl ester).
Psilocin.
Racemethorphan.
Racemoramide.
Racemorphan.
Thebacon.
Thebaine.

Trimeperidine.
4-Bromo-2,5-dimethoxy-α-
methylphenethylamine.
4-Cyano-2-dimethylamino-4,
4-diphenylbutane.
4-Cyano-1-methyl-4-phenyl-
piperidine.
N,N-Diethyltryptamine.
N,N-Dimethyltryptamine.
2,5-Dimethoxy-α,4-dimethyl-
phenethylamine.
1-Methyl-4-phenylpiperidine-4-
carboxylic acid.
2-Methyl-3-morpholino-1,
1-diphenylpropanecarboxylic acid.
4-Phenylpiperidine-4-carboxylic
acid ethyl ester.

(*b*) any compound (not being a compound for the time being specified in subparagraph (*a*) above) structurally derived from tryptamine or from a ring-hydroxy tryptamine by substitution at the nitrogen atom of the sidechain with one or more alkyl substituents;

(*c*) any compound (not being methoxyphenamine or a compound for the time being specified in sub-paragraph (*a*) above) structurally derived from phenethylamine, an *n*-alkylphenethylamine, α-methylphenethylamine, an *n*-alkyl-α-methylphenthylamine, α-ethylphenethylamine, or an *n*-alkyl-α-ethylphenethylamine by substitution in the ring to any extent with alkyl, alkoxy, alkylenedioxy or halide substituents, whether or not further substituted in the ring by one or more univalent substituents.

2. Any stereoisomeric form of a substance for the time being specified in paragraph 1 above not being dextromethorphan or dextrorphan.

3. Any ester or ether of a substance for the time being specified in paragraph 1 or 2 above not being a substance for the time being specified in Part II of this Schedule.

4. Any salt of a substance for the time being specified in any of paragraphs 1 to 3 above.

5. Any preparation or other product containing a substance or product for the time being specified in any of paragraphs 1 to 4 above.

6. Any preparation designed for administration by injection which includes a substance or product for the time being specified in any of paragraphs 1 to 3 of Part II of this Schedule.

Class B drugs [Part II]

1. The following substances and products, namely:

Acetyldihydrocodeine.
Amphetamine.
Cannabis and cannabis resin.
Codeine.
Dexamphetamine.
Dihydrocodeine.
Ethylmorphine (3-ethylmorphine).

Methylamphetamine.
Methylphenidate.
Nicodicodeine.
Norcodeine.
Phenmetrazine.
Pholcodine.
Propiram.

2. Any stereoisomeric form of a substance for the time being specified in paragraph 1 of this Part of this Schedule.

3. Any salt of a substance for the time being specified in paragraph 1 or 2 of this Part of this Schedule.

4. Any preparation or other product containing a substance or product for the time being specified in any of paragraphs 1 to 3 of this Part of this Schedule, not being a preparation falling within paragraph 6 of Part I of this Schedule.

Class C drugs [Part III]

1. The following substances, namely:

Benzphetamine.
Chlorphentermine.
Mephentermine.

Methaqualone.
Phendimetrazine (not used).
Pipradrol (not used).

2. Any stereoisomeric form of a substance for the time being specified in paragraph 1 of this Part of this Schedule.

3. Any salt of a substance for the time being specified in paragraph 1 or 2 of this Part of this Schedule.

4. Any preparation or other product containing a substance for the time being specified in any of paragraphs 1 to 3 of this Part of this Schedule.

The *Misuse of Drugs Regulations 1973* permit the free possession and use of codeine preparations up to a strength of 2.5%, cocaine up to 0.1%, morphine up to 0.2% and diphenoxylate up to 2.5%, provided they are not for injection. Ipecacuana-and-opium preparations of not over 10% (each) in an excipient are also permitted without restraint. Otherwise:

1. **Import or export** is prohibited.
2. **Persons authorised to possess** controlled drugs, unless by prescription for treatment:

(*a*) Registered medical practitioners, dentists, sisters in charge of a ward or theatre, veterinary surgeons.
(*b*) Certified midwives in practice (restricted to medicinal opium, tincture of opium and pethidine) bearing an order from 'the appropriate authority'.
(*c*) Authorised sellers of poisons (pharmaceutical chemists).
(*d*) Registered pharmaceutical chemists employed in hospitals, health centres, dispensaries, etc.
(*e*) Persons in charge of laboratories used in research or instruction and attached to a university or hospital—or otherwise approved by the state.
(*f*) Public analysts, sampling officers, inspectors of drugs. The master of a ship that does not carry a medical officer is also permitted to possess controlled drugs and supply them to the crew. Farmers are allowed nearly 1 kg (32 oz) of tinct. opii on certificate from the police.

Doctors must report to the Home Office addicts to the following:

Cocaine
Dextromoramide (Palfium)
Diamorphine (heroin)
Dipipanone (Diconal)
Hydrocodone
Hydromorphone (Dilaudid)
Levorphanol (Dromoran)
Methadone (Physeptone)

Morphine products
Opium
Oxycodone pectinate (Proladone)
Pethadine (Pethilorfan)
Phenazocine (Narphen)
Piritramide (Dipidolor)

and thereafter may not supply them with such drugs.

3. **The form of prescription** for ordinary patients must comply with the following regulations:

(*a*) It must be in writing or typewriting, dated, signed by the person giving it and, except for NHS or official prescriptions on the proper form, must add the address of the person giving it. It must specify the name and address of the person for whose treatment the prescription is given.

(*b*) It must state the dose to be taken, and the form—e.g. tablets or capsules—and the strength of the preparation, thus enabling doctors to prescribe proprietary preparations where preferable. The total quantity or number of dose units—written in words *and* figures.

(*c*) The prescription must be marked with the date on which it is dispensed and, except in the case of National Health prescriptions, must be retained by the pharmacist supplying the drug.

4. **The special records of receipt and supply** require compliance with the following provisions. Records must be kept in an official form, and made indelibly in a special register on the day the drugs are obtained or supplied; details of both receipt and supply must be filled in. A doctor now has to keep a record of *all* drugs prescribed under the Regulations, administered personally or under his direction while he is present, unless these have been ordered by prescription. The Secretary of State may withdraw the authority of the doctor to obtain and prescribe the listed drugs if he has reason to believe that they are being given otherwise than is properly required for medical purposes. A dentist or midwife, since they may only administer such drugs personally, have no reason to keep a register.

The form of register is as follows:

(*a*) *Entries to be made in case of drugs or preparations obtained*

(The class of drugs and preparations to which the entries relate to be specified at the head of each page in the register.)

Date on which received	Name Address of person from whom obtained	Amount obtained	Form in which obtained

(b) *Entries to be made in case of drugs or preparations supplied*

(The class of drugs and preparations to which the entries relate to be specified at the head of each page in the register.)

Date of trans- action	Name	Address	Authority of person to whom article supplied	Amount supplied	Form in which supplied	In case of supply on a prescription, the ingredients of the prescription
	of person to whom supplied					

Any correction or cancellation of the entries must be made by marginal notes which are dated, and not across the original entries. A separate register or a separate part of the register must be used for each class of dangerous drug or preparation.

If a doctor keeps a day-book in which details of the drugs dispensed by him to his patients are made and which includes the name and address of the patient and the date of supply, he need only record in the scheduled drug register an appropriate reference to his day-book. Records must be available for inspection and must be preserved for 2 years.

A registered pharmacist may deliver drugs to a messenger on the production of a signed authority from a doctor or dentist provided the pharmacist is satisfied that the authority is genuine. Telephone orders from medical practitioners may be accepted, but the written order must follow within 24 hours, and preferably upon delivery of the drug.

Doctors are from time to time reminded that dangerous drugs carried about during practice visits 'must be kept in a locked receptacle'. A car is not, in the view of the law, a receptacle, but a locked boot or bag is.

The advisory council set up under the provisions of the Misuse of Drugs Act 1971 is charged with the duty of keeping the Minister of State informed of developments in the field of drug abuse and its social consequences in a way that will, it is hoped, keep abreast of the pharmaceutical—and social—times. Simplification of the regulations, the *ultima thule* of all doctors as well as students, is not always amenable to law.

19

General facts about poisons

Poisoning is a very common clinical problem, about 120 000 people per annum being admitted to hospital for treatment; so it is important for the doctor to be familiar with the commoner poisons, ready to recognise their effects and able to combat them. The common domestic medicaments, barbiturates, tranquillisers, or analgesic aspirin or paracetamol compounds, mixers' and solvents—or household products containing

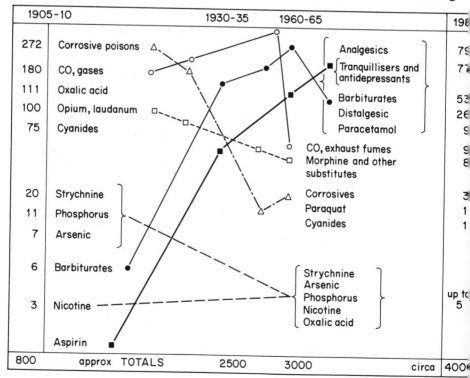

Fig 19.1 Trends of poisoning in the UK.

them—are the everyday poisons of social and domestic existence. The less common—to which correspondingly less space will be given—are seen in industry, scientific trades and the occasional mishaps of therapeutics.

The law has wisely never attempted to define a poison in precise terms, requiring only that when applied to the body or administered internally it will cause harm. In the Offences Against the Person Act 1861 the crime of giving or causing to be taken 'any poison or other destructive or noxious thing' is set out clearly enough to cover any kind of substance capable of causing bodily harm.

The various sections of this part of the Act deal with the intent—and general effect of poisoning:

1. intent to murder
2. intent to enable the poisoner (or assist any other person) to commit an indictable offence such as rape or procure abortion
3. endangering life or inflicting grievous bodily harm, burning, disfigurement, etc.
4. injuring, aggrieving or annoying,

so covering all kinds of bodily hurt from death to mere sickness.

The vast majority of poisonings are suicidal or accidental. Murder by poison is rare: the Crippens, Seddons and Armstrongs are sensational, but it is not to such lurid colour that the doctor's eye should be trained.

Everyday suicides, missing pills and capsules, and the day-to-day accidents with household solvents and cleaners, often among toddlers, are the mundane experience of both the practising doctor and the pathologist. Over 100 000 poisoning cases were admitted to hospitals in England and Wales in 1980. *Some 15 000 of these were children under 5 years of age.*

This is not to say that the GP and the hospital casualty officer should not be alert to the possibility of crime. Widows like Mrs. Merryfield may mix phosphorus bisque for money, and trusted chauffeurs like William Waite may be disposing of unwanted wives with slow arsenic. Thallium caught doctors napping in 1970 in Hertfordshire.

A laboratory assistant whose wife was dying of pulmonary tuberculosis (too slow for his liking) in a Surrey Hospital sent her fruit pies and bottled fruit drinks into which he had introduced potassium arsenite—sufficient, in fact, to kill her under the very noses of the staff who had not the slightest suspicion murder was being committed. A certificate of death from natural causes was stopped only when a succession of chance happenings brought the real facts of light (see Fig. 21.1).

Suspicion of poisoning from food is often aroused because symptoms have followed upon the taking of a meal, and although this is naturally likely to be the course of events when the food does, in fact, contain some poison, such cases often prove to have simple explanations; gastroenteritis is most often bacterial.

An old gentleman who had formed a sudden affection for a foreign parlour-maid and expressed a desire to alter his will substantially in her favour, to the bitter disappointment of his faded wife, suddenly developed a bout of vomiting which continued in spite of medical attendance until his death 4 days later. Two doctors in attendance were unable to suggest the cause of the vomiting and prostration, and when the parlour-maid (and her brother) made allegations of poisoning by the wife it was considered advisable to inform the police as well as the coroner. Autopsy revealed a tense swelling in the right groin from a several days' strangulated inguinal hernia, undetected in life. Analysis failed to reveal any poison.

Almost every event in our life follows upon a meal. It can hardly be otherwise since we eat every 3–4 hours, but this should not of itself be permitted to arouse suspicion of poisoning. When only one member of a party of several at a meal suffers afterwards, poisoning is less likely than some natural disease.

When, however, suspicion is not without grounds, even if only circumstantial grounds, it would be wise to take materials at autopsy for preservation and for analysis even if some natural cause for death is found. There have been cases of narcotic and of CO poisoning with coronary thrombosis, and acute lobar pneumonia as final precipitating causes when, in fact, poisoning was the material cause of death.

Some of the general facts with regard to the action of poisons are no more than plain common sense.

Amount taken

It is to be expected that the more poison taken the more severe the reaction to it, and this is so except where the immediate result of taking some large dose by mouth is to vomit part of it. It is surprising how uncommon this event is. Many poisons entering the body in small quantities repeatedly are broken down or excreted whilst exercising their effects, and chronic poisoning will be likely to occur only where there is some (*ac*)*cumulative action*, as with arsenic and lead.

Route of administration

Poisons may enter the body through the skin or vagina, by intramuscular injection, by stomach or rectum, through the lungs or by injection into veins, and will become circulated with a rapidity increasing in the order of entry stated. Grease on the skin or food in the stomach may interfere with absorption.

Form of poison

Gaseous and dissolved or fluid poisons will naturally enter the circulation with greater ease than a solid poison. The speed of absorption of prussic acid fumes is striking in its immediate ill-effects, and CO or sewer gases (H_2S, etc.) are equally rapidly absorbed. A mixture of corrosive sublimate in alcohol (used for killing worm in furniture) is more rapid in action than a solution in water, the poison being less soluble in water. Some poisons have a surface corrosive action, like lysol, or, by causing vomiting, like aspirin, may reduce their own absorption thereby.

Tolerance and idiosyncrasy

The most remarkable tolerance to some drugs such as morphine may be acquired by subjects taking them regularly over long periods of time. De Quincey, in his classic book *The Confessions of an Opium Eater*, described the daily taking of quantities of the tincture of laudanum with no more than the desired euphoria and relief from worldly cares; and the case of Dr Bodkin Adams in 1957 revolved to some extent around the need among elderly patients in distress for doses of morphine preparations far above the normal owing to their acquiring tolerance.

The contrary reaction of exaggerated response shows some subjects to possess an idiosyncrasy towards such drugs as aspirin, bromides, cocaine, penicillin and many others. Violent circulatory phenomena, skin rashes, vertigo and vomiting are common symptoms of this intolerance, and death may follow from sudden reaction to doses within ordinary therapeutic limits.

It is little more than common sense that in cases of illness, especially where the function of the liver or kidneys is interfered with, the effects of any given dose of poison will be more grave. A minimum lethal dose is stated for healthy subjects. Similarly, with a few exceptions, children are more susceptible to small doses of poison.

> In one case a child of 13 months, slightly scalded, was given about 5 mg heroin on being taken to the doctor's surgery in a pram. It was dead when taken out of the pram on arrival home 25 minutes later.

Signs and symptoms

These will be detailed as each poison is considered, for the reactions to poisons are as legion as the signs and symptoms of disease, and great care may have to be exercised to avoid confusing one with the other. Sometimes both exist together, as, for instance, when a patient suffering from gastric ulcer swallows a corrosive poison, or a drunken subject develops a cerebral haemorrhage. Certain broad groups of poisons may be defined by their common mode of action, and poisons are sometimes roughly classified in this way as follows:

1. *Corrosive*—strong mineral or organic acids, alkalis, cresols, etc.
2. *Irritant*—metallic (As, Sb, Hg), and vegetable irritants (e.g. castor oil), phosphorus, irritant gases (e.g. ammonia, SO_2), etc.
3. *Hypnotic or narcotic*—barbiturate, morphine, chloral, paracetamol, etc.
4. *Deliriant and convulsant*—cocaine, strychnine, aconite, etc.
5. *Paralytic and anticholinesterase*—coniine, curare, nicotine, etc.
6. *Abortifacient*—ergot, quinine, pituitary hormone, etc.

7. *Irrespirable* (e.g. CO, H₂S) *and poisonous* (e.g. HCN, arsine, tetrach-lorethane) *gases or vapours.*

Many poisons have compound actions; oxalates, for instance, are both gastrointestinal irritant and neurodepressant, mercuric chloride is irritant and nephrotoxic, and phosphorus is both an irritant and a liver poison.

Specific elections for tissues are also shown by some poisons. Strychnine affects the spinal cord, prussic acid (HCN) the tissue oxidases, arsine gas (AsH₃) the red cell. No classification can possibly encompass the multitudinous actions of so many poisons, and only a broad outline of arrangement into groups can be made.

Drug interaction

The majority of serious drug interactions fall into three groups:

1. Drugs with a small therapeutic ratio and which are extensively metabolised and protein-bound; relatively small changes in the kinetic balance can cause a major change in effect. Examples are phenytoin and the oral anticoagulant warfarin.

2. Drugs which alter brain function and whose effects are additive (e.g. phenothiazines, chlormethiaxole, benzodiazepines, antihistamines, tricyclic antidepressants and lithium. The interaction of alcohol with these drugs is of particular importance.

3. Drugs which alter neurotransmitter metabolism, transport or storage: some antihypertensive drugs such as bethanidine; tricyclic antidepressants; centrally acting pressor amines such as tyramine and appetite suppressants; and MAO inhibitors.

It must be kept in mind also that:

1. Drug interactions generally result in an increase or a decrease of the effects of the object drug, not in new features.

2. Patients taking a large number of drugs are more at risk.

3. Prescribing by trade names only, without knowing the chemical identities of the drugs, increases the risk.

4. Knowledge in practice of the adverse effects and basic pharmacology of the drug being used decreases the risk.

Doctor's duties in cases of poisoning

Poisoning is certain

Where poisoning is certain and its nature is known, the principles of immediate treatment are dictated by common sense. The subject is removed from the source of the poison, as much of it as possible washed or otherwise removed from the body—by stomach wash-out or oxygen ventilation—and an antidote is given where one exists. The circulation may be restored by raising the foot of the bed, and the respiration maintained by cuffed intubation. Elimination by sweating and through the kidneys may be encouraged, and fluid administration with periods of dialysis will be beneficial.

The stomach tube   must be used with some care for corrosive or spirit solvents, as the oesophagus or stomach may already be softened by corrosive action and perforation may follow the introduction of the tube. Little good can follow the use of the tube at a late stage or where a large amount of corrosive has been taken, for only minutes are required for substances such as the strong mineral acids and lysol to cause irreparable harm.

In cases of hypnotic or tranquilliser poisoning, far more good is likely to follow upon patient and thorough stomach wash-outs. All too often a single wash is given, and when death follows, autopsy shows surprisingly large quantities of crystalline, powdered or even fragmented pill matter still present in the stomach. The procedure must be repeated. At least 4.5 litres (1 gallon) of warmed water should be used in 0.5-litre (1-pint) lavages. These may (after a preliminary aspiration, preserved for analysis) contain a neutralising agent or antidote. The air passages should be protected by a cuffed tube.

Emetics   such as syrup of ipecacuanha are safe and helpful if given soon enough—as are careful gastric washouts—but the older emetics such as saline or copper sulphate solution can be lethal, and have lost favour for this reason.

Antidotes   and antagonists are of variable practical value. Some, such as atropine, nalorpine or thiosulphate, are more reliable than others. Direct chemical actions such as those between acids and alkalis are likely to neutralise excess poison, but cannot repair the damage done.

Methods of combating poison must be ready and immediately effective to be of value, and few attain this objective. The preparation of fresh ferrous hydroxide is likely to be going on long after the critical phase of acute arsenical poisoning is passed. Potassium permanganate, with its powerful oxidising effect on morphine and other alkaloids, does no more than deal ineffectually with the poison lying in the stomach.

Simple physical antidotes such as paraffin or olive oil for corrosives, charcoal adsorbent for alkaloids (including strychnine), and egg albumen in cases of mercury poisoning (so that the insoluble albuminate is formed) are likely to have a more practical value. Where the doctor is in doubt he may telephone one of the National Poisons Centres that have been developed to give information and advice.

Whatever the value of such measures, the doctor cannot afford to stand inactive. No effort may be spared to save the life of a wretched would-be suicide, likely as he may well be to try again, for fear of criticism that 'the doctor did not do everything in his power' to avert a fatal issue. It is not a doctor's duty to decide whether a suicide's life is worth saving.

Poisoning is suspected

Where poisoning is suspected there can be no doubt of the advisability of sending a patient to hospital for observation.

1. In a previously healthy subject, the onset, sudden or slow, of symptoms which do not conform to ordinary illness should raise suspicion.

2. A careful sifting of the statements of the patient and persons present during the material times should be written down; some trivial detail, easily forgotten, may later prove vital.

3. If the source is suspected to be food endeavour to obtain samples of it: trace other persons who partook of it and who should suffer in the same way if it were a source of poison.

4. Keep any vomit, stomach wash-out, faeces, urine or CSF which come to hand; seal them and affix labels. Analysis may later prove vital.

5. If the symptoms clear up on removal from the house and recur on return, suspect deliberate poisoning, and take steps to obtain evidence of it. Samples of suspected food and of urine, faeces and hair may confirm such suspicions.

6. A doctor may, at his own discretion, warn persons concerned that he suspects poisoning, and should inform the police without delay when he has unmistakable proof of it being wilful.

7. On death, the coroner must be informed.

It is well to have a suspicious mind where poisoning is concerned. The most disarming personality may be a cultured veneer to a black soul. Let the evidence which accumulates speak for itself.

Food poisoning

Although both suspected and recognised cases of food poisoning have medico-legal aspects, their investigation and bacteriology are the province of the public health and epidemiological expert, and no detailed survey will be attempted here.

The medico-legal aspects of the subject are:

1. That bacterial food poisoning should be clearly distinguished from toxic reaction due to:

(*a*) Contaminant metals such as arsenic, lead or tin.

(*b*) Toxic vegetable and substances such as muscarine or amanitin from fungi, or myelotoxin from mussels.

(*c*) Allergic reactions to food.

2. That in the event of death the coroner should be informed. Even if bacterial food infection were considered a natural event (e.g. typhoid infection from oysters) it would be likely that allegations of negligence and perhaps civil action would follow.

Bacterial food poisoning by staphylococci or the Salmonella group of organisms will be given no space here, but something must be said of non-bacterial food poisoning by contaminant metals, vegetable and animal alkaloids, and of allergy in relation to food.

Metallic contamination   is probably more common than dangerous. Arsenic contamination of iron pyrites, used to prepare sulphuric acid with which to convert starch to sugar, has caused poisoning of beer, confectionery and baking-powder 'boosted' with acid calcium phosphate. Fruit sprayed with arsenic has also caused symptoms.

Tinplate containers soldered with lead sometimes dissolve in acid fruits, lemonade or cider and may cause symptoms. Peaty water, being acid and therefore 'plumbo-solvent', may collect enough lead in passing through supply pipes to do the same.

Copper salts are sometimes added to peas to preserve their colour, and regular cooking in copper utensils may, rarely, cause harm.

Enamels containing antimony caused an outbreak of poisoning in 65 nurses who drank fresh fruit lemonade.

Aluminium has no toxic effect, and for this reason has become accepted as a standard luxury metal for cooking utensils.

Preservatives and dyes which used to provide sources of metallic poisoning in food were eliminated by the Public Health (Preservatives in Food) Regulations 1925–40, which scheduled certain harmless colours and limited the preservatives to benzoic and sulphurous acids and sodium nitrite in limited quantity.

Toxic substances   occur in mushrooms and mussels, and although the gastroenteritis, prostration and delirium of *Amanita phalloides* and *A. Muscaria* are likely to be attributed (correctly) to mushroom eating, particles often being found in the vomit or stomach washout, symptoms of the same kind after eating mussels must be carefully distinguished from bacterial infection.

Allergic reactions   also occur after eating mussels and are common enough to have become called 'musselling' in the North of England, urticarial skin blebbing and flushing being outstanding features. Similar reactions with oedema of the glottis and 'asthmatic' seizures may follow from many articles of food, notably shellfish, eggs, tomatoes and strawberries. Subjects of these are usually so painfully aware of their sensitiveness to protein matter that they are likely to present a diagnosis ready-made, merely asking for treatment. The antihistamine drugs have solved this problem.

20

Corrosive poisons

A corrosive poison does more than irritate the surface it touches: it fixes, destroys and erodes it. The common corrosives are:

1. *Acids*—mineral, such as HCl, HNO_3, H_2SO_4 or HF and the fluorides; or organic, such as oxalic, acetic and carbolic acid (phenol), cresols such as a lysol.
2. *Alkalis*—caustics such as NaOH (lye), KOH, CaOH (lime), ammonia, or the alkaline or chlorinated household bleaches and detergents.
3. *Heavy metal salts*—chlorides of Sb, Zn or Hg, and Zn or ferrous sulphate.

Most metal polishes are corrosive, acid or alkaline, and so also are many household cleaners for carpets. Toilet cleansers such as sodium hypochlorite (Parozone or Brobat) and sodium acid sulphate (Harpic) are particularly destructive.

Some corrosives have a double action, both oxalic and carbolic acid being also CNS poisons; and some, such as mercury salts, harm the kidneys in excretion. Danger is not averted by merely washing the skin or lavage and dilution of the stomach contents.

General symptoms

General symptoms of corrosive action are common to all. Soon after swallowing the poison there is a burning sensation in the mouth and throat and intense abdominal pain. Difficulty in swallowing rapidly ensues and grey or brownish corrosive burns of the lips and adjacent skin may be seen. Vomiting is not long delayed, and thirst ensues. The vomit may smell of some poison such as lysol and is often darkened by altered blood.

Choking and dyspnoea are common since the glottis is itself likely to have become corroded. Traces of poison also find their way into the trachea, and fuming acid or ammonia may become inhaled. Collapse follows, the pulse becoming irregular and weak and the colour ashen from circulatory and respiratory failure. Death usually follows within a few hours, but when the quantity of poison swallowed is small it may be delayed until hypostatic pneumonia develops; or recovery, with some complication such as stricture, ensues.

Dangerous dosage

Quantities which might well be fatal if taken by mouth are approximately:

Inorganic acids—HCl, HNO$_3$, H$_2$SO$_4$, HF	10–25 ml
Organic acids—phenol (carbolic acid)	2.0 ml
oxalic, acetic	5–10 g
Alkalis—Ammonia (25%)	30 ml
Na, KOH	10–15 g
Calcium oxide (lime), hydroxide	50 g
Fe, Zn or Na sulphate	10 g
Acid sulphates (e.g. Harpic)	30 g
Hg, Sb, Zn chloride	1 g

(Nb. 1 g = 15 gr; 1 ml (cc) = 16.9 min; 1 drachm = 3.5 ml)

General autopsy appearances

The lips, and often also the adjacent cheeks, chin and neck, are likely to be stained by corrosion (Fig. 20.1). The fingers are seldom 'burned'. The difference in shape between a bottle orifice and the horizontal level of a cup brimming with poison may sometimes be defined at the lips. Corrosion may extend through the mouth and throat, down the glottis, and into the stomach, where it varies in extent according to the amount of poison taken, sometimes reaching into the small bowel. The amount taken varies from the vast gulpings of plainly suicidal acts to the sips or spoonfuls taken in mistake for some medicine.

With the fuming mineral acids such as nitric, hydrochloric or hydrofluoric, and with ammonia, fumes are certain to be inhaled. Serious

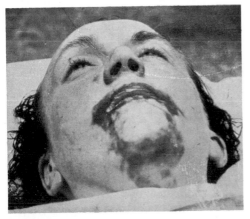

Fig 20.1 Corrosive burns of the lips, running down over the chin on to the neck. Suicide by drinking lysol from a cup.

irritation of the air passages ensues at once from even small quantities, and, in spite of temporary improvement, pneumonia is almost certain to follow.

In a refrigeration plant explosion, two men were exposed for several minutes to concentrated ammonia fumes bursting as a jet of liquid ammonia from a split jacket. Intense conjunctivitis and bloodshot swelling of the mucous membranes of lips, mouth, fauces and glottis developed almost immediately, accompanied by a distressing difficulty in breathing. In one case pulmonary oedema and pneumonia caused death some 4 hours after the accident; the other man recovered, having been farther away from the burst pipe at the time.

The alkalis cause a slimy corrosive change with copious excesses of mucus and much puffy swelling of the tissues.

The colour changes in the corroded skin or mucous membranes are given in Table 20.1.

Table 20.1

Hydrochloric acid (spirit of salt)	Grey—becoming *black* from blood.
Sulphuric acid (vitriol)	Grey—becoming *black* from blood.
Nitric acid	Brown—remaining so.
Hydrofluoric acid	Reddish-brown, bleeding.
Caustic alkalis and NH_4OH	Greyish-white—mucoid.
Oxalic acid and oxlates	Grey blackened by blood.
Carbolic acid (phenol)	Greyish white.
Cresols	Brown—leathery.
Zinc chloride	Whitish.
Mercury chloride	Bluish-white—blood-streaked.
Chromic acid ⎫	
Potassium chromate ⎭	Orange—leathery.

Perforation of the oesophagus or stomach is most common with sulphuric, hydrofluoric and hydrochloric acids, but the danger of perforation upon instrumentation exists with all forms of corrosives; washing-out is risky.

Some special remarks must be made on two organic acids since they have somewhat more complex effects, exerting both local (corrosive) and remote (neurodepressant) action.

Oxalic acid   (and potassium quadroxalate—salts of sorrel or salts of lemon). Fatal dose about 5 g.

The acid is used by shoemakers, bookbinders, brass polishers and straw-hat makers and for domestic metal cleaning. Its value lies in its ability to remove stains, especially stains of blood (which the potash salt also does equally well). Both oxalic acid and potassium quadroxalate look like Epsom salts and may be swallowed in mistake for these white crystals.

In 1956 two mental patients in a Scottish hospital died when oxalic acid was given to them in mistake for Epsom salts. In the absence on holiday of the dispenser, the matron and a sister had replenished the ward supply from a package that was unlabelled.

Signs and symptoms The outstanding feature of oxalic acid poisoning is the rapid onset of its neurodepressant symptoms, a sequel irrespective of the corrosive quality of the material swallowed. Even diluted acid will have grave remote effects. Collapse and prostration follow within a few minutes of the burning sensation and bloody vomiting which ensue upon swallowing the poison. The pulse becomes thin and irregular, the skin clammy, respirations shallow; numbness and tingling, or convulsions, may indicate the effects on the nervous system. Death commonly follows in 15-20 minutes, and is rarely delayed more than an hour.

Treatment So rapid a course of events leaves little time for treatment. As soon as confirmation of the poison taken is reasonably sure—inspection of a bottle or cup will often show crystals in the dregs or adherent to the walls—a tube may be gently passed and a wash-out commenced. Plain water, saccharated lime, or chalky or plaster-treated water is best, the calcium oxalate so formed being insoluble. Prostration and circulatory or respiratory collapse must be countered vigorously. Intravenous calcium chloride or gluconate may be given.

The kidneys will not bear 'flushing', for the drug has already caused grave renal damage.

Carbolic acid (phenol), phenolic disinfectants, such as cresol (methylphenol), lysol (cresol and soap solution); Izal, Jeyes' Fluid; Dettol (chloroxylenol).

These substances, which are in such common domestic use, are more common than the other swallowed corrosives, for the public has no difficulty in buying them, and when the impulse to commit suicide arises they are ready to hand.

Phenol, the pure carbolic acid, consists of long colourless or pinkish crystals having a sweet taste and a distinct odour. Although termed an acid, it has no action on litmus, depending for its local corrosive effect on its destructive and 'fixing' qualities. It is the simplest—and the most poisonous—of a group of related phenolic substances which form the basis of creosote and of Izal, Jeyes' fluid, Dettol, and many other well-known trade products used as germicides.

Lysol is made by mixing equal parts of commercial cresol (cresylic acid) with linseed or castor oil saponified by the addition of KOH or NaOH; it is a mixture of cresol and soap.

Mixtures of cresols with soap and xylenol have a much reduced poisonous action, especially local corrosive action, and the manufacturers of one such product have even labelled it 'non-poisonous'. This, of course, cannot be, although the poisonous effects may be remarkably reduced. Recovery from taking Jeyes' fluid or Dettol is more likely than from a similar dose of crude commercial cresol, but none of these products could be described as 'non-toxic'. It is often said that cresols are about one-eighth as poisonous as carbolic acid itself, and this is probably a fair generalisation.

Signs and symptoms   Lysol and phenol burns are commonly present on the lips and may extend over the face and neck as corrosive fluid trickles away. They are light brown in colour and may be missed in artificial light, but the smell of the breath, even the odour in the mouth of the dead, is usually strong and unmistakable.

A burning pain, mollified slightly by the anaesthetic action of the phenols, is felt in the mouth and down the gullet. Froth, coloured brown, accumulates in the glottis and cyanosis follows. Shock ensues rapidly and is grave, both local (corrosive) and the more remote (central nervous depressant) action of phenol being rapidly established. The skin is pale, ashen where cyanosed, and clammy, the pulse thin and barely perceptible, the temperature subnormal, and breathing stertorous and laboured. Vomiting is uncommon owing to the soothing anaesthetic action of the poison. Death is seldom delayed more than a few hours. Soiling of the air passages and pneumonia are common complications.

Weak solutions have little or no corrosive action, exerting the central nervous depressant action only, whereas solutions of over 30-40% (the cresols sold retail are usually 40-50%) cause the most intense corrosive change. Wrinkled greyish leathery hardening of the oesophageal mucous membranes and a softer flaking brown corrosive fixation of the gastric mucosa are present.

The urine is concentrated and darkens on exposure to air, owing to the presence of hydroquinone or derivatives of this substance.

No special method of treatment is available, and although the most vigorous general measures are undertaken they are only likely to end in recovery when comparatively small amounts of lysol have been swallowed.

One other form of carbolic acid poisoning merits attention. The poison may be absorbed through the skin, through wound surfaces, mucous membranes or the cervix, and its remote action on the nervous system may cause sudden collapse. Most cases of collapse on the application of local poisons such as cocaine and phenol, although often attributed to their poisonous effects, have in fact more to do with functional circulatory collapses—mere faints—than with reaction to a poison.

Chromic acid   (and bichromates), although occasionally seen as gastric corrosives, are more frequently encountered in industry as the cause of painless 'chrome ulcers' in chromium-plating, anodic oxidation or the manufacture of bichromates. Numerous cases are reported to the Inspector of Factories every year. The hands and nasal septum are common sites, but epithelioma does not develop as a consequence.

Metallic salt irritants   possess a slight corrosive action, but are predominantly 'irritant' and will be considered in detail in the next chapter. 'Corrosive sublimate' (mercuric chloride) is an intense irritant with an important specific effect on the kidneys.

One form of antimony chloride in veterinary use is intensely corrosive as a result of the salt being dissolved in strong HCl solution; when swallowed, it causes the most intense gastric corrosion with the black surface colour characteristic of HCl.

Fluorides, notably sodium fluoride which is sold as a cockroach killer, cause intense erosive as well as some corrosive change, bleeding being an outstanding feature (see p. 291).

21

Irritant poisons

Metallic irritants

In recent years deaths from poisoning by arsenicals, antimony, chrome, lead and mercury compounds amounted to only some 0.2 per cent of the total deaths from poison. The Chief Inspector of Factories is notified of all clinically diagnosed cases of industrial intoxications on a list of 'prescribed' diseases for National Insurance purposes, and the irritant poisons, chrome and lead commonly appear as causes of illness but seldom of death.

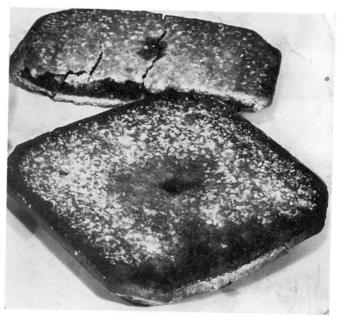

Fig. 21.1 Food poisoned with arsenic for murder. Tarts found to contain 162.5 mg of potassium arsenite sent into sanatorium by husband for wife dying (too slowly) of pulmonary tuberculosis. Death was accelerated by acute arsenical poisoning.

278

In some other countries—Egypt, India and Africa—the arsenical salts, phosphates or thallium are more frequently encountered.

These are not, thus, the everyday experience of either the practising doctor or the pathologist. Nevertheless, the heavy metals, their salts, fumes and gases, comprise an important as well as historic place in toxicology. Like all uncommon happenings they may be easily overlooked.

A woman under treatment for pulmonary tuberculosis in a Surrey County sanatorium in 1949 was poisoned by her husband (Radford) by means of food and drink brought into hospital for her. Pies were found—after her death—to contain 162.5 mg of sodium arsenite. None of the hospital staff had realised that murder was being committed 'under their very noses'. Symptoms typical of arsenic had been attributed to natural disease.

In 1970 a Midlands chauffeur successfully disposed of his wife by giving her repeated small doses of arsenic, causing skin lesions, loss of weight, bouts of vomiting and neuritis that were treated as natural diseases in life.

Arsenic

Arsenical substances are used extensively in industry, in agriculture and husbandry and in medicine. The chief forms are listed in Table 21.1.

The mode of action is by irritant, fixing and combining actions, the

Table 21.1

Industry

Smelting and refining ores, alloys	As_2O_3 (white oxide)
Impurities in minerals, glass, ceramics and 'mineral' acids	As_2O_3, As_2O_5
Plating, dross-laying	AsH_3 (arsine gas)
Taxidermy, skins, furs, hides	As_2O_3
Colouring and dyeing pigments, wallpapers, paints, etc.	Cu arsenite (Scheele's green) As bisulphide (red realgar) As trisulphide (yellow orpiment)

Agriculture and husbandry

Sheeps dips	As_2O_3, K or Na arsenite
Insecticides, fruit sprays	Na arsenite, Cu acetoarsenite (Paris green)
Weed-killers	Cu arsenate, Na arsenite
Rat and ant pastes	Na arsenite

Medicine

Inorganic forms

Fowler's solution	Liquor arsenicalis (1% As_2O_3)
Donovan's solution	Liquor As et Hg iodide (1% ea)
Pasta arsenicalis (dentistry)	As_2O_3 et cocaine HCl
Mist. potassium bromide	Containing liquor arsenicalis

Organic forms

Sodium cacodylate	Dimethyl arsonate
Tryparsamide, stovarsol	Aromatic As compounds
Arsphenamines, neo-, sulph-, oxo-phenarsines.	

last—with the sulphhydrine (SH) enzymes—interfering with cell metabolism. Arsenic is stored for long periods in the body—permanently in
hair and nails—and is easily detected. It is the more remarkable that so
many murders by poison, the Maybricks, Seddons, Armstrongs of the
crime calendar, should have chosen it. Recurrent bouts of vomiting, loss
of flesh and unexplained ailing health must always raise suspicion of
arsenic poisoning in a doctor's mind.

Accidents may always happen:

> A farmer brought home some weed-killer and foolishly put it in a bottle
> labelled 'Symon's Cyder' in the pantry. His wife returning home from a
> shopping trip, took a long cool drink straight from the bottle. Almost at once
> she complained of a burning sensation, gripped her throat, retched and vom-
> ited. She died 4 hours later.

Suicides by arsenical preparations usually resort to weed-killer or insecticide preparations in overwhelming quantity.

> A woman of 63, subject to delusions of religious figures haunting her, went
> to an outdoor lavatory with a full tin of 80% As_2O_3 concentrated weed-killer
> and was found there unconscious, dying $2\frac{1}{4}$ hours later. She had swallowed
> some 450 minimum lethal doses of the fluid.

Arsenical compounds are now eliminated from many of their older
sources. Colours for wallpaper and toys are now usually aniline or synthetic, and fly-papers are smeared with adhesives or impregnated with
DDT. Arsenic poisoning is a rare event. It is a dramatic personality
whose occasional criminal appearances are sensational. Nevertheless its
rarity must not lull the doctor into forgetfulness.

Signs and symptoms

Acute poisoning   If there is sufficient oxide of arsenic in food, there
may be some burning in the mouth. A short interval follows, then symptoms of intense gastroenteritis develop quite suddenly, with nausea, pain
in the abdomen, burning regurgitations into the throat and vomiting.
There is great prostration with the last and this is made worse by the
diarrhoea which follows, the stool quickly becoming watery, often
bloody.

The natural results of this loss of fluid—thirst, oliguria or suppression,
and sometimes cramps in the limbs—develop soon after, and the pulse
grows weak, collapse deepens to literal prostration, and with muscular
twitchings and sometimes convulsions as death supervenes. A few hours
or several days may see the course of these changes, depending on the
amount swallowed.

In chronic poisoning   a classic state of ill-health results, usually from
the repeated absorption of small doses of arsenic as in the traditional
homicides. The outstanding features are:

1. *Loss of appetite* and vague nausea.
2. *Occasional vomiting*, sometimes slight jaundice.

3. *Loss of weight*—general malnutrition and anaemia.

4. *Skin eruptions*—eczema, keratosis of the hands (palms) and feet (soles). Brittle nails. Hair falling out. Later brown pigmentation (Fig. 21.2) of the skin (melanosis), relieved by patches of leucoplakia.

5. *Peripheral neuritis*—notably of hands and feet, with itching, tingling paraesthesia, and sometimes painful swelling (erythromelagia).

6. *Cachexia*, myocardial degeneration, intercurrent infection, death.

Treatment   for the acute forms is effected on general lines. An antidote in the form of fresh ferric hydrate (formed by adding alkali to tincture of ferric chloride) is available (though irritatingly slow to prepare). BAL or dimercaprol has proved of value in the treatment of chronic cases—in 3 mg/kg body weight dosage.

Fatal dose   Some 130–195 mg of arsenious oxide is the minimum fatal dose, although recoveries may occur after larger doses because of vomiting or early treatment. Over a long period larger total doses may be tolerated as part is being excreted.

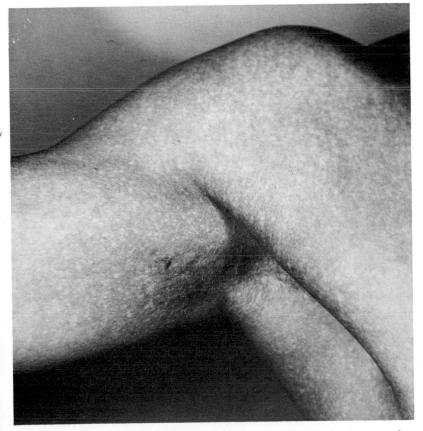

Fig. 21.2 Chronic arsenical poisoning pigmentation showing 'raindrop' pattern of melanosis.

Autopsy findings In *acute forms* the stomach and upper parts of the small intestine are highly inflamed, the mucous membrane having a typical velvety appearance, coloured bright red and puffed up by inflammatory oedema. Stray particles of white oxide may still remain adherent to the wall, sometimes in erosions caused by their presence, and bleeding from these erosions often tinges the vomit.

The liver may show patchy fatty degenerative change and, less frequently, necrosis with jaundice, and the heart muscle and kidney parenchyma may show a similar acute fatty degeneration. Decomposition is not significantly retarded by the presence of the arsenic.

In *chronic poisoning*, on the contrary, retardation of decomposition may sometimes be seen. Long-standing absorption of the poison will have resulted in great loss of flesh, anaemia and fatty degenerative changes in the heart muscle, liver and kidneys. Microscopy may disclose peripheral neural degenerative changes. The skin changes have been described.

Samples of hair and nails should be taken for analysis as the poison is stored permanently in them. The taking of urine and faecal samples should also be part of the autopsy, although in fact these analyses are more applicable in life. Some 2 weeks is usually sufficient to eliminate a single dose of arsenic from all except hair and nails, but prolonged administration will result in the appearance of traces of the poison for many months after in both the urine and the faeces. It is remarkable that poisoners should accept these hazards and still, as they do, turn to arsenic.

Arseniuretted hydrogen (AsH_3, arsine) must be considered separately, for it is encountered only industrially and accidentally. Only eight cases were reported to the Factories Department of the Home Office between 1935 and 1950; it is now rare. The gas is evolved as a contaminant when metals such as zinc, tainted with traces of arsenic in their natural state, are used to generate hydrogen, and is common only in the plating trade.

The gas is extremely poisonous, one part in 20 000 being sufficient to cause symptoms. It is absorbed through the lungs and, circulated in the blood stream, causes lysis of the red cells, haemoglobinuria and a breakdown of kidney function ending in uraemia.

'Spot' tests for arsenic, antimony, mercury, etc.

The older *Reinsch* and *Gutzeit tests* are reliable in expert hands. As a preliminary test they may assist the perplexed doctor or pathologist in calling for—or abandoning—further analysis.

Reinsch test A small piece of clean copper foil is placed in a beaker. Equal parts of water and strong HCl are added and the mixture is heated for 20 minutes. If the copper remains bright the reagents may be taken as pure. The suspected material, heated with nitric and sulphuric acid to destroy organic matter, is added, and the heating repeated. The following deposits, if formed on the foil, may be heated in a sublimation tube and the sublimate examined microscopically:

Arsenic: grey deposit—octahedral crystalline sublimate
Antimony: purple deposit—amorphous powder sublimate
Mercury: silver deposit—metallic globules of mercury sublimate
Bismuth: grey deposit—amorphous powder

Gutzeit test The material under test is dissolved in dilute arsenic-free HCl or H_2SO_4 and the addition of zinc permits the generation of gas. After filtration through a roll of lead acetate paper, the gas is diffused through a disc of mercuric chloride paper. A yellow to brown stain, of an intensity proportional to the amount of arsenic present, results. It turns brick red on immersion in HCl. Antimony gives only a grey stain. The test is delicate and can be made quantitative.

The *Marsh–Berzelius test* is for the expert analyst, as is the delicate *neutron* (atomic pile) *activation method*.

Antimony

If it were not for the famous case of R. *v.* Chapman (Klosowski) the amount of space devoted to antimony poisoning would be small indeed, for it is rare.

Sources *Tartar emetic* (antimony potassium tartrate), the most common antimony drug, has few uses and is so unpleasant to take that is is rare. '*Butter on antimony*' (liquor antimonii chloride), used in veterinary practice and furniture polishes, is a solution of the trichloride in strong hydrochloric acid, being even more unpalatable. The former is irritant, the latter corrosive.

Stibine (S_6H_3) is an irritant gas, like arsine, developed by the acid treatment of alloys and platings for mordant purposes. The mode of action is identical with that of the closely similar arsenicals.

Fatal dose An amount of 650–975 mg of tartar emetic and two or three teaspoonfuls of the chloride 'butter' are sufficient to cause death, though if vomiting is immoderate, as is likely with the emetic, survival may follow upon the taking of larger doses.

The Chapman case is worth quoting because it is historic and shows that even the most skilled medical attendants, in that case the staff of Guy's Hospital, may be decieved by homicidal poisoning.

> A woman named Maud Marsh was admitted to Guy's Hospital in July 1902 suffering from recurring bouts of sickness with abdominal pain and diarrhoea. She was diagnosed as a case of tuberculous peritonitis. She left the hospital after a month and remained well until a recurrence of the illness 2 months later, followed, after 12 days' treatment from a local doctor, by her death. She had been seen by another doctor in consultation 2 days before this, and as the cause of death was obscure these doctors performed a private autopsy. Since nothing was found to account for death, material was sent to a chemist, who found antimony. The coroner was informed, and on his instructions Sir Thomas Stevenson repeated the analysis, finding antimony in all parts submitted.
>
> A man named Chapman, with whom Maud Marsh had been living, had bought 28 g (1 oz) of tartar emetic 5 years before, at Hastings, and inquiries

revealed further that he had twice previously been married, his first wife, Isabella Spinks, dying 5 years previously (just after he had purchased the tartar emetic) and the second wife, Bessie Taylor, dying 3 years later.

The first wife was said to have died of 'consumption' according to the death certificate, but exhumation revealed no trace of it.

The second wife, dead some 2 years, was in a state of good preservation. The cause of death, as stated on the death certificate, after four doctors had seen her for vomiting, abdominal pain and diarrhoea, was 'intestinal obstruction, vomiting, and diarrhoea'.

Large amounts of antimony were found in both bodies, and Chapman was found guilty and executed.

The case will remain a classic example of the need to keep a constant *qui vive* (or *qui meurt*) for poisoning, but it must not be allowed to give the impression that arsenic or antimony poisoning is common.

Mercury

Although mercury is used in many industries, and is easily obtained, it is an uncommon poison. The metal itself is not poisonous. The soluble salts are interfering with the—SH enzymes like other heavy metals.

Sources   Two forms of salts, the mercuric and mercurous, exist; as the former are more soluble they are the more poisonous. *Mercuric chloride* or *perchloride* (corrosive sublimate) is by far the commonest mercurial poison owing to its general use in medicine as an antiseptic in solid tablet or solution form. The volatile diethyl and dimethyl mercury compounds are used in the treatment of seeds: they are dangerous.

It is not always realised how dangerous a strong solution of mercuric perchloride—even more so a tablet left in the vagina for germicidal or contraceptive purposes—may be; death will almost certainly follow.

Mercuric cyanide, a less irritant fungicide, and mercuric iodide provide other sources of poisoning.

Mercury is also in use among thermometer and barometer makers, and among mercury vapour lamp artisans, in explosive factories (Hg fulminate) and in the felting of hats and furs (Hg nitrate).

The mercurial diuretics such as mersalyl, now seldom used, are occasionally responsible for poisoning, even in medicinal dosage; the introduction of BAL checked this unwelcome reaction.

Signs and symptoms   in *acute poisoning* do not at first vary materially from those of arsenic and antimony. The taste is perhaps more strikingly metallic and the violence of the purging as grave as with any of this group of poisons. On the second or third day, however, salivation develops, the gums becoming swollen and inflamed and the breath foul. Some loosening of the teeth may follow. A renal lesion soon becomes established, and oliguria with much albumen or even complete suppression follows. Dehydration, thirst, collapse, twitching or minor convulsions may all precede death—after several days as a rule.

Chronic forms of Mercurial poisoning, recorded in 1948 in seven Lancashire policemen using mercury powder for finger-print examinations, included loss of appetite and flesh, occasional vomiting and diarrhoea, and progressive cachexia and anaemia. But there are certain special features of chronic mercurial poisoning which distinguish it from the group members. These are:

1. *Salivation*, foul gingivitis (often with a bluish-black mercurial line), loosening of the teeth, and sometimes necrosis of the jaw.

2. *Mercurial palsy*, with intention tremor of the tongue, the face, the arms and legs, usually in this order ... called 'hatters' shakes' in the hat industry. *Erethism*—a nervous 'touchiness'—may also occur.

3. *Chronic nephritis*, due to the elimination of the mercury through the kidney. The most striking feature is an intense catarrhal necrosis of the tubular epithelium (and in the handling of mercury fulminate—skin itch).

Treatment   of acute poisoning includes the giving of albumen, as white of egg, to form the insoluble albuminate. This is soluble in excess of albumen and must be removed without delay by lavage. Charcoal is just as effective. Sodium formaldehyde sulphoxylate is a real chemical antidote, reducing the perchloride to metallic mercury.

Fatal dose   Some 195–325 mg of corrosive sublimate constitute an average fatal dose though vomiting may encourage recovery after much larger doses. A single tablet (0.5 g) left in the vagina is ample to cause fatal changes. One such tablet swallowed by a nurse with suicidal intent caused death in some 38 hours, with nephritis and grave oliguria already established.

Autopsy appearances   reflect the signs and symptoms described above. The corrosive and irritant effects involve the throat, gullet and stomach, the mucous membranes being white, wrinkled and toughened, and the underlying tissues oedematous and inflamed. As mercury is excreted via both the colon and the kidneys, each may develop signs of irritation. The colon may ulcerate, even slough, and the kidneys become swollen from tubular necrosis.

Tests have been described on page 282. All mercuric salts give a scarlet precipitate with KI soluble in excess. H_2S gives a white, yellow, then black precipitate as more gas is bubbled through; it is insoluble in ammonium sulphide.

Lead

Here is a poison which, though less in evidence in criminal history than arsenic or its attendant antimony, is of infinitely greater importance owing to its industrial incidence.

Industrial lead, mercurial, arsenical and phosphorus poisonings are in the group of poisonings notifiable to the Chief Inspector of Factories, Home Office, under the Factories Act of 1961 (p. 158).

Sources   The only common medicinal lead preparations are lead acetate (sugar of lead), which is used as lotio plumbi č opio as an astringent and local sedative for strains, and diachylon plaster, a crude oleate of lead used in medicine for lumbago plasters. Machine-spread plasters and substances containing less than 4% lead acetate are exempt from the restrictions. Petrol additives are also a major environmental source.

No doubt whatever exists among industrial hygienists that the respiratory route is by far the most significant, although compound absorption is usual.

Accidental posionings have occurred in the past owing to contaminated water (peaty water being plumbosolvent), to the use of lead solder in cooking utensils, and in breaking up car batteries.

Precautions taken in the lead industries resulted in a fall in the notifications from over 500 in 1910 to some 50–70 every year from 1950 to 1960. Exhaust ventilation, wet pulping of white lead, hosing of scrap metal and enclosure of vaporising processes in machines have almost eliminated such cases. Insoluble lead bisilicate is now used in modern pottery glazing. Paints, the mixing of which provided a source of danger, now seldom contain lead in absorbable form, sandpapering of coachwork must be done wet, and a waxed sandpaper has been devised. Plumbism is no longer a grave menace to industry, although it is unlikely it will die out owing to the innumerable surprise sources. A barrel cooper may be at work on wood smeared with lead oxide previously stored in it, and a rubber compounder may add oxides of lead to crude rubber in preparation for vulcanising. No metal trade is absolutely safe from contamination.

In industry the poison may be absorbed:

1. *From the hands and mouth*—Type-setting, plumbing, accumulator work, glazing pottery.

2. *By inhalation*—manufacture of white lead, smelting oxyacetylene ship-breaking, diamond-cutting, file-making, turning, car-welding and polishing.

3. *Through the skin, hands, mouth,* and *lungs*—painting, coach-building, lacquering, tinning, vitreous enamelling, colour and dye manufacture and use.

Signs and symptoms   of *acute forms*, usually by lead acetate, are very similar to those of acute arsenical, antimony or mercurial poisoning, except that diarrhoea is replaced by constipation and the stool is blackened by the sulphide of lead and is offensive. Kidney damage has been observed in outbreaks of plumbism in Queensland, Australia, where the paint on fences and verandas, dried by the sun, flaked and powdered off and was swallowed and inhaled by thunb-sucking and playing children. Many deaths occurred at an early age from lead palsy and nephritis proper; of 34 studied by Nye, who had had lead palsy in childhood, 29 had well-established renal insufficiency and some showed renal dwarfism and hypertension, with low urea concentration.

Treatment   in acute forms consists of magnesium sulphate stomach washes instituted as soon as possible, 60 g of sulphate to 9 litres of water (2 oz to 2 gallons), being repeated if necessary; the insoluble lead sulphate is formed. In the chronic forms EDTA (edathamil)—also called 'versenate'—has proved a good chelating agent.

Chronic poisoning accounts for the vast majority of cases, and these usually arise from industrial exposure.

Lead which enters the body is not excreted at the same rate through the colon and kidneys, a cumulative process resulting. The metal is stored in the liver and as triple phosphates in the bones. Variations in acid–base equilibrium of the blood, of diet and in parathyroid activity may mobilise it from time to time, causing renewed circulation and excretion; this may be controlled therapeutically.

The classic features of chronic poisoning are:

1. *Anaemia*, with punctate basophilia.
2. *Colic*—of an intense character, and constipation.
3. *Blue line* (lead sulphide line) on the gums near the gingival margin— when infection and teeth are present.
4. *Wrist drop*, with paralysis, muscular atrophy and tremors of extensor and supinator muscles of forearms (except supinator longus).
5. *Encephalopathy* (especially from tetraethyl lead), causing convulsions, confusion, tremors of the eyes, tongue and fingers, with incoordination. Loss of vision.

Colic—the most common manifestation of plumbism—basophilia and a blue line afford strong presumptive evidence of lead poisoning. Palsy or encephalopathy will clinch the argument.

Unfortunately there are also two other conditions which are commonly associated with lead posioning of long standing, *both of which may also occur quite naturally*—sclerosis of the kidneys and hypertension. Proof of their association with lead is usually lacking, mere circumstance suggesting a connection—as if no lead-worker could develop hypertension and renal changes like his office fellow. These conditions alone afford no kind of scientific proof of plumbism. A specific renal change does occur during the acute phases of plumbism, and chronic renal sclerosis (and hypertension) may follow. The incidence of hypertension, arteriosclerosis and cerebral vascular catastrophe does not seem to be significantly higher in adult workers in lead; the figures afford little convincing evidence in either direction.

Mobilisation of stored lead by inducing acidosis with ammonium chloride, a low-calcium diet and parathyroid hormone may cause diagnostic exacerbations of plumbism—blue line, colic, punctate basophilia and paresis of the forearm extensor and supinator muscles—and the output of lead on a fixed diet may be measured. Urine should show over 0.2 mg/litre, a 24-hour faecal total over 0.3 mg, and the blood 0.08 mg/100 g or more in a well-marked case of plumbism. The corresponding normal figures are 0.02 mg, 0.03 mg and 0.03 mg. Samples of bone may be analysed: as wide a normal range as 12–140 parts per million occurs, and in plumbism the figure may be several hundred parts. The lead is stored in the lamellar and cortical bone, not the marrow. Popular belief that the formation of red cells is embarrassed by the presence of lead in the marrow is false; the effect of lead on the blood results from changes wrought on the red cell in its circulation.

Fatal dose   is difficult to assess, even with acute forms. It is probably some 2 g as a single dose of the acetate. A woman recovered after developing a acute plumbism due to taking some 7 g over a period of a month for abortion.

Some 1–2 mg of lead absorbed through the lung daily is enough to cause chronic poisoning. It has already been emphasised that the respiratory route is undoubtedly the most rapid and dangerous.

Autopsy appearances   are not specific in the acute irritant forms except for black colour of the stool; the renal changes are not specific. In chronic forms the findings after death are likely merely to confirm or dispose of the clinical features described. Anaemia, colic, a blue line, hypertension and renal sclerosis have other causes. A long bone should always be preserved in case analysis becomes desirable.

Tests   Dilute sulphuric acid gives a white precipitate insoluble in nitric but soluble in hydrochloric acid or ammonium acetate.

Sulphuretted hydrogen gives a black precipitate insoluble in ammonium sulphide but soluble (as $PbSO_4$) in hot nitric acid.

Potassium iodide solution gives a bright yellow precipitate soluble in excess hot water, from which it will crystallise in brilliant yellow crystals on cooling.

Copper

Poisoning by copper salts is uncommon, for they are too brightly coloured to be used for criminal purposes or to be taken in mistake for some other bland substance. Copper sulphate (blue vitriol), sometimes swallowed by children attracted by the colour, and the subacetate (verdigris) are the only sources encountered. The latter is sometimes taken for abortion purposes. Symptoms are those of an irritant poisoning.

Iron

Iron salts are, in the main, inert, but in recent years the widespread use of Tab. Ferr. Sulph. Co.—a compound tablet of ferrous, copper and manganese sulphate for anaemia—caused a small number of cases of acute poisoning in young children. Production of the attractive green Fersolate tablets has now ceased.

Symptoms of acute gastrointestinal irritation may develop almost at once, and deaths have followed in infancy where as few as 3–5 tablets had been swallowed. The iron salt was shown to be chiefly responsible.

Zinc

The chloride and sulphate of zinc both cause serious ill-effects when swallowed, the chloride being the more corrosive of the two. The phosphide is used as a rat poison and is particularly dangerous.

Occasionally symptoms follow the taking of food cooked in galvanised vessels. Some 200 people suffered nausea, burning in the throat, diarrhoea and collapse in 1923 after eating fruit cooked in galvanised stew pans, but no deaths followed.

Tin

The only likely source of poisoning by tin—a mild acute metallic irritant—is canned food, usually acid fruits or fruit juice, which has acquired a metallic taste from the tinplate: it is astringent.

Thallium

Thallium salts, notably the acetate, have been used as depilatories, but have proved too dangerous. The widespread use of rat-killers such as Zelio-paste or Thalrat also introduced thallium to the murderer. The principal clinical features are depilation, stomatitis, loss of energy and of weight, together with polyneuritis—but above all the classic loss of hair: all these are delayed, and can be reduced by giving Prussian blue as a chelating agent by mouth.

Barium

All soluble salts of barium are poisonous. The chloride, nitrate and carbonate—all constituents of certain rat poisons—are highly irritant and prostrating. Accidents with these soluble salts, given for x-ray investigations in mistake for the insoluble sulphate, occur from time to time in spite of strong warnings of the danger.

The symptoms are those of other metallic irritants, tingling, paralysis and convulsions being rather more frequent than with other acute heavy metal poisonings; fatalities may follow from 1 g.

Bismuth

Poisoning from salts of this metal is rare owing to their insolubility except in strong acid, but the subnitrate may be mentioned conveniently here as, in addition to the irritant action common to the more soluble bismuth salts, it may cause methaemoglobinaemia. This is due to the conversion of subnitrate into nitrite.

Potassium nitrate (saltpetre) and **potassium chlorate,** commonly used for a gargle or throat tablets, may act in the same manner. Renal damage may ensue and the urine may become concentrated, containing methaemoglobin in addition to albumen and red cells.

Non-metallic irritants

Pyrogallic acid

Although in common use as a developer in photography, for hair dyes, marking inks and as an ointment or caustic, pyrogallic acid is an uncommon poison.

It may be absorbed through the skin or by swallowing, and the symptoms and signs are very like those of potassium chlorate and bismuth subnitrate, haemolysis and methaemoglobinaemia being features more pronounced than the mild gastric irritation which first develops.

Phosphorus

Although seldom encountered in practice in the UK, phosphorus poisoning is striking owing to its unusual characters. In 1955 Mrs Merryfield used it to murder a widower by whose will she stood to profit.

Sources Yellow phosphorus, the luminous waxy form, kept in sticks under water to prevent oxidation, is the only poisonous form; it gives off dense white fumes of phosphoric and phosphorous acids on exposure. The red amorphous form has none of these qualities.

Yellow phosphorus, once used for match-heads, but now prohibited for this purpose, had one domestic form—rat paste, which contained 1–4 per cent of the poison.

Industrial exposure occurs in the making of phosphate fertilisers from bones, and in the manufacture of the commercial stick.

Hydrogen phosphide, accumulating from wetted ferrosilicon cargoes in ships' holds, is an irrespirable gas which is considered under that heading (p. 333).

Signs and symptoms *Acute forms*, which are usually the result of swallowing a poisonous dose of rat paste or phosphorus stick, result, after several hours' interval, in signs of irritant poisoning, burning sensations, in the throat and gullet, nausea, eructations flavoured as of garlic, and vomiting. The vomit is darkened by blood, has a garlic odour and is usually luminous in the dark. Diarrhoea follows, with similar darkened luminous evacuations. Collapse and death may follow, but intermissions lasting even several days are more common, after which the original symptoms are renewed and, in addition, jaundice and some distension of the abdomen occur as a result of enlargement and necrosis of the liver; purpura and nose-bleeds may follow. The urine becomes scanty and concentrated, coloured by bile pigments and containing albumen, casts and occasional red cells. Death from hepatic and renal insufficiency follows a period of increasing uraemia, with significant nervous restlessness.

In *chronic poisoning*, which is industrial and rare, more vague and intermittent gastric symptoms occur, and the breath comes foetid and garlicky, the mouth showing sloughing of the gums and loosening of the teeth. Necrosis of the alveolar bone of the jaw (phossy jaw) may develop from this. Anaemia develops and a milder form of hepatic necro(bio)sis may cause jaundice.

Treatment   should be instituted without waiting for symptoms (which may be delayed for hours). The stomach must be washed out repeatedly with a 1% solution of potassium permanganate. Liquid paraffin may retard absorption, but no other oily or fatty substances—even milk— should be given, as phosphorus is dissolved in them and its absorption thereby hastened.

Fatal dose   About a boot-polish-sized tin of the paste containing 1–4 per cent phosphorus will be likely to prove fatal. The fatal dose is about 130 mg, although, as with all gastric irritants, vomiting may permit recovery from far larger doses.

Autopsy appearances   reflect the signs and symptoms described. The outstanding features are: (1) luminous blood-tinged or blackened gastric and intestinal content, with garlicky smell; and (2)—more usually since death is likely to be delayed some days—necrobiosis of the liver, which is swollen and yellow, with jaundice and purpura. Fatty degenerative changes are also present in the heart muscle and kidneys. Haemorrhagic erosions may still be present in the stomach.

Tests   The luminous character and garlicky odour are characteristic. The former may be accentuated by acidifying the gastric contents or evacuations with H_2SO_4, connecting the flask with a condensing tube and warming in the dark. Luminous globules may be seen passing down the tube. One part per 100 000 may be detected by this method.

Organic phosphates

The development, during the 1939–45 war, of a number of phosphorus compounds as insecticides introduced several dangerous new poisons. Hexaethyl tetraphosphate (HEPT), tetraethyl pyrophosphate (TEPP), and Parathion (diethyl *para*-nitrophenyl thiophosphate) are all powerful inhibitors of cholinesterase and have, thus, toxic effects like those of nicotine. Their use on a large scale in spraying crops has caused a number of deaths. In tropical countries they are a common suicidal agent.

Anorexia, nausea, vomiting, muscular twitching and cramps, sweating and collapse are the usual events. Atropine relieves the parasympathetic effects but not the ganglionic. The newer antidotes such as PAM are more effective.

Fluorides

Hydrofluoric acid, a highly irritant gas which is dangerous even in dilutions as low as 50 parts per million, can erode marble and porcelain enamel, but is not a significant industrial poison.

The use of sodium fluoride as an insecticide (mainly for cockroaches) has, however, put it into the hands of the ordinary public. In 1942, 263 people were poisoned by a scrambled egg mixture made up in the Oregon

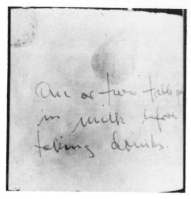

Fig. 21.3 Label giving advice to take contents as a medicine. Death ensued, for the contents were of sodium fluoride, sold as shown with a printed label. A charge of murder followed.

State Hospital with sodium fluoride mistakenly used as powdered milk. Occasional suicidal deaths have also occurred.

In 1954 a girl who arrived home drunk after a party was reproached by her mother. Saying, 'If you want to see what I *can* drink', the girl took a glass into which she poured some cockroach powder and water, and swallowed the contents. She survived some 4 or 5 hours, vomiting and purging without remission. Autopsy showed only an intense haemorrhagic gastrointestinal irritation due to the fluoride.

Sodium fluoroacetate is also a dangerous poison, as little as 65 mg being fatal. It is used as a rodenticide. Monoacetin (60% glycerol monoacetate) is a useful antidote.

Paraquat, diquat (bipyridilium compounds)

A contact herbicide in general use (as Gammaxone or Weedol), paraquat is toxic to the conjunctivae, skin and the liver—and, after some hours' delay, to the lungs. A remarkable proliferative thickening of the lining endothelium of the alveolar membranes causes profound cyanosis and dyspnoea. The condition is irreversible and almost always fatal when the poison, taken by mouth, has been absorbed. Early deaths are usually due to liver necrosis and renal failure, delayed deaths to lung damage.

No effective treatment has yet been discovered for paraquat poisoning—partly owing to the 'latent' period before symptoms develop: by the time they have, it is too late. Fuller's earth may delay absorption, after gastric lavage.

22

Analgesic, hypnotic, tranquilliser and narcotic poisons

Analgesics—aspirin, phenacetin, paracetamol (Panadol, Distalgesic), perphenazine (Fentazin), dichloralphenazone (Welldorm), phenylbutazone (Butazolidin).

Hypnotics—chloral, paraldehyde, barbiturates, glutethimide (Doriden).

Sedative and tranquilliser—chlorpromazine (Largactil, Sparine), diazepam (Valium), chlordiazepoxide (Librium), meprobamate (Equanil, Miltown).

Antidepressants—impramine (Tofranil), amitriptyline (Tryptizol), monoamine oxidase inhibitors, phenelzine (Nardil), tranylcypromine (Parnate).

Anticonvulsants—troxidone (Tridione), phenacemide (Phenurone), primidone (Mysoline), phenytoin (Epanutin).

Narcotics—opium alkaloids, morphine, heroin, and other synthetic substitutes.

Under the perpetual tensions of current times the 'civilised' peoples have turned for relief to drugs—analgesic, sedative, hypnotic, narcotic or, more insidiously, 'tranquillising'. Pharmaceutical preparations have poured out and doctors, themselves harassed, have acceded to their wide distribution. As a result, poisoning by these substances have risen at an alarming rate (see Fig. 19.1). Anything the parents have about the house is at hand for inquiring toddlers' fingers, and a WHO review of poisoning in children showed over 55 per cent of all cases to be due to medicines (35 per cent in the above groups).

Analgesics

Aspirin

Aspirin and simple compounds of this basic drug with phenacetin and caffeine (APC) or codeine (Veganin) are in everyday household use and can be obtained without restriction. Aspirin and its more soluble forms in medicinal dosage causes a reaction in some intolerant people, but to most adults the fatal dose is huge—something in the region of 25 g.

A girl who had attempted to cut her jilting fiancé's throat with a razor was 'wanted by the police' within an hour of his arrival at hospital. She was found unconscious, lying on her bed with seven empty 100 tab. (325 mg) aspirin bottles beside her. White powdered matter lay in the vomit which trickled from her lips. She was dead on arrival at hospital some 15 minutes later.

Autopsy revealed the stomach to be filled by a solid cast of undissolved aspirin.

Those who are sensitive to aspirin may quickly become dizzy or faint, grow pale and sweat, breathing with air-hunger and with a shallow irregular pulse. Some may vomit, for the drug irritates the stomach and often causes erosive bleeding. Otherwise the course of events is much the same as for any mild analgesic—only the codeine compound adding a hypnotic factor. The acid-base balance is severely disturbed and sweating, hyperventilation, cyanosis, delirium and coma rapidly ensue on the taking of large doses.

Acrid-smelling vomit darkened by altered blood may soil the lips or bed-linen. The urine quickly gives a strong ferric chloride (deep purple) reaction as salicyclic acid is rapidly excreted.

Treatment by gastric lavage, infusions of sodium lactate and 10-mg doses of vitamin K and artificial or assisted respirations are usually effective, but the blood pH may be seriously disturbed for some 24 hours. Levels of plasma salicylate above 50 mg per cent are dangerous.

Acetanilide (antifebrin), **paracetamol** (Panadol, Distalgesic), **phenazone** (antipyrin), **amidopyrine** (Piramidon), **phenylbutazone** (Butazolidin), **dichloralphenazone** (Welldorm)

These synthetic antipyretic and alagesic drugs are in wide use for rheumatic and other painful joint conditions, for headache and neuralgia, often in combination with aspirin, caffeine, dextropropoxyphene, codeine or barbiturates. *Veganin* (aspirin and codeine), the BP *tab codeine* Co. or APC—aspirin and caffeine are in everyday use without restriction. Phenacetin is no longer prescribed in compound tablets owing to its tendency to cause kidney damage.

Idiosyncracy is not uncommon, especially with acetanilide and phenyulbutozone (Butazolidin). Rashes, circulatory collapse with faints and air-hunger, occasionally oliguria, are faint rumblings of the thunder of real intolerance. The pyrazolones amidopyrine and phenylbutazone in particular have caused fatalities from agranulocytosis, marrow aplasias and, rarely, leukaemia. Methaemoglobinaemia is of little consequence. Phenacetin can, over long periods, cause kidney damage.

Dosages of 5 g have often caused serious reactions, sometimes fatalities, but the likely single lethal dosage is several times this. Four or 5 days' survival from an acute reaction usually presages recovery, but the doctor who prescribes these useful drugs runs the risk of an action for negligence if he fails to warn his patient of their well-known complications—or, worse, is caught napping by the dreaded 'anginal' throat infection of an established agranulocytosis.

Distalgesic

A proprietary mild analgesic sedative, consisting of paracetamol (325 mg) and dextropropoxyphene (32.5 mg) in a white tablet, Distalgesic has become a popular 'safe' analgesic, supplanting aspirin/codeine tablets in use. Some 5 million prescriptions for this drug were written in the UK in 1982. The opioid dextropropoxyphene is the more dangerous component, tending to accumulate even on medicinal dosage, and although naloxone acts as a detoxifier it is not very effective.

Hypnotics

Choral (trichloracetaldehyde), *chlorhexadol* and **Paraldehyde** (paracetaldehyde

These are old but still popular hypnotics, both rather disagreeable, but curiously addictive. Neither can be regarded as dangerous by modern sedative standards, but alcoholics are particularly susceptible to either, and may develop the disturbing symptomatology of the alcohol–disulfiram mixture. Dangerous dosage is in the region of 4–6 g of chloral and 100–150 ml of paraldehyde, coma and respiratory failure ensuing. Chloral is the more hepatotoxic.

Metacetaldehyde is a solid fuel, sold in oblong white tablets stamped 'Meta'. It is also a useful slug bait. Children sometimes mistake it for sugar or a sweet, and as the double tablet contains 5 mg, fatalities may ensue. The outstanding symptoms, after a short interval, are nausea, abdominal pain and vomiting, followed by twitching and convulsions.

A girl of $3\frac{1}{2}$ who ate unwashed strawberries that had been treated with Slogan (meta) slug spray developed typical symptoms, lost consciousness, but recovered after 48 hours' resuscitation.

Formaldehyde though in common use as a 40% (formalin) solution, is too rare a poison in practice to deserve mention here.

Barbiturates

These synthetic derivatives of malonyl urea and, later, the closely related 'straight-chain' ureides, poured in vast quantity into the statistics of poisoning. However, stringent voluntary restriction in their prescribing, because of the danger of overdosage, has dramatically reduced fatalities in recent years in Britain.

A wide variation in rapidity of action and duration of effect, and their almost complete freedom from the dangerous side effects, made them the most popular hypnotic for the harassing pace and anxieties of current times.

It is of practical use to divide the barbiturates into groups according to their rapidity of action and duration (Table 22.1).

Fatal dosage Barbiturates with a short action are quickly metabolised, mainly by the liver, so that unless the liver is degenerate the amounts recoverable from the body or appearing in the urine may be very small. It is possible for a fatal blood barbiturate level (2–3 mg/

100 ml for the faster acting, 4–8 mg for the slower) to be achieved without measurable amounts being excreted; renal dysfunction will increase the probability. The ordinaty lethal dosage is set out in Table 22.1; a minimum lethal dose is commonly about ten times the therapeutic dose. Often it is found after inquiry that the patient was taking some other preparation—chlorpromazine, a synthetic 'tranquilliser', or an alcoholic drink—which may add dangerously to the hypnotic effect of the barbiturate, reducing the minimal lethal dosage very substantially. Wines and spirits such as gin or whisky have a well-recognised 'adjuvant' or 'additive' effect.

Table 22.1

			Fatal dose
Ultra-short action—anaesthetic duration			
Thiopentone sodium	Pentothal, Intraval	White powder or	1 g
Methohexobarbitone	Brietal	solution	
Short action—effect from $\frac{1}{4}$ to 2–3 hours			
Cyclobarbitone	Phanodorm	White tab.	
Hexobarbitone	Evipan	White tab.	1 to
Quinallbarbitone	Seconal	Red caps.	1·5 g
Secobarbitone+ amylobarbitone	Tuinal	Red/blue caps.	
Intermediate action—effect from $\frac{1}{2}$ to 5–6 hours			
Amylobarbitone	Amytal	Blue caps.	1·5 to
Butobarbitone	Soneryl	Pink tab.	2·0 g
Pentobarbitone	Nembutal	Yellow caps.	
Long action—effect from 1 to 8–10 hours			
Phenobarbitone	Luminal	Small white tab.	2 to
Methylphenobarbitone	Prominal	Small white tab.	4 g

Mandrax (methaqualone 250 mg, diphenhydramine hydrochloride 25 mg) is no longer marketed in the UK. Most victims can be allowed to sleep off the effects of any mild hypnotic under supervision, but monitoring is advisable.

Tests   All barbiturates except thio-compounds give a violet colour with copper isopropylamine reagents and with cobalt isopropylamine. Minute quantities can be both detected and measured in protein-free blood and tissue fluid extracts by ultra-violet spectrophotometry.

Treatment   The deepening hypnotic sleep or coma which results from overdosage of barbiturates is best treated on the basic principles.

1. *Maintain respiration*—artificially, with oxygen and, if it appears desirable also with stimulants such as amphetamine sulphate (10 mg). Tracheostomy may also appear necessary to clear the airways of accumulating mucus or pus. Antibiotics should be given to hold pneumonitis at arm's length.
2. *Stimulate the circulation* as with a noradrenaline (Levophed) 12 mg per minute infusion. The more specific analeptics such as bemegride

in 50-mg dosage repeated at 10-minute intervals either have a striking effect within the half hour or none at all.

3. *Remove the poison*—if it has been recently taken—by emetic or gastric lavage. The latter is inadvisable unless the air passages are sealed by cuffed intubation. Diureis or the artificial kidney are also useful.

Glutethimides and the ureides

The only common glutethimide since the tragic failure of thalidomide is Doriden.

The straight-chain ureides carbromal and bromvaletone which are closely related to the barbiturates have the same hypnotic action and greater dangers: they are also habit-forming, and were commonly responsible for blood dyscrasies. As a consequence, they have been removed from the pharmacopoeia.

Tranquillisers

Before dealing with the sedative and psychotherapeutic tranquillisers classified in the chapter heading on p. 293, mention must be made of the spasmolytic rauwolfia, and antihistamine drugs such as antazoline (Antistin), diphenhydramine (Benadryl) and mepyramine (Anthisan), that may, in larger dosage, sedate—sometimes with preliminary disturbances of vision, hallucinations or confusion.

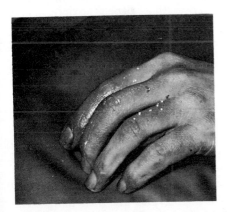 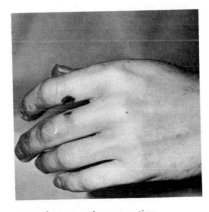

Fig. 22.1 Clues of hypnotic poisoning. (*a*) Granules of a spansule preparation adherent to sweaty fingers. (*b*) Cigarette burn between 'unconscious' fingers.

Doses in the region of 1 g are dangerous. The antihistamines are often taken without due regard for their dangers by patients depressed by heavy colds or hay fever, and their effects are heightened by alcohol or the more everyday sedatives.

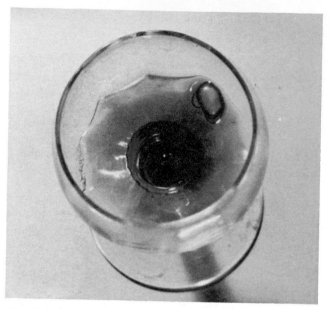

Fig. 22.2 A clue by the bedside. Wineglass containing a residue of whisky and a methylpebntynol capsule: to be preserved with care by the doctor for the police.

Chlorpromazine (Largactil)

Chlorpromazine and phenothiazine derivatives of the same type are in common use as potentiators of analgesic and mildly hypnotic drugs, having a distinct 'psychic inhibitor' effect that dispels anxiety. Their danger, like that of the antihistamines, is that they are often taken in combination with alcohols, sedatives, hypnotics or tranquillisers whose effect they enhance. Liver damage has been reported as well as the more likely marrow depressions, and toxic reactions are as common as 4 or 5 per cent. Brain damage has resulted in parkinsonism.

Sedative tranquillisers

Other related sedative tranquillisers with a chlorpromazine-like effect are diazepam (Valium), chloridiazepoxide (Librium), the meprobamates (Equanil, Miltown) and nitrazepam (Mogadon).

Antidepressants are in wide use in psychiatric treatment: many in larger dosage have a mildly sedative action, and are then dangerous, especially with other sedative drugs or alcohols. The more common are imipramine (Tofranil), amitriptyline (Tryptizol) and a group with monoamine-oxidase-inhibiting action—phenelzine (Nardil), tranylcypromine (Parnate) and isocarboxazid (Marplan).

Since all these elevate states of depression, overdosage is sometimes featured by agitation and hallucinations that may break out in hypomania.

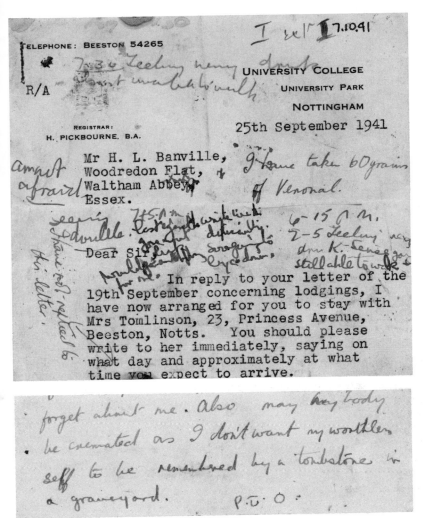

Fig. 22.3 Personal remarks upon the sensations of a student who swallowed 'almost 4 g of Veronal' (barbitone) at about '6.15 p.m.' '7.5 Feeling very drunk. Senses gone. Still able to walk ... etc. Further notes for 7.30 (above) and 7.45 may be deciphered.

A woman of 34 was found in a scene of great disorder in her home at Aylesbury—her clothing torn off, the brassiere dragged to the waist, furniture disarranged and curtains drawn, although it was daylight. She lay on her face, partly suffocated, on the kitchen floor, and the body bore multiple bruises. An intruder was suspected, but routine analysis for drugs revealed the equivalent of 50–80 25-mg of Tofranil in the body. A state of hypomania was concluded to be responsible. Criminal investigations were fruitless.

Toxic changes of the monoamine oxidase group inxclude hypertensive crises that are especially dangerous: they result from the ingestion of foods—especially cheeses—rich in tyramine.

Anticonvulsants

The anticonvulsants trimethadione (Tridione), phenacemide (Phenurone) and primidone (Mysoline), phenytoin sodium (Epanutin, Dilantin) all have a mildly sedative and hypnotic effect, but are not likely to be dangerously depressant.

Opium alkaloids and the synthetic narcotics

To be 'narcotic' a drug must be able both to dull pain and to reduce consciousness. Opium, the dried juice of the poppy *Papaver somniferum*, contains several natural narcotic alkaloids, morphine, noscapine, papaverine, codeine (methylmorphine) and dionin (ethylmorphine), and from these have been derived the synthetic diacetyl morphine (Heroin) and dihydrocodeine (Dicodid)—and the structurally similar nalorphine (Lethidrone), the morphine antagonist.

Most of the legitimate commercial production of opium is converted to codeine, which if under 1.5 per cent is not restricted, used widely as a safer analgesic and cough suppressor—often in combination with other drugs such as aspirin and phenacetin. Heroin has not been officially banned, although its very strong habit-forming character is as vicious as any: it had strong therapeutic support although it is well known to be the most dangerous habit-forming drugs in 'popular' use among traffickers.

Opium juice contains about 10 per cent morphine, 6 per cent noscapine and 1 per cent papaverine, together with smaller proportions of thebaine. Only morphine has powerful narcotic action.

The more important pharmacopoeal forms of opium and morphine are:

Papaveretum (Omnopon)	50%
Pulv. opii	10%
Tinct. opii (laudanum)	1%
Inj. morph. hydrochlor., sulph.	10–20 mg
Tinct. ipecac. et morph.	0.7 mg in 10 ml
Linct. diamorph.	3 mg in 5 ml
Tinct. opii camphorata (paragoric)	0.05%

Trade forms exist in the form of Nepenthe (0.84% M) and Chlorodyne (0.81% M—less than the 0.2 per cent which would make it subject to poison regulations). Codeine under 1.5% strength is exempt from regulations.

In the endeavour to avoid the habit-forming disadvantages of morphine derivatives, a large number of synthetic substitutes have been developed. The most used of these are pethidine, levorphanol (Dromoran), Methadone (Physeptone) and dipipanone, and there is no doubt that the most seriously addictive of these is pethidine—not least among nurses who have access to it in midwifery. Methadone is commonly used to wean addicts from heroin, but of course they become converts to it.

Fatal dose   Although the adult is in danger only with doses exceeding

200 mg, children are very much more susceptible and may succumb to very small doses. The case of a child slightly burned who died in its pram on the way home after being given some 5 mg heroin has been quoted earlier.

In another case, a child of 6 years who was given about 10.8 mg morphine hydrochloride in mistake for antitoxin, died in coma within some 5 hours.

There is another factor which may qualify the amount. Tolerance to both morphine and heroin is quickly acquired, and it is not uncommon to find addicts used to taking 1–2 g a day. De Quincey, famous for his *Confessions of an Opium Eater*, described the taking of a vast quantity of the tincture of laudanum per day, and the evidence given in the case of R. *v.* Dr. Bodkin Adams at the Old Bailey in 1957 made it clear that elderly patients whose minds have deteriorated, as well as those in pain, commonly need doses of morphine or similar narcotics in dosage much in excess of normal maximal dosage. Some degree of addiction is inevitable, and the fatal dose becomes individual.

Signs and symptoms   Simple narcosis passing into stupor and deepening cyanotic coma with free sweating are the usual events preceding death. Occasionally, as with most narcotics, a slight cerebral excitement with quickened pulse and flushed features precedes this. Thebaine is the only alkaloid in opium having this effect markedly, so it is more likely with crude opium than with purer extracts.

The pupils are small, usually so contracted that they almost deserve the classic description 'pin-point', the pulse slows, the body grows cold, respiration becomes less frequent and, after a period of Cheyne–Stokes breathing, death ensues from central respiratory depression. Sometimes opium may be smelled in the breath, and this and a subnormal or normal temperature best serve to distinguish a morphine coma from that of a pontine haemorrhage.

Treatment   is likely to be rewarded, if continued with patience, even from deepest coma. Controlled respiration should be started and oxygen given: the effects of this alone may be striking, but washing out of the stomach may also be done with advantage, preferably with the help of an anaesthetist to seal off the glottis. Dilute (0.05%) potassium permanganate in the wash-out fluid will help oxidise any alkaloid. Even if the drug was taken hypodermically this procedure has some value, for morphine is excreted into the stomach and lower intestine. *N*-Allyl morphine (nalorphine, Lethidrone), a morphine isomer, has a direct antagonistic action and is of real value in 10-mg repeated doses intravenously.

Tests   Morphine gives a blue colour with ferric chloride and a yellow to orange-red colour with strong nitric acid with increasing proportions of the drug. A portion of dry residue, touched with a drop of equal parts of concentrated H_2SO_4 and formaldehyde, will turn purple instantly and change rapidly to blue if morphine is present.

Addiction to drugs

In the past, the 'morphine habit' was commonly acquired as a result of its medical use for the control of pain, and the term 'registered addict' became applied to those in whom increasing dosage demanded special medical authority. Some were taking up to 1 or 2 g of morphine a day,

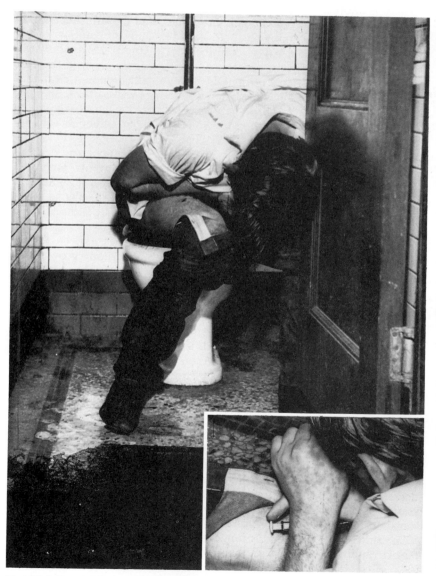

Fig. 22.4 Drug addiction. Accidental death from heroin injection causing a vomit reflex. Syringe needle in vein (inset).

and had sunk, in consequence of their loss of interest in food, into wretched states of emaciation and self-neglect.

The craving for drugs engendered deceit, dishonesty, moral degradation and a detachment from social life. Death followed from either injection infections or some intercurrent disease taking a hold on a wrecked body.

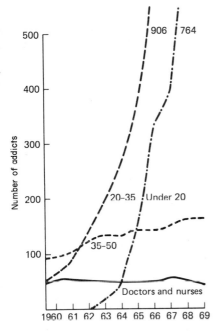

Fig. 22.5 Graph showing the marked increase in drug addiction in youth during the period 1960–70. The figures remained high throughout the seventies.

Times have changed. The 'morphine habit' has given way to a wide variety of addictions, from glue-sniffing to heroin or methadone indulgence. The term *drug dependence* came into official use to cover the wider spectrum of cravings and addictions. Young people, drifting into the wrong company in coffee bars and discotheques, have swollen the ranks of habitual drug-takers to disturbing proportions. Starting on nothing more than a 'reefer' cigarette of marijuanha 'weed' (cannabis), they have sought 'kicks' in stimulants such as the amphetamines, the hallucinogens such as the imipramine, phenelzine or amitriptyline tranquillisers, or lysergic acid diethylamide (LSD), and subsequently the frankly 'hard' drugs such as heroin (diamorphine), methadone or cocaine.

The statistics show a continuing alarming rise in young addicts, and a New York review showed that 86 per cent of 'hooked' hard drug addicts had started on the otherwise relatively harmless cannabis. The meaning of this must, however, be qualified by lack of knowledge as to how many cannabis smokers go no further. Maturity often brings wisdom. *The Misuse of Drugs Act 1971* was designed to limit the supply, possession and use of all the addictive drugs to professional persons and their genuine patients. By Regulations of 1973 addicts had to be *notified* and the *supply* of the two worst drugs, cocaine and heroin, was limited (so far as addicts were concerned) to their treatment in Home Office treatment centres.

Methadone (Physeptone) has proved a useful weaning drug, but is itself a dangerous substance, liable to isuse and dependence by young people. And as with so many addictions, drugs are often mixed—amphetamines and LSD or cocaine and heroin, seldom with drink. The adolescent who has got 'high' on a stimulant or 'blocked' by 'joy-popping' or 'main-line (vein) shooting' on 'hard stuff' suffers badly on being deprived of his drug. 'Coming down' is anguish, and to be avoided at all costs—by return to the drug.

Life is menaced by:

1. Infection of injection sites, or hepatitis from shared or dirty needles.
2. Return to the drug after abstinence—which may cause vomiting and asphyxia.
3. Accidental overdosage—or ignorance of the dangers of adjuvant drug or drug/alcohol action.

The expectation of life of an 18-year-old addict is only some 5 years—a tragic fact that few will face.

23

Stimulants, excitants and convulsant poisons

Amphetamines

Adolescent 'drifters' took to the amphetamines dexamphetamine (Dexedrine; or Drinamyl, with amylobarbitone) and methylamphetamine (Methedrine) for 'kicks' in the 1950s and tended to move on to cannabis and LSD in the 60s. The amphetamines were in legitimate use as appetite controllers as soon as they appeared on the market, but their dangerous misuse led to their being included with the 'hard' drugs in Class A of the Misuse of Drugs Regulations 1973.

Atropine (*dl.* hyoscyamine)

Atropine, derived from belladonna (deadly nightshade) and other allied plants, and hyoscyamine are isomeric and almost identical in action.

Poisoning is quite common, although fatalities are rare. Children who eat the deadly nightshade berries suffer but do not often die, whereas accidental swallowing of belladonna liniment and the deliberate suicidal taking of larger quantities of it are likely to be fatal unless early treatment is undertaken. Fatalities amount to less than 1 per cent of poisonings, but 125 mg of atropine or 5–7 mg of the liniment might be fatal. Some 20–30 berries would be dangerous to a child. Lomotil, the atropine-containing anti-diarrhoeic tablets or fluid, can be dangerous to children.

The symptoms are primarily excitative, restlessness, mental excitement, incoherence, even mania, accompanying the flushing and dry skin which mark the early stages of poisoning. The mouth and throat are so dry that speech is husky and swallowing difficult. The pupils are widely dilated. Depression soon follows, and the respiration and pulse, which have been fast, become slowed, coma and respiratory failure ensuing.

Treatment by lavage is important, using 1 in 5000 potassium permanganate, as for all alkaloids. Neostigmine (2.5 mg i.v. every 3 hours) is the natural antidote. Mild hypnotics are better than morphine for the excitement, since depression is going to follow.

Autopsy may reveal nothing but a state of narcosis with conditions of (central) respiratory depression and failure. In children, berries and leaves may occasionally be found.

Hyoscine (scopolamine)

Hyoscine derived from the same group of plants, principally from *Datura*, is far less deliriant in action than atropine and hyoscyamine: indeed it is much used in the control of motion sickness. The form usually prescribed in medicine, the hydrobromide, was used by the infamous 'Dr' Crippen, an agent for patent medicines, to kill his wife. It was estimated that 32.5 mg or rather more was present. The usual dose was 0.32–0.65 mg.

Camphor

Children sometimes eat camphor, and the BP camphor liniment is sometimes drunk. Vomiting, excitement, convulsions and then respiratory depression may follow in quick succession, coma preceding death. The odour is unmistakable.

A woman of 62, who was unable to read the label on any of three medicine bottles, drank lin. camph. from one in error. She became flushed, confused and delirious, and died 4 hours later.

Turpentine   from which camphor may be prepared, may cause very similar symptoms.

As little as 15 ml of either may kill a child, but some 100 ml constitute the fatal dose for an adult.

Eucalyptus oil and oil of wintergreen (methyl salicylate)   also have toxic action. Each is readily recognised by its smell.

Cocaine

Sources   Cocaine is derived from the dried leaves of *Erythroxylum coca* plant. It is methyl benzoylecgonine, this being the other alkaloid included with cocaine in the Misuse of Drugs Act 1971. The white crystal may be powdered, dissolved in water, spirit or oil, or taken as snuff with menthol.

Two per cent solutions in oils may be used for the eye or ear, and 4–10% aqueous solutions for local anaesthesia. Infiltration methods and perithecal injections utilise the various synthetic substances closely allied to cocaine, such as procaine (Nupercaine) and many others.

Signs and symptoms   The toxicology of cocaine must be set out in two distinct forms:

1. Accidental overdosage or violent intolerance to proper medical use.
2. Deliberate regular use—cocaine addiction.

Overdosage (or intolerance) is marked by sudden collapse, with pallor, dilated immobile pupils, convulsions, rapid feeble pulse, and in fatal cases a rapid central respiratory failure.

The onset is rapid and the course of events disturbingly fast also. Owing to the tendency of excited nervous subjects to react over-violently to any injection (even of water), excitative stages—with talkativeness, flushing, rapid pulse and exaggerated responses—are all too easily regarded as due to cocaine. It is not until real mental confusion, motor spasms, tingling and numbness of the limbs and irregularity of heart beat ensue that diagnosis becomes more assured. The dilation of the pupil is not, like that due to atropine, accompanied by loss of the light reflex.

In one fatal case seen at autopsy, a stolid man of 40 had become flushed, complained of dizziness and tingling of the fingers within 1½ minutes of the throat being sprayed with a 10% aqueous solution of cocaine hydrochloride. He became excited and delirious, made several convulsive movements of the arms and legs, and collapsed. The pulse was thin and irregular, the breathing slow and sighing; death took place some 6–7 minutes after the application. A 2% solution would have sufficed.

Fatal dose   About 500 mg cocaine by mouth is, in the absence of some special sensitiveness, a fatal dose, but as little as 30 mg may, on application to raw surfaces or mucous membranes or by injection, cause fatalities. If the victim survives half an hour, recovery will probably follow.

Chronic poisoning is always due to addiction, and like the morphine habit it results in the most degrading spectacle. Mentally and morally, the subject lapses into a low state which precludes living in harmony with society. The mental exhilaration and erotic well-being of the excitatory phase gives way to delusions, misleading hallucinations of sight and hearing, and the feeling of creeping things or 'grains of sand' in the skin.

The same loss of appetite as is seen in the morphine habit is common and serious wasting may ensue.

Treatment   for the excitative phases usually demands only sedatives. Convulsions may be controlled by intravenous barbiturates. A stomach wash-out—or a nose or throat wash, where suitable—and controlled respiration, together with procainamide (10% v.v.) to steady the heart, provide the other general methods of control. The principles of treatment for addiction are much the same as those for morphine, but there are seldom any 'withdrawal' troubles.

Convulsant poisons

Strychnine

Owing to the stringent regulations which further restrict the sale of strychnine to trading, export, scientific education, doctors and veterinary surgeons—and for killing seals or moles—strychnine poisoning is rarely met except among scientific and professional men. It may be sold to the public only as an ingredient of a medicine. Dr Palmer used it to murder his victim Cook—for money—in 1856.

Vermin-killers containing strychnine provide occasional cases: an Army officer who died after a series of convulsive seizures at Aldershot was found to have been poisoned by a pheasant so killed. The use of strychnine outside medicines is now limited, by the 1971 Poisons Rules, to those possessing written authority from the Ministry of Agriculture.

Sources   The alkaloid comes from the seeds of *Nux vomica* and is marketed in colourless crystal form as the hydrochloride or sulphate. It has a bitter taste, and is not likely to be taken in pure form except suicidally. But Easton's syrup (syr. ferr. phos. c. quinin. et strych.) contains 1.5 mg of strychnine in each 5 ml, and tablets of the two strengths are marketed. These provide the only common 'domestic' sources of poisoning, being restricted only by sale in proper form at a chemist's.

Strychnine is precipitated in an alkaline medium, and may settle to the bottom of a bottle of medicine in this event. Failure to observe this fact or to shake the bottle sometimes results in accidental overdosage.

Fatal dose   Some 30–60 mg is sufficient to cause death, although individual variation is considerable. A boy of 3 years died after putting two or possibly three Easton's tablets—2–3 mg—in his mouth.

A woman, who was given a 180-ml (6-oz) bottle of Easton's syrup to be taken in 4-ml (1-drachm) doses, felt so much better after her first two doses that she drank the rest (containing about 94 mg strychnine) in one dose. She walked into the accident department with stiff gait and arched back some 10 minutes later, and within several minutes was having a convulsion. Recovery followed upon prompt treatment.

Signs and symptoms   The bitter taste is usually noticed, although it may be deliberately obscured when the poison is used for murder. Within 5–15 minutes twitching of the muscles and 'catching' of the breathing develop; the chest feels tight. Quite suddenly a rigid stiffening of the body takes place, the back becoming arched (opisthotonos) and the chest more or less fixed so that cyanosis ensues. It is this fixation of the chest which best serves to distinguish strychnine convulsions from those of tetanus. Tetanus spasm is most pronounced in the jaw. The face is fixed in a grim sardonic smile (risus sardonicus). After a minute or two the whole body relaxes and the wretched subject lies exhausted, gasping for breath. Some minutes later the seizure suddenly grips the body again, often 'fired off' by some trivial stimulus—sometimes a mere touch of the clothing. The mind remains clear till death follows from exhaustion an hour or two later.

A veterinary student was found in his room at a YMCA hostel in London, frothing at the mouth, with the back arched and breathing suspended, the colour a dusky blue. A fellow medical student thought he was in a 'status epilepticus', but he died on the way to hospital, and search later revealed a small packet of strychnine crystals screwed up and tossed away in his locker. He had been robbed by a pickpocket on docking at Tilbury from Australia.

Treatment   is difficult if convulsions are already established. It is hopeless to try to introduce a stomach tube until the victim has been narcotised, for any such attempt will immediately excite another convulsion. Sedation with paraldehyde, or an intravenous diazepam, if the spasms permit, should be effected, and the stomach then washed out with water, paraldehyde being left in its place. Anaesthesis may be continued if desirable.

Haggard and Greenberg have suggested that phenobarbitone has also some direct antagonism for strychnine, and narcosis with this drug may therefore be tried.

Tests are simpler than for most alkaloids, and made the easier by the resistance of strychnine to decomposition. A drop of strong H_2SO_4 is added to the crystal and the edge of the solution is touched with a crystal of $K_2Cr_2O_7$. A purple colour forms instantly and, changing from crimson and rose, finally fades away. Physiological tests on the frog may also be tried.

Aconite

The alkaloid aconitine is one of the fastest poisons known; no specific antidote is available. The root of the flowering plant, the monkshood, has been mistaken for horseradish.

Sources The only natural sources are the plants *Aconitum napellus*, the common 'monkshood' garden flower, and *A. ferox*, the Indian aconite. The extract is a white powder, and the BP tincture colourless.

The only common medical form of the poison is the liniment ABC (aconite, belladonna and chloroform in olive oil).

> A man was found unconscious in his City office a few minutes after a distasteful interview, dribbling froth, with slow laboured respirations ceasing before medical assistance arrived. He had drunk about 60 ml (some 2 oz) of ABC liniment.
>
> A woman of 87, given a teaspoonful of lin. ABC in mistake for medicine, was given a gastric lavage and, unfortunately, sent home. She was readmitted 7 hours later, unconscious, grey and breathing faintly, dying some 2 hours later.

Fatal dose is probably about 4–5 mg, or 3–4 ml of the liniment: aconite is a deadly poison.

Signs and symptoms usually appear within a few minutes, and develop in a classic order. First there is tingling and numbness of the mouth and a feeling of constriction in the throat. Pain in the stomach, vomiting and salivation follow quickly, the pulse becomes slow and irregular, and collapse follows. The victim loses power in all voluntary muscles—arms, legs, speech, breathing all becoming embarrassed and respiratory failure ensuing. The mind usually remains clear.

Treatment Gastric lavage should be effected without delay, using milk or the 'universal' antidote, and digitalis may be given as a stimulant. Atropine has a weak direct antidote action, and 1–2 mg may be given and repeated within 20 or 30 minutes.

Tests for aconite are confined to biological assay—the tingling and numbness of the tongue, and the effect on the frog on injection; both are dependent upon isolation of aconite for test from the body, a matter of great difficulty, for it is destroyed by putrefaction.

Veratrine contains the mixture of alkaloids in cevadilla or sabadilla, the hellebore species of plant, and has an action similar to that of aconite.

Picrotoxin, derived from *Anamirta cocculus* (Levant nuts), is a poison more closely similar to strychnine in its convulsant effect, and acting primarily on the medulla rather than the spinal cord.

Cicutoxin, derived from the water hemlock (*Cicuta virosa*) is, unlike the spotted hemlock poison coniine, a convulsant like picrotoxin.

Yew, with its toxic alkaloid taxine in leaves and scarlet berry seeds, and the common laburnum bark and seed, containing cytisine, have actions of a similar character.

Gelsemium, derived from *Gelsemium nitidum*, contains a mixture of alkaloids having a weak strychnine-like action.

24

Paralytic, anticholinesterase and antihistamine poisons

Coniine

Coniine, from the common spotted hemlock, has ancient traditions. The cup of hemlock used to execute criminals sentenced to die, and Socrates' use of it, gives it historic interest. Its toxic properties are due to coniine blocking neuromuscular transmission, first of the legs, then the rest of the body: respiration fails. **Aethusia,** from dog parsley, has the same action.

Curare

Curare—mainly tubocurarine—have been developed from the native gourd poisons used as arrow venoms. They paralyse neuromuscular action, and have thus been put to good use in anaesthesia; gallamine (Flaxedil) and pancuronium (Pavulon) are in common use. Since they are usually in capable hands, danger is remote. Neostigmine is the natural antidote.

Nicotine

Nicotine poisoning is increasing a little in frequency, owing to the development of preparations for husbandry.

Sources Tobacco is chewed among seafaring men in many parts of the world, and swallowing the decoction or, worse, the wad, may cause toxic symptoms. More common sources are the commercial nicotine preparations made for rose sprays and vermin-killers. Some such solutions contain as much as 95% nicotine, and are very dangerous even when in contact only with the skin, for they are rapidly absorbed and highly toxic.

A factory girl spilled 8 ml (2 drachms) of a 95% insecticide on her overall sleeve. She collapsed a few minutes later, but was revived after the poison had been washed away with soap and cold water.

Another girl, who rushed to her bedroom after a quarrel with her fiancé, drank several drachms of a 34% nicotine rose spray. She collapsed on the floor and was dead when her parents broke in a few minutes later.

311

Fatal dose   Three or four drops of the pure alkaloid (or a teaspoonful of insecticide) are sufficient to prove rapidly fatal.

Symptoms and signs   consist mainly of faintness, sudden collapse, convulsive movements, feeble disorderly action of the heart and respiratory paralysis, and in quick succession. Lavage is vital.

Anticholinesterases

In recent years, a number of substances having eserine- or prostigmine-like action have been elaborated as systemic insecticides, mainly for aphids and red-spider (see 'Organic phosphates', p. 291). Their principal effects are lachrymation, salivation, cramps, twitchings of muscles, weakness, and then paralysis and circulatory failure.

Antihistamines

A group of synthetic drugs designed to combat the effects of histamine and thus restrict the distressing features of allergic conditions such as hay-fever and eczema have been found useful also in the treatment of drug intolerance. The proprietary preparations Benadryl, Dramamine and Antistin are well known, and both toxic reactions and deaths have been reported. There are no specific features but disorientation, tremors and hyperthermia, with disordered heart action, often occur.

Drowsiness is a common side effect, but coma rare. All antihistamine drugs that are prepacked for use in the prevention of sea or air sickness must be labelled 'Caution. This may cause drowsiness', for they are no longer subject to the restrictions of Schedules 1 or 4. Anyone may receive samples through the ordinary post.

Treatment   by lavage and resuscitation usually suffices, noradrenaline being useful in the maintenance of blood pressure. It is important to avoid stimulants.

25

Gaseous and volatile poisons

The removal of carbon monoxide from domestic gas has radically altered the situation of former years, where most suicides in Britain were caused by domestic coal gas. In 1982 there were 4279 suicides in England and Wales (2781 male, 1498 female), of which only 712 were by means of carbon monoxide. Motor exhaust fumes accounted for the majority of these (491 male, 41 female), other forms of monoxide suicide totalling 180.

Ammonia fumes (NH₃)

As a result of the widespread installation of ammonia refrigerators, accidental exposure to ammonia has become common. Experience was unfortunately increased by a war operations incident in East London when a large number of shelters in a brewery cellar were suddenly exposed to ammonia gas escaping from a refrigerating system burst by a bomb.

> Of 47 cases admitted to hospital, six with moderate and seven with severe exposure died. Irritation of the conjunctival and respiratory mucous membranes is intense, and reddening and swelling follow with dangerous rapidity. Of the fatal cases in this shelter incident all died of pulmonary oedema with 36 48 hours, or of bronchopneumonia during the succeeding few days.

Choking sensations, hoarseness and coughing develop with alarming rapidity, and dyspnoea and cyanosis may be aggravated by the production of copious frothed mucoid oedema fluid in the main air passages. Inflammatory changes quickly become established and bronchopneumonia rapidly ensues. The prospects in severe cases are gloomy. Maximal air concentration is 100 p.p.m.

The gastrointestinal changes from ingestion of ammonium hydroxide are the same as with alkalis (p. 272).

Treatment consists of eye-washes of saline, throat-straying and atropine 0.5-1 mg 2-hourly. A weak vinegar or paraffin gargle gives relief to the throat. Gastric lavage may also include vinegar.

Hydrocyanic (prussic) acid (HCN) and cyanides

Sources   Hydrocyanic acid is encountered as the colourless solution in water, the BP acid at 2% strength and Scheele's acid at 4%. The last is more common in veterinary use. The commercial cyanide (KCN and NaCN) or the pure potassium cyanide are commonly used in photography, engraving, electroplating and biochemical laboratory procedures. The solid cyanide is used to kill wasps and vermin, and to 'put down' domestic animals, for the poison is very rapid and virtually painless. The oil of bitter almonds (oleum amygdalae amarae) contains some 2–10% hydrocyanic acid. The kernels of various fruits and cherry-laurel contain about 0.1%. Cyanamide is in use as a fertiliser, but does not release HCN.

Fumigation of trees and fruit and of vermin by HCN is common, and dangerous owing to the vast quantities and concentrations used.

> After a ship's hold had been processed with HCN in an East India dock, when fugitives from Nazi persecution were numerous, examination of the hold after fumigation revealed a number of dead rats—and two German stowaway fugitives who had been hiding to escape arrest and deportation.

Chemists and laboratory assistants are sometimes overcome by the sudden evolution of HNC following the pouring away of cyanide solutions into sinks already containing strong acid residues.

Suicides by means of both hydrocyanic acid and the commercial cyanides are among the common poisonings, the cyanide being about three times as common as the acid owing to its more common domestic usage in the garden and in photography.

> A chemist's father was found dead of potassium cyanide poisoning on the edge of a pond, a stoppered stock bottle in his pocket. The poison should have been kept in a separate part of the premises; indeed, the chemist's son 'kept them under lock and key and never left the premises without slipping the key in his pocket'. Asked to produce it at the inquest, he fumbled in his pocket and shamefacedly admitted he had forgotten it. A police officer found it in the shop cupboard lock!

Lethal dose   One part in 2000 of the gas will quickly produce symptoms under industrial conditions. Something like 1 ml of the '2%' acid—according to the degree to which it has lost strength by volatilisation—and about 300 mg of the cyanide provide minimum fatal doses. Cyanides deteriorate when kept, and dosage becomes unreliable.

It must be remembered that the cyanide is more or less harmless until it comes into contact with the ionising acid in the gastric juices—though even the carbonic acid gas in the air will cause it to volatilise traces of HCN. Should the victim suffer from chronic gastritis as Rasputin probably did, he may swallow many times the fatal dose and escape the fate an ordinary subject would quickly meet.

Signs and symptoms   When the acid is taken the train of events is lightning in rapidity: the subject may literally 'drop dead'. With the cyanide there is likely to be a period of 10–20 minutes' suffering before death supervenes, depending upon the factors described above.

A commercial laboratory assistant was seen by one of his fellows to drink from a standard 20 ml bottle of 25% BP acid, and to fall to the ground as the bottle was lowered from his lips, before being able to replace the stopper. He ceased to breathe within a matter of seconds.

A university teacher walked out of a toilet in a London Underground station, stood with fellow passengers for 'some minutes', and then, as a train approached, threw himself in front of it. A bottle of cyanide, stoppered, was found in the toilet upon search, after autopsy had revealed cyanide to be present in the stomach.

The acid has a powerful action on the tissues after its rapid absorption and circulation in the blood plasma. It inhibits the cytochrome oxidases and thus prevents the tissues using the oxygen circulating in the blood; the saturation of oxyhaemoglobin rises steadily and at death the blood is bright pink. Cyanhaemoglobin is not formed in life and the blood has no characteristic spectrum.

Where there is any lapse of time before death the symptoms include dizziness, loss of muscular power and collapse, with rapidly supervening unconsciousness. The skin is flushed by capillary paralysis and dilation, and the tissues become suffused and pink owing to the rising oxygen tension. The pulse is thin and respirations quickly become irregular; the breath smells distinctly of 'bitter almonds'. Convulsions or twitchings may precede death from central respiratory and circulatory paralysis.

Where the cyanide is taken, vomiting is more likely owing to the time elapsing and the slight irritant and corrosive action of the carbonate (formed by air decomposition during storage).

Treatment Lavage by stomach tube is an urgent necessity, and the use of a mixture of ferrous and ferric hydroxides (forming Prussian blue) or of sodium thiosulphate (as a detoxicant) should be performed without an instant's delay. Stimulants such as methylamphetamine may be given, and the respirations sustained by artificial means. It has been suggested that methylene blue administered intravenously is of value, but this is not so. A 25% sodium thiosulphate infusion is preferable.

It is, of course, of no value whatever to give oxygen, for the tissues are already incapable of using oxygen owing to the action of the cyanide on the cell oxidases.

Autopsy appearances The head and neck are congested and suffused a pinkish cyanotic tint peculiar to hydrocyanic poisoning. The livid marks are patchy, pink and pronounced, for the blood remains largely fluid. The mouth smells distinctly of bitter almonds, and this sweet, penetrating smell should instantly give away the form of poisoning. One's sense of smell for it quickly becomes dulled: entry into the mortuary, or re-entry from the fresh air of another room—or, better, the open air—are the favourable moments for catching this unmistakable odour. As the skull vault is lifted off, or the chest or abdomen are opened, fresh waves of stronger smelling gas emerge for detection.

A coroner's officer called by a doctor to take particulars of the unexpected collapse and death of a public school headmaster noted the smell instantly on entering the premises—outside the room—and to the chagrin of the doctor made a confident diagnosis, and upon search found a re-stoppered bottle of cyanide in a sink cupboard of a room adjoining. The headmaster, 'respected by all, loved by none', had obtained it from his school laboratory for the purpose of suicide.

The blood is bright red, the pink livid stains being correspondingly tinted as described: cyan haemoglobin is not formed in life; the colour of the blood is due to the failure to utilise the oxygen it carries, and the tinge of cyanosis often seen to pulmonary oedema and respiratory embarrassment.

The stomach is coloured, like all other tissues, by this striking tint, and if the cyanide has been taken it may also show a shreddy brown corrosive change from the presence of alkaline carbonates. Cyanhaemochromogen formation may follow.

Tests a watch-glass moistened with silver nitrate and inverted over the stomach contents or even the tissues and body cavities will become cloudy from the formation of a white precipitate of silver cyanide, insoluble in nitric acid. Evaporation with ammonium sulphide and a touch of ferric chloride results in a brilliant red solution.

Carbon dioxide (CO_2)

Failure to recognise serious respiratory depression from rising CO_2 levels provides a number of unexpected deaths under anaesthesia. One source of excess CO_2 is a depleted oxygen cylinder and a new CO_2 supply working through a common union feed (set at the same position as with the low pressure CO_2 cylinder just replaced).

Almost all the other sources of CO_2 are industrial. 'Choke-damp' (a mixture of CO and CO_2) collects at the bottom of mines, and CO_2 in vats, pits, ships' holds, and from the burning of lime, wood and coal. Respiration, decay, fermenting processes and the 'fizzy' mineral-water industry provide other sources of exposure. After explosions and war-blasting or firing procedures it is present in the atmosphere, often in dangerous proportions.

It is an irrespirable gas proper, preventing the elimination of CO_2 from the lungs so that anoxial changes follow. Three per cent in the atmosphere will cause headache, drowsiness, giddiness and loss of muscle power; this last is always a dangerous element as it prevents escape—first increasing, then depressing, the respiritory movements.

In 1954, 189 cotton growers died overnight in a single Sudanese barrack room—later referred to as the 'Black Hole of Kosti'—following riots over the selling price of cotton. The room measured only about 18 × 6 metres (60 × 20 ft), and 300 men had been locked in it, without relief, from 9.30 p.m. until 5.30 next morning. No one had room to lie down, and there was no ventilation, the two doors and eighteen windows available having been closed to prevent escape. Heat, exhaustion and extreme deprivation of oxygen—with

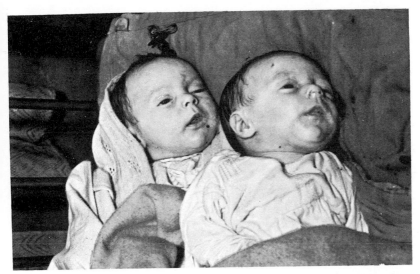

Fig. 25.1 Anoxial (CO$_2$) death. Twins of 2 months found dead as seen, cyanosed, lips soiled with vomit. Mother and father, twins and three older children slept together in a room measuring roughly 3 × 2.75 m (10 × 9 ft) without ventilation, windows and door having been sealed to exclude cold.

accumulation of carbon dioxide—all played parts in the causation of death. Only 111 prisoners survived.

The minimum fatal concentration is 25–30%, and high concentrations of 60–80% may, as with other irrespirable gases, cause instant collapse and death. Tissue anoxia is the cause of death.

Carbon monoxide (CO)

In former years the main source of toxicity from carbon monoxide was the domestic gas supply, called 'coal gas', which contained between 7 and 15 per cent of monoxide. In most countries the gas supply is now provided by natural petroleum gas which, although it cannot sustain life, is not actively poisonous.

Carbon monoxide is odourless when unmixed with other fuel gases, and may accumulate in lethal proportions long before its presence is recognised. The gas is rapidly absorbed according to its proportion in the atmosphere inhaled, and forms carboxyhaemoglobin (HbCO) which is some 300 times as stable as oxyhaemoglobin. It has a rapid cumulative action for this reason.

Although the domestic gas supply no longer contains any monoxide, toxicity and fatalities still occur from gas appliances used in the home. This is due to the fact that when any hydrocarbon fuel gas is burned, restriction of an adequate oxygen supply will prevent total combustion to the inert carbon dioxide, and accumulation of the dangerous monoxide. Faulty adjustment, blocked flues, restricted ventilation and any

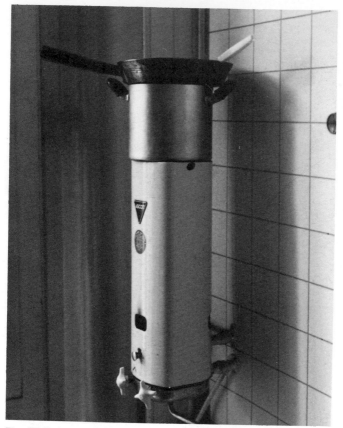

Fig. 25.2 A clue to the cause of death in a lodger—using a water heater to warm soup and slow-cook food—but obstructing thereby the proper flow of air from below into the burner area ... and the ventilation. Poor combustion resulted in the fumes containing a high CO and this was ill-ventilated. There was no cowl or vent pipe.

cause for incomplete combustion will lead to the very real danger of monoxide accumulation.

Other sources of CO are also common. They may be listed as

Car exhaust fumes	4–7 per cent CO	
Producer gas	25 ,, ,,
Water gas (production of hydrogen)	30–40 ,, ,,
Blast furnaces	25–30 ,, ,,
Coke ovens, charcoal fires	15–20 ,, ,,
Fire-damp (mines)	0.5–1 ,, ,,

Their effects will naturally depend largely upon the size and ventilation of the premises in which the gas accumulates. The air of a small garage would be made lethal by a car running for 5 minutes if doors and windows were shut, whereas a number of cars running in a large garage with fair passive ventilation develops only three or four parts per 10 000.

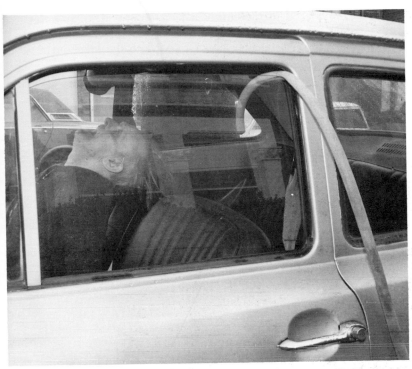

Fig. 25.3 CO poisoning by car exhaust fumes carried from the rear through an open window—a carefully planned suicidal act.

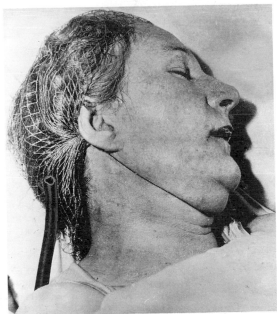

Fig. 25.4 Suicide or murder by carbon monoxide. Woman found dead in bed with gas tube lying by head. Such circumstances require careful investigation.

A coke brazier placed in the entrance to a night-watchman's hut is a serious menace, and workmen have been overcome in cellars or pits while attending to coke-burning boilers, owing to the inadequate ventilation.

The use of butane gas for heating or cooking in inadequately ventilated caravans or holiday cruisers is dangerous: even oil heaters can become lethal in closed rooms.

Lethal dose Owing to the stability of HbCO, which continues to accumulate as the blood absorbs proportionate saturations of the gases in the alveoli, remarkably small proportions of the gas—not immediately dangerous—may eventually prove fatal; 0.1% CO may after some $2\frac{1}{2}$–3 hours result in a blood saturation of 55–60% Hb (a minimum lethal proportion); 1% can cause unconsciousness in 15–20 minutes. The 7–15% of CO in coal gas is likely to be fatal, in spite of some ventilation, in some 2–5 minutes. Exercise, causing faster breathing, and children's more rapid respirations quicken the process. Most persons dying of uncomplicated CO poisoning show blood saturations of about 65–75% at death, provided they are physically fit. The 'debilitated, diseased or drunk' may succumb to lower saturations.

Signs and symptoms Examination of groups of persons working in New York have shown symptomless proportions of 1% (average living) to 3% (street cleaners) of the gas. Smokers may acquire as much as 3–5%. Haldane, in one of his many classic observations on respiration,

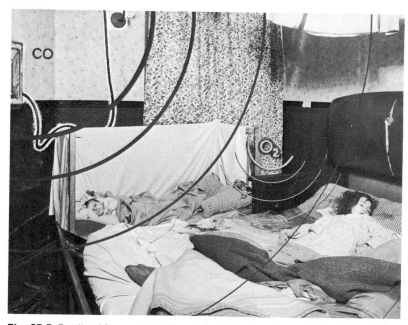

Fig. 25.5 Family of five poisoned by accumulating fumes of gas burner and gas fire in a closed room. Only the mother and one of the babies in the cot–close to an ill-fitting window admitting air—survived.

found that symptoms seldom occur until the saturation reaches 20%, when upon exercise slight shortness of breath and giddiness occur.

30%   causes dizziness, headache, malaise.
40%   „   inco-ordination, staggering, mental confusion.
50%   „   'drunkun gait', slurred speech, weak, aimless inco-ordi-
          nate voluntary movements, exhaustion, flushing,
          vomiting.
60%   „   unconsciousness.
70%   „   death.

Weakness may come on suddenly owing to muscular hypoxia, and prevent escape from the dangerous atmosphere, leading to collapse, sometimes with injury, and death.

The striking resemblance of the symptoms ensuing from saturations of 40–50% to those resulting from drunkenness is important, for persons driving cars with faulty floor-boarding may be overcome by exhaust fumes leaking into the interior of the car and may drive and behave under observation like persons under the influence of drink. It is important to bear the possibility in mind, so that if such a defence is later raised it may be disposed of by quoting the HbCO analysis. Bona-fide cases of this kind are rare indeed, but inability to dispose of the suggestion when raised by defending counsel is surprisingly common.

When recovery follows upon a period of unconsciousness from CO poisoning its completeness varies with the depth of anoxia and the length of time during which the brain suffered. Confusional states are common and disorientation or amnesia sometimes occur. Symmetrical softening of the basal nuclei, due to prolonged anoxia, may cause Parkinsonism, or other brain softening syndromes.

Treatment It may seem needless to emphasise the importance of the removal of the subject to a fresher air before commencing artificial respiration. When breathing is poor, a mixture of oxygen (93–95%) and carbon dioxide (5–7%) will facilitate revival of the respiratory centre. Orthodox stimulants and warmth are of help, and blood transfusion may prove vital in grave cases.

Autopsy appearances As there is a combination of carboxyhaemoglobinaemia and hypoxia from interference with respiration, the post-mortem appearances include evidence of both, varying with the importance of each element in the causation of death. Frank respiratory obstruction may have increased the asphyxial features.

In one case seen, a youth had asphyxiated himself by lying with his neck over the edge of the oven—before more than 20 per cent of CO had been aborbed. The appearances in this case were those of uncomplicated asphyxia.

From carboxyhaemoglobinaemia, the blood, which often fails to clot, becomes tinted a bright cherry-red, and colours the organs, the musculature and the *post mortem* livid stains the same bright red colour; the last become more pronounced than usual owing to the blood remaining fluid. Much the same colour is mimicked by the bright red of high oxygen saturation in HCN poisoning, by nitrite poisoning, and by exposure to cold as in bodies recovering from the river of lying exposed in cold weather, and analysis alone can prove the condition to be due to CO absorption. The colour, seen much better on dilution, becomes marked at saturations of 35–40%—well below that of the minimum lethal saturation, except in the aged who may die at this level.

From the asphyxial element, the face becomes suffused and the veins of the neck congested. The lungs and the right heart are engorged and froth pours into the air passages. This may add to the asphyxial element, and intrapulmonary haemorrhages of varying size may follow upon the struggle to breathe. The capillary permeability is increased and petechiae are common in the lungs, conjunctivae, skin and in the brain.

Where the element of anoxia has been prolonged by unconsciousness for several days after removal from the gas, symmetrical necrosis of the basal nuclei of the brain may develop.

The gas is eliminated fairly rapidly from the blood by breathing a clean air, and a mere trace only will remain after 6 hours. If death is delayed until hypostatic pneumonia supervenes (upon the state of respiratory depression) no CO will be likely to be found remaining in the blood. An early sample is important to diagnosis.

It must be remembered also that in elderly or unfit persons exertion alone may prove fatal.

> In one case an old gentleman had died as a result of the endeavour to climb up upon a table on which he had prepared a 'gas-bed' for himself: the gas was not yet turned on and blood analysis was negative.

Tests   Both chemical and spectroscopic tests are available.

The two (D and E) absorption bands of carboxyhaemoglobin remain unaffected by reduction with ammonium sulphide, but as affected blood always contains oxy- and carboxyhaemoglobin in varying proportions the coalescence of bands may be difficult to judge. A scaled spectrometer enables one to show that the two principal bands of carboxyhaemoglobin absorption lie a little closer to the violet end of the spectrum than those of oxyhaemoglobin, and a 'reversion' spectroscope has been designed to throw these two spectra close together so that this 'shift' may be measured; it is proportionate to the saturation of HbCO. The method is easy, reliable and fairly accurate.

The student and doctor in practice will not be expected to be familiar with practical details of these laboratory methods.

More sophisticated analytical methods are now in use but require special equipment.

Alcohols and glycols

Methyl alcohol (CH_3OH)

Methyl alcohol in any form is poisonous. Several commercial forms of methylated spirit provide common sources for poisoning. The 10% commercial methylated spirit contains 10% crude wood spirit, pyridine, acetone, bone oil, paraffin and traces of aldehydes. It is an intoxicating spirit, and the introduction of colouring matter (methyl violet) has done nothing to restrict its use among degenerate drinkers. Indeed, filtration through charcoal or a half loaf of bread extracts the colour and leaves a highly toxic clear fluid for which a poor-quality red wine—originally the unwanted Lisbon cask residues—provides a 'vehicle'. The result is the well-known 'Red Lizzie' or 'Red Biddy' or 'Flaming Lizzie'.

> In one case examined after death from the effects of several months' 'Biddy' drinking, inquiry showed that the wretched victim had frequently aerated the red wine with a lump of calcium carbide, producing acetylene gas (and traces of both phosphoretted and arseniuretted hydrogen).

Ethyl alcohol (C_2H_5OH)

The lay use of the word 'alcohol' often enough refers to any intoxicating drink, but a doctor would be wise to avoid such a loose general term. The common sources of ethyl alcohol are:

Whisky	(40%)	Liqueurs	(35–40%
Brandy	(45%)	Sherry and port	(15–20%)
Rum	(50–60%)	Wines	(10–15%
Gin	(40%)	Beers	(2–6%)

A large whisky in England measures approx. 47 ml ($1\frac{2}{3}$ fl oz), in Scotland 70 ml ($2\frac{1}{2}$ oz). A 'tot' ($\frac{5}{6}$ oz, approx. 23 ml) of spirits is the equivalent (in alcohol content) of $\frac{1}{2}$ pint of beer (300 ml).

Three forms of poisoning occur: acute (fatal) alcoholic poisoning, 'drunkenness' (insobriety) and chronic alcoholic poisoning (chronic alcoholism).

Acute (fatal) alcoholic poisoning

Distinction between lethal intoxication and grave drunkeness is justified by the occurrence of poisoning among bottlers of spirits, dockers, cellarmen, and others with access to unlimited liquor.

> A rum-bottler was found at 3 p.m. unconscious under his bench, stertorous, suffused in the face and livid, though with clammy skin, smelling strongly of rum. It was not the first time this had occurred, and his father was called to remove him by taxi to his home, where he was dumped fully dressed on his bed to sleep it off. He was left lying on his back, deeply unconscious, and was found at 7.30 a.m. the next morning dead in the same position.

Paralysis of the respiratory centre by alcohol, inhalation of vomit and suffocation on the face are common ends to such bouts of drinking. Blood alcohol levels are likely to be between 400 and 500 mg/100 ml.

Drunkenness

Drunkenness is an offence only when it endangers others. To be hopelessly drunk in the club or at home is to be a nuisance, and occasionally a danger to oneself; but it is when the safety of children at home, of pedestrians, motorists, public vehicles and ships at sea are at risk that the law must step in: it becomes a serious offence.

'Drunk and disorderly', 'incapable' or 'using abusive language' usually mean so drunk that the matter can safely be left in the hands of the police. Doctors are likely to be called only when injury or some uncertainty about real illness has arisen. The doctor is called to assess the real substance of the physical condition, in someone who has plainly been drinking, rather than to confirm drunkenness. Diseases such as migraine, Ménière's syndrome and multiple sclerosis can mimic the signs and symptoms of drunkenness, and the combination of a lesion such as a 'stroke' or a cerebral contusion and drunkenness may make either most difficult to assess.

Any doubt should always be resolved in hospital where, in the patient's best interests, he should be detained for observation until next day. Every now and again a 'dead drunk' is put in a police station cell to sleep it off, only to be found dead a few hours later—a tragic mistake that clouds the reputation of both the police and their doctors.

The Transport Act 1981 and drunken driving

From May 1983, new statutory provisions (the Transport Act 1981) has replaced the blood and urine tests previously in force. It is now an offence to drive a vehicle with more than 35 micrograms (μg) of alcohol per 100 ml *of breath*. This is approximately equivalent to 80 mg/100 ml in the blood, but the law now makes the breath content the vital issue. A screening test is performed at the roadside and, if positive, a definitive test on a meter which delivers a written print-out is used in the police station by a police officer—*not a doctor*.

No action is taken on levels up to 39 μg, but 40 μg and over leads to automatic conviction. If the level is between 40 and 50 μg, the driver has the option to request a blood or urine test.

As no 'defence specimen' is available in breath testing, a duplicate copy of the print-out is given to the driver. The test is always performed twice and the lower of the two readings is used in evidence.

Thus the police surgeon or other doctor now has no part to play in the procedure, unless the police request a blood sample where the driver opts for a check on a 40–50 μg breath reading. Although theoretically the clinical standards set by the old law relating to 'fitness to drive' still operate, they are now practically never invoked. They naturally must be used where suspicion of other drugs exists.

Under the 1982 Act there is no opportunity for a doctor to examine the driver for illness or head injury which might qualify the effects of alcohol. It is, nevertheless, still possible for an accused to request—and have—the benefit of an examination by his own doctor or a specialist if he is fit to make the request. The offence remains one of having a breath level above the statutory 35 μg.

Some drivers have, in the past, avoided early tests of their breath or blood levels by making their way to the safety of their homes. The police now have authority to make entry to any place where a driver has taken refuge, provided that an accident has caused injury to a third party. Another old evasive trick—'totting up' from a hip flask or in a nearby public-house 'to steady the nerves' after an accident—is less easy to work since an accused now has to produce evidence of the fact.

Signs and symptoms

Individual variations in reaction to given doses—even the same individual's reactions to the same dose—vary according to the following.

1. *The rapidity of absorption* Food matter, especially if fatty, tends to delay the process, and 'an empty stomach' to hasten it. A warm alcoholic drink which dilates the gastric mucosal capillaries will act with greater speed than an iced one of the same calibre. Chronic gastritis, with its excess mucus barrier to absorption, is one of the explanations for the tolerance of the habitual drinker.

2. *The dilution of the alcohol* On the whole, very concentrated forms of alcohol are absorbed more rapidly than similar total doses in weak strength, but it appears that about 20% is the optimum for rapid effect. The popular 'chaser system' of taking spirits, then beer, or the reverse, and of repeating the process is rapidly intoxicating for this reason. Of course the 'washing through' of more concentrated forms of alcohol by weak beer at later stages tends to reduce the effect.

3. *The ability of the body to metabolise alcohol* Normally, the body can metabolise some 10 ml of absolute alcohol every hour. This lowers the blood alcohol at the rate of some 12–15 mg per hour—say, the equivalent of 300 ml ($\frac{1}{2}$ pint) of beer or 23 ml (one tot) of spirits per hour.

4. *The tolerance of an individual*—his reactions to a given dose absorbed in a given period are variable. They are undoubtedly improved by training, and the fact must be borne in mind in estimating the effects of a given blood alcohol.

The blood alcohol in states of marked drunkenness is usually 200–400 mg/100 ml; the lower is the equivalent of some 3 litres (5$\frac{1}{4}$ pints) of ordinary beer or 252 ml (9 fluid ounces) of whisky, the higher double these figures. Anything over this is likely to be associated with complete stupor. Under 100 mg/100 ml is seldom associated with more than the gay abandon of one's inhibitions, the vivacity of the average cocktail-party guest. The blood alcohol level is related to the amount taken on fairly straight lines, subject only to the conditions affecting the rapidity of absorption and other less important factors described above. The urine is about 4:3 the concentration of the blood, but in absorption stages the blood is higher than the urine. Equilibrium (4:3 urine/blood) develops in about an hour, then the blood figure falls away.

But individuals do vary greatly in their reactions to given blood con-

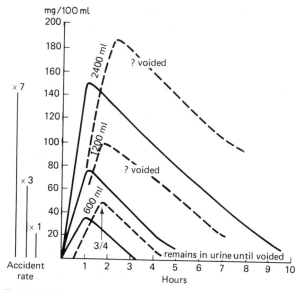

Fig. 25.6 Theoretical blood and urine levels of alcohol after drinking (1, 2, 4 pints of beer; 2, 4, 6 tots).

centrations. The stages of intoxication may be divided into three distinct periods.

1. *Excitement*—loquacity, vivacity, a sense of well-being often fostered by the light-hearted jocular conversational stimulus of friends, a tendency to lose emotional restraint, to forget animosities, converse with abandon, to be less critical (of oneself and others) and to lose control over one's moral integrity. Feeble jokes and easy affection mark the hour. But the ability to 'pull oneself out of it', to 'sober up' by force of will, still exists.

2. *Confusion*—a tendency to come to grief over longer words owing to slight inco-ordination, to slur speech, to lose control of finer movements—buttoning up one's clothes, visual concentration—blurring of sight, an inability to perform co-ordinated acts such as writing or driving a car with the usual quick appreciation of danger. Confusion of mind also exists over any problem requiring concentration and clear thinking (for even the stage makes fun of muddled drunken concentration). Emotional upsets become more marked, boasting, loud laughter and indulgence in coarser jesting alternating with anger and violence. Again it is largely the stimulus of surrounding persons who stir these emotions into fire.

3. *Stupor*—this is the 'dead drunk' stage which is roused into response only by the strongest stimuli. To be 'anaesthetic' or unfeeling to injury, to lie in a snoring stupor with flushed face and dribbling lips, is the last stage of helpless inebriety. This is the stage which is likely to be simulated by cerebral disease or head injury, and given such a lesion and a smell of alcohol, no skill can ensure a certain diagnosis. The coexistence of

drunkenness *and* a head injury is common enough to justify detaining all such cases for observation pending a satisfying diagnosis.

Clinical tests   A doctor may be summoned:

1. To exclude illness or injury.
2. To indicate whether on clinical test, under the Road Traffic Act 1972, there is evidence of unfitness from drink or drugs.
3. Merely to take blood in support of a positive breath test (obtained by the police) under the Transport Act.

The police may have formed the view that, although the breath tests on the road and in the station were below the statutory limit, the driver was nevertheless unfit to be in charge of the vehicle.

'a person shall be taken to be unfit to drive if his ability to drive properly is for the time being impaired' . . . through drink or *drugs.*

A clinical examination—excluding disease or injury—will be necessary to press a charge under the Act; it is seldom requested.

It must be accepted that whether or not the blood alcohol level is over 80 mg/100 ml, a poor capacity for drink and drugs—or drugs alone—can cause unfitness to drive. This was the purpose of the 1960 Road Traffic Act, and of the 1962 Act provision calling for an alcohol estimation.

The wording of the 1962 Act is of importance, for this is the standard the doctor is being asked to set when called to examine a driver for fitness to drive under that Act. *He is not being asked to say whether the driver was 'drunk'.* The law has recognised the difficulty of setting a standard by which to judge drunkenness, and first defined it as being 'unfit to drive through drink or drugs' and then as unfit because 'his ability to drive properly is for the time being impaired'. These are the words a doctor should be ready to quote when giving evidence of his examination of the case under the 1962 Act. He should be prepared to state:

1. The accused's own medical history, the story of his drinks and the subsequent course of events.
2. An opinion with regard to natural disease, fits, injury or other drugs influencing the conditions observed.
3. Whether or not, in his view, at the time of examination the ability of the accused to drive properly was for the time being impaired.

The time at which the examination took place should be carefully noted, and the length of time elapsing between the alleged offence and the examination should be stated in the report which is made.

Where concussion or grave head injuries were sustained in an accident the doctor should be most wary of giving an opinion at all, knowing how the effects of such injuries might qualify the evidence of drunkenness (see p. 116). The effect of drugs—any kind of pill, insulin, etc—is entirely on a par with the taking of alcohol so far as the law is concerned.

The importance of carbon monoxide in its power to simulate the signs and symptoms of drunkenness has been overemphasised: it is a more common excuse than is justifiable, and the doctor would do well to find out whether it has any substance before giving evidence.

The British Medical Association published a report on 'The Recognition of Intoxication' in 1958, in which it was said:

> 'That there is no simple test by itself which would justify a medical practitioner in deciding that the amount of alcohol consumed had caused a person to lose control of his faculties to such an extent as to render him unable to execute safely the occupation on which he was engaged at the material time. A correct conclusion can only be arrived at by the result of the consideration of a combination of several tests or observations such as:
> General demeanour.
> State of the clothing.
> Appearance of the conjunctivae.
> State of the tongue.
> Smell of the breath.
> Character of speech.
> Manner of walking, turning sharply, sitting down and rising, picking up a pencil or a coin from the floor.
> Memory of incidents within the previous few hours, and estimation of their time intervals.
> Reaction of the pupils.
> Character of the breathing, especially in regard to hiccup.'

In 1960 the BMA published a further report 'The Drinking Driver', in which it was stressed that clinical examination, in the absence of chemical tests, is neither sufficiently sensitive nor reliable enough to detect deterioration in driving ability unless it is considerable. This undoubtedly resulted in the 1962 Act, which—for the first time—incorporated blood tests.

Where the doctor has been called by the police he is likely to be asked to express his opinion as soon as his examination is over. When he has been called in defence by the accused or his solicitor he may reserve the information he has elicited, and his views. He may also consider the wisdom of delaying his examination so as to see his patient in as favourable a state as is possible, but his evidence will lose value as the length of time elapsing between the alleged offence and the examination increases. The British Medical Association recommended that a person be seen 'if he so desires'—i.e. in his defence—within half an hour of the time at which he is charged. Too long a delay will invalidate the findings.

The elaboration of complicated tests is to be avoided, and each doctor will find that he gradually comes to adopt a standard routine of his own. It will be likely to include:

1. Admission by the subject as to the kind and amount and the timing of the drinking.
2. An account of the subsequent course of events leading up to arrest, and especially of injuries sustained to the head.

3. An estimate of temperament—whether calm, or excited and unduly emotional.

4. The smell of the breath—no index of the quantity of alcohol, but of assistance as to its kind.

5. Examination for visual defects, artificial limbs, deafness and other disabilities which might affect a person's behaviour or reactions. Accounts of fits, black-outs, etc.

6. Observations on suffusion of the face and conjunctivae, flushing and tachycardia. The state of the pupils, and their reactions.

7. Observations on tremor of the lips, tongue, hands.

8. Writing or drawing (patterns only).

9. Visual tests—as seeing the time across a 6 m (20 ft) gap, or deciphering print of smaller sizes. A person unable to see 6/15 is unfit by law to drive.

10. Co-ordination tests—e.g. walking, lighting a candle or cigarette.

11. Speech and spelling tests of an everyday kind.

12. Blood (or urine) alcohol estimations. The doctor may take the specimens—sufficient to afford 2 ml of fluid for test, sealed and placed in refrigeration—but had better leave analysis to the laboratory biochemist. A preliminary breath test may already have been taken.

Nothing is more unfair than an exacting test which includes demands the doctor or the police officer themselves might find too much. Try yourself to say 'the sinking steamer sank' several times without pause, or to spell words such as gullibility and eroticism, to stand bolt upright with your eyes shut or walk a white chalk line even in your sober moments. Add, say, a recent motor-car accident after a trying day when you have sought relief in a glass of sherry, picking yourself out of the wreckage of your car to be taken against your wishes and at great inconvenience to a police station, even by a courteous police officer, and you will determine to impose only the fairest and most reasonable tests for 'drunkenness.'

Never allow sympathy for a fellow-doctor who is unquestionably drunk to divert you from your usual standards. If a person is a menace because of drunkenness, then the more so if he has professional responsibilities in his drunken hands.

Casualty officers often forget, when dealing with drivers or pedestrians in street accidents, that to take blood or urine for alcohol may be vital, not only to diagnosis but also to justice. However, the sample must *not* be given to the police without the patient's consent.

Chronic alcoholism   is characterised by a gradual physical and mental deterioration. The subject loses appetite and, more particularly in spirit drinkers, becomes thinner, although seldom developing the apathy towards food that is so striking a feature of 'dangerous drug' addiction. The musculature becomes soft and fatty, the heart muscle and the liver developing grave fatty degenerative changes which may cause death. The mental changes of chronic alcoholism have already been described. Vitamin B deficiency may cause a peripheral neuritis.

Although cirrhosis may be seen in chronic alcholics it is, alone, no evidence of addiction, being a common natural disease with a variety of causes.

Methylpentynol (Oblivon), an acetylenic alcohol which acquired a considerable popularity as a 'sedative', had an action similar to those of the higher alcohols, allaying anxiety and creating a feeling of euphoria.

Although safe when administered under medical control, its comparative innocuousness was a source of danger, for it inebriates. Methylpentynol, itself an alcohol, worsens the effects of alcohol and hypnotics. Its production in the UK has ceased.

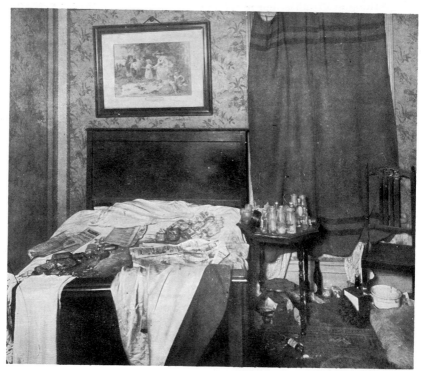

Fig. 25.7 Scene of discovery of woman, aged 52, dead of acute alcoholic poisoning. She had lived for many weeks on a daily milk supply of one half-pint of milk. Thirty-seven empty brandy bottles lay around her on the bed, the bedside table, and the floor.

In 1955 a man consumed a quantity of methlypentynol and pentobarbitone (Nembutal) capsules, apparently in order to commit suicide. He died within the hour. Analysis of the viscera indicated that a dose of the order of only 9 capsules of methylpentynol and about 0.5 g of Nembutal had been consumed. Such a dose of either would not be expected to have a fatal effect: their combination was fatal.

The glycols

This group of chemical solvents includes three which are already known to have toxic effects in man—ethylene chlorhydrin, diethylene dioxide (dioxan) and diethylene glycol.

They are in wide use as solvents for resins, shoe-creams, waxes, varnishes, lacquers, paints, etc. Dioxan is also commonly used as a wool degreaser, ethylene glycol as an antifreeze mixture.

A man of 33 was seen to drink some 200 ml ($\frac{1}{4}$-$\frac{1}{2}$ pint) of antifreeze solution consisting of almost pure ethylene glycol. Five hours later he became drowsy and appeared ill. He was put to bed and slept—or was comatose, for on the next day he could not be roused. He made a temporary partial recovery 8 hours after this, but then became delirious, developed twitchings and a rise in temperature, and died of suppression of urine on the twelfth day.

The symptoms of poisoning are very like those of ethyl alcohol, but pulmonary oedema is a feature. Diethylene glycol and dioxan have also caused a form of nephritis indistinguishable from the cortical necroses of pregnancy. Oxalic acid is one of the metabolites of the glycols, and calcium gluconate is, therefore, a useful antidote.

26

Industrial gaseous and volatile poisons

Sulphur gases

Sulphuretted hydrogen This is the chief dangerous constituent in sewer gas. It is highly toxic, concentrations of 0.05% being sufficient to cause symptoms and 0.1% being fatal within a very short period of time. It is colourless, smells of 'rotten eggs', and, being heavier than air, tends to settle in the bottom of pits and cellars or sewers. It is generated in the decomposition of organic sulphur-containing matter—animal or vegetable decay—and therefore tends to accumulate in sewers, cesspools, tannery vats, etc. It also becomes formed in the chemical manufacture of glue, gas, petroleum distillates and artificial rayon, and from the use of carbon bisulphide in making artificial silk.

Symptoms following exposure to strong concentrations of H_2S consist simply of dramatically sudden collapse, literally instantaneous, with immediate unconsciousness. Weaker concentrations cause irritation of the eyes and air passages, nausea, dizziness, muscular weakness and respiratory collapse.

The gas combines with haemoglobin mainly after death, but in life it may convert oxyhaemoglobin extensively into methaemoglobin and embarrass respiration as a result. The importance of methaemoglobin has probably been overestimated in the past. It must be remembered, too, that sulphaemoglobin forms naturally as *post mortem* decomposition sets in.

Tests Spectroscopy will show absorption bands between C and D and—an ill-defined zone—between D and E, rather like methaemoglobin, but with the C—D band remaining unaffected by reducing agents.

Filter paper moistened with lead acetate will turn black if sulphuretted hydrogen is in the air.

Sulphur dioxide

This is not as toxic as H_2S. It is almost equally irritating to the eyes and respiratory tract, but there is resemblance ends. No further harm ensues unless the concentration is such as to add an anoxic element or the gas is hot enough to burn, as it is in a number of heavy industry processes.

Carbon bisulphide

A volatile liquid whose gas is rapidly absorbed through the lung, carbon bisulphide is in wide use as a solvent for rubber and in vulcanising processes. Poisoning is usually the result of exposure of some standing and is characterised by nausea, headache, giddiness, with visual disturbances and sometimes mental excitement. Peripheral and retrobulbar neuritis may also occur. The changes are not unlike those of the refrigerant methyl chloride poisoning.

Nitric oxide

High-pressure oxypropane or oxyacetylene arc welding or ship-breaking may cause nitrogen dioxide poisoning from atmospheric nitrogen, and nitric fumes also occur in explosive factories. The toxic effects are concentrated mainly in the respiratory apparatus, dyspnoea, cyanosis and pulmonary oedema being outstanding.

Sixty-four men on HMS *Phoebe* suffered from spasmodic cough, constriction of the chest, cyanosis and painful dyspnoea when a torpedo exploded amidships in 1942, releasing nitric fumes.

Hydrogen phosphide
(Phosphoretted hydrogen)

Ferrosilicon may, when brought into contact with water, liberate both phosphoretted hydrogen and arseniuretted hydrogen (p. 282). The onset of symptoms is rapid and the changes are much the same as those seen in poisoning by nitric oxide.

Petroleum distillates
(Petrol, benzine, paraffin, kerosene, diesel oil)

The common error of confusing benzine (from petroleum) with benzene, better called benzol (from coal tar), must be avoided. The former is far less toxic.

Inhalation or swallowing of these distillates is followed by nausea, vomiting headache, vertigo and, sometimes, coma. Unconsciousness may supervene rapidly, especially when choking with petrol causes dyspnoea and cyanosis. Fatalities may occur in children drinking petrol or kerosene, and even after apparent immediate recovery residual mental confusion may be present.

Cases of petroleum poisoning occasionally follow from persons attempting to suck petrol out of car tanks through rubber tubing and being choked by a sudden rush of petrol into the mouth and throat.

Few fatalities occur, but bronchial irritation and oedema or inflammatory consolidation of the lungs may ensue.

The aromatic compounds

The number of aromatic coal-tar derivatives on the market is so large that it is quite beyond the scope of the student's requirements in forensic medicine to consider more than those whose toxic action in man has provided important medical problems in industry.

Benzene, the basic member of the group, is, owing partly to its chemical form and partly to its high volatility, less toxic than other members. The addition of nitro- and nitroso-groups to the benzene ring tends to increase the toxicity, and reduction to amine form, as with the reduction of nitrobenzene to aniline, tends to diminish the poisonous action. Sulphonation almost eliminates their toxicity. These generalities provide a basis for the introduction of safer solvents and plasticisers in industry and for the reduction of illness from industrial exposure.

Benzene

Sources   Benzene or benzol, a colourless liquid with distinctive odour, is met in the coal-tar distilling and motor-fuel blending industries in bulk, usually in apparatus, and as a solvent in the processing rubber, aeroplane paint, linoleum, celluloid, varnish, printing ink and cellulose lacquer.

The fluid is highly volatile and is rapidly absorbed through the lungs. Acute forms of poisoning occur from breakages of distilling apparatus and in cleaning out vats and tanks, but the more common forms are due to prolonged exposure in handling the fluid for solvent purposes or the material in which the benzene is soaked, and from which it is constantly evaporating. Ventilation is the key to safety in such processes: the industrial safe maximum is 25 p.p.m.

Symptoms   The symptoms of acute forms are mainly cerebral and nervous, with excitement, incoherency, headache, giddiness, nausea, insomnia, paraesthesiae in hands and feet, and—if severe—narcosis and ultimate death. The death rate is high as 10 per cent.

The more common chronic forms have a classic feature which is virtually confined to benezene among the hydrocarbons—anaemia. This is not, as was first thought, a simple aplastic form of anaemia due to benzene poisoning the bone marrow. It is due to haemolysis, for the plasma bilirubin is raised and there is haemosiderosis of the reticuloendothelial tissue. The bone marrow may be aplastic, especially in women, but is more commonly overactive, pouring reticulocytes into the circulation. No other aromatic compound causes such a change. In addition, some evidence has accumulated to suggest that benzene may cause the development of leukaemia.

Naphthalene

Naphthalene, the moth repellent, is also a coal-tar derivative. The solid moth-ball is swallowed by children and as little as 2 g may be fatal owing to rapid absorption, haemolysis and renal tubular damage. Early lavage and alkaline diuresis with sodium bicarbonate are essential.

Nitro- and amino-benzenes

Sources of the various aromatic benzene derivatives are shown in Table 26.1. They are, without exception, industrial.

Table 26.1

Chemical form	Industrial forms and uses	Toxic changes
Nitrobenzene (oil of mirbane)	Manuf. of aniline dyes and explosives. Solvent for shoe and floor polish. Cheap odorant for soap and perfumery.	Met. Hb anaemia
Dinitrobenzene	Manuf. of dyes and explosives (*Cheddite* and *Roburite*).	Met. Hb anaemia
Nitroglycerine	Vasodilator. Explosive.	Hypotension
DNP and DNOC	Insecticide and weed-killer. Explosive.	Raised BMR. Toxic jaundice
Trinitrotoluene (TNT)	Explosive (*Amatol—č.* ammonium nitrate; and *Ammonal—č.* ammonium nitrate and aluminium).	Jaundice, anaemia, dermatitis
Aniline and nitroanilines	Manuf. of dyes, explosive, perfumes, pharmacy, photography, paints, dyes, varnishes.	Met. Hb anaemia

This tabulated outline of the predominant poisonous effects shows the outstanding feature to be conversion of circulating haemoglobin into methaemoglobin. The significance of this is now recognised to be considerably less than was first thought. Although the blood may become browner and the skin assume the classic lilac hue, the oxygen-carrying capacity of arterial blood is still likely to suffice for life, even mild exercise. *meta*-Nitrotoluene may be excreted in the urine, darkening it.

Nitrobenzene, oil of mirbane, is probably the most dangerous of all the aromatic group to handle, for it is readily absorbed through the skin from soiled or splashed clothing.

Hamilton recorded the case of a man who spilt a little oil of mirbane on his trousers whilst carrying a 5-gallon can of the fluid. He became shaky and, in collapsing, spilt a lot more over his clothes; they were not removed till he arrived in hospital, where he was found to be unconscious, with slow irregular breathing, small fixed pupils and pale grey-blue skin. Some blood withdrawn from a vein was 'as brown as chocolate'. He died 1 hour after admission.

The nervous system suffers gravely—fatigue, headache and vertigo, with muscular weakness and numbness, being common symptoms. Loss of consciousness may follow with slowed respirations but remarkably good pulse till near the end. Methaemoglobin is formed, giving the blood a brown tint and the cyanosis a 'lilac' tint. Jaundice and anaemia may also develop after a few days, and the latter is the prominent feature of subacute and chronic forms. The remedy lies in ventilation, the use of closed apparatus and change of occupation.

Nitroglycerine   an oily explosive fluid, used in a 1% solution in medicine as a vasodilator, is absorbed, even through the skin, with great rapidity and may cause fatal hypotension. Men in the armed services have swallowed the impregnated gun-cotton in order to obtain a medical certificate that will ensure a few days' leave.

Dinitrophenol (DNP) and dinitro-orthocresol (DNOC)   were long ago discarded as weight-reducing drugs owning to their toxic effects, but a new danger became evident with the reintroduction of DNP as a timber preservative and DNOC as an agricultural insecticide and selective week-killer. Exposure to the large-scale spraying of fields causes loss of weight and—expecially during hot weather—crises of thirst, sweating, hyperpyrexia, tachcardia and sometimes jaundice which may pass rapidly to coma and death.

A man of 27 who had been working with DNOC for 5 weeks, complained of 2 days' headache and tiredness, then developed a high temperature and thirst. The blood DNOC was 55µg/ml; BMR 275. He had neglected to wear a mask when filling tanks or spraying. He recovered.

The fine spray is rapidly absorbed through the skin and also by inhalation, and great care has to be exercised in both the manufacture and the spraying processes: the men engaged in handling it are all too often unaware of its highly toxic nature.

Trinitrotoluene   is a pale yellow crystalline substance handled as an explosive in blocks which exude oily impurities. It is this feature which hastens its absorption through the skin, and as vast quantities of it are handled during times of war the incidence of poisoning rises sharply over these periods. TNT was responsible for nearly 80 per cent of all forms of poisoning by volatile aromatic substances returned to the Factories Department of the Home Office in 1943—a war year.

The outstanding features are dermatitis, gastritis, cyanosis and anaemia—and toxic jaundice. The hands and sometimes also the face are stained orange with TNT, and the combination of lilac cyanosis with this forms one of the striking facies in industrial medicine.

Toxic jaundice, although much publicised by pathologists and experimental workers, is in practice a rare complication. Hunter remarked that 'if cyanosis occurs in 1 in 10 of the workers, jaundice attacks 1 in 500'. It may be many weeks after exposure to TNT has ceased that the systemic complications, in particular anaemia and toxic jaundice, make their appearance. No antidote is known.

Aniline   is a colourless oily liquid, with a distinctive aromatic odour, in widespread commercial use—dyes, perfumes, pharmaceutical products, photography, explosives, calico-printing, varnishing and rubber processing all demanding its use. It is a lipoid solvent and absorbed mainly through the skin, often from soiled clothing. An American infant was poisoned by a napkin stamped with an aniline hydrochloride dye.

The onset of symptoms—flushing, throbbing and violent headache, weakness, dizziness and tinnitus, cyanosis of classic lilac tint—is rapid and, unlike that from nitro-aromatics, rapidly evanescent, 24 hours usually sufficing whereas several weeks may be necessary for nitrobenzene changes to become resolved.

The methaemoglobinaemia is accompanied by severe anaemia with punctate basophilia, and these latter features may be the only pronounced changes in more chronic forms.

Other aromatic amines besides aniline have a direct association with papillomata of the bladder, but 'aniline cancer', as it was called, was among the first observed chemically induced tumours. The impurity naphthylamine is the cause.

Phenylenediamine, which is in use for hair dyeing and in the fur dyeing trade, carries much the same menace as aniline. Toxic changes are commonest in the skin. Anaemia and lesions in the liver or kidneys are uncommon.

Chlorinated hydrocarbons

The growth in the use of plastics and the necessity for devising some means of using the chlorine byproduct of the alkali industry has increased the sue of the halogenated hydrocarbons. They are non-inflammable, non-combustible and non-explosive, but cause no little harm to the body on absorption. Chlorinated hydrocarbons have also increased their use for refrigeration (methyl chloride), dry-cleaning (trichlorethylene and carbon tetrachloride), fire extinguishers (carbon tetrachloride and tetrachlorethane), cellulose solvents (tetrachlorethane), rubber, wax varnish, grease ssllents and wax insulation (chlorinated naphthalene). Many have also come into use as insecticides in spray or powder form. The principal sources of exposure are shown in Table 26.2.

All are in common industrial use, and unless workers are properly protected from both inhalation and skin contact—even corneal exposure—they may suffer serious damage to the liver and kidneys. Dichlorethane is by far the most dangerous, and trichlorethylene (Trilene) the least toxic of these compounds.

The skin suffers by reason of the strongly fat-solvent character of the group as a whole, but this, although the most common, constitutes the least serious of the ill-effects.

Workers with a past history of jaundice, and pregnant women, should not be given sedatives such as chloral hydrate or anaesthetics such as halothane nor exposed by occupation to the chlorinated hydrocarbons in view of their tendency to damage the liver. Liver necrosis with jaundice is the outstanding single sign of poisoning by members of this group, with the sole exception of trichlorethylene.

Table 26.2

Methyl chloride Methyl bromide	Refrigerant. Fire extinguisher. Insecticide. }	Cerebellar-type and ocular brain lesions
Carbon tetrachloride (tetrachlor- methane)	Rubber, chemical, grease and wax solvent, 'dry' cleaning, *Pyrene* fire extinguisher, *Thawpit* cleaner. Insecticide (fumigant). }	Liver and kidney necrosis
Ethylene dichloride (dichlorethane)	Oil, fat, wax, resin, gum, rubber solvent. Insecticide. Household cleaning fluid.	Serious liver and kidney damage Narcotic
Acetylene tetrachloride (tetrachlor- ethane)	Plastics, wax and resin, camera film, safety glass, artificial silk. Dry cleaner.	Liver and kidney damage Strongly narcotic
Trichlorethylene (Trilene)	Rubber, grease, oil, fat solvent. Enamel, paint, dye solvent. Dry cleaner. Insecticide.	*Less liver damage.* Acute narcotic. Anaesthetic
Chlorinated naphthalene	Insulating wax for wiring, plating.	Acne. Liver necrosis
DDT BHC	Insecticides.	CNS stimulant, convulsant. Liver damage

The ordinary doctor need not know more about these substances, and only a few lines will be added to help fix an association and add a little colour to the dry formal background of the table set out above.

Methyl(ene) chloride

This is a gas whose use in industry leapt into prominence with improvement in refrigeration. Twenty-nine cases, with ten deaths, occurred in Chicago in 1929 due to a refrigerator factory leakage, and 96 milder cases were described in 1927 and 1930 among the employees of refrigerator firms. Even travelling refrigerator salesmen fell prey to its ill-effects. It rapidly became clear that the slightest exposure might, if repeated or continued over a period of time, causing dizziness, vertigo, staggering gait, weakness and vomiting—a cerebellar syndrome—with delayed diplopia and misty vision.

Research by industrial chemists has found a better refrigerant for domestic use in dichlordifluoromethane, which appears to be far less harmful.

Methyl bromide

Similar to methyl chloride in its toxic effects and equally highly poisonous, methyl bromide is in use as a fire extinguisher and also as a potent insecticide. It penetrates clothing, even leather, and rubber with great rapidity, blistering the skin and mucous membranes. Ataxia, muscular inco-ordination, twitching and other nervous symptoms follow upon absorption.

Carbon tetrachloride

In common domestic use as both a stain-remover (Thawpit) and fire extinguisher (Pyrene), carbon tetrachloride is also widely used as a commercial solvent. Although a liver-necrosing agent, it is less harmful than tetrachlorethane in this respect. The more common clinical features are headaches, nausea and vomiting, with grave impairment of renal function.

In 1931 six members of a Swiss family were taken ill with nausea, headache and malaise after 3 days' floor waxing with a hot wax thinned out by carbon tetrachloride. The father, who had been most exposed, became confused and developed oliguria, but all recovered.

Cases have also followed from the use of fire extinguishers in confined spaces in British warships, and of leaky dry-cleaning machinery, but the trivial risks of careful use in no sense outweigh the value of the liquid for fire-fighting, cleaning and as a solvent. Far more lives have been saved from fire than were ever endangered by carbon tetrachloride. Phosgene is formed by the decomposition by fire of carbon tetrachloride.

Tetrachlorethane

Tetrachlorethane first came into prominence as a liver poison in 1914, when aeroplane fabric was treated with a cellophane 'dope' thinned out by tetrachlorethane to make it waterproof; the process was dangerous and was abandoned. The fluid still provides the best 'plasticiser' for films, plastic glass and pearls, and artificial silk.

It is about nine times as toxic as carbon tetrachloride, its effect being predominantly narcotic, although prolonged exposure is more likely to present itself as a toxic jaundice. Between 1914 and 1917 when aeroplane 'doping' ended, 70 cases of toxic jaundice were reported in England, with 12 deaths. Germany had forbidden its use within a few months of early 1914, when the first cases were reported, and no serious trouble ensued during the war.

Cases present themselves with predominant gastrohepatic symptomatology, often with early jaundice, or with an outstanding nervous lesion—usually polyneuritis, the hands and feet being more commonly affected. Artificial-pearl workers are particularly liable to the latter.

Chlorinated naphthalenes

Used as waxes in the electrical insulation industry chlorinated naphthalenes usually cause no more than acne-like skin eruptions, but liver lesions very occasionally complicate the issue.

DDT (dichlorodiphenyltrichlorethane, dicophane)

This insecticide, though falling into disuse, may be purchased without restriction either as a dusting powder or dissolved in a variety of solvents, more commonly kerosene, acetone or cyclohexanol.

The lethal dose for man is estimated to lie between 15 and 20 g, and several fatal cases have been reported from exposure of the skin to dissolved forms or as a result of swallowing the fluid poison. The solvents are sufficiently harmless to have played relatively little part in the causation of the symptoms which have followed and there can be no doubt that DDT may readily be fatal. Liver damage may occur.

Inco-ordination, tremor, spastic paresis of the legs and convulsions, preceding respiratory failure, appear to be the outstanding symptoms. Gastric lavage is worth doing for an hour or so after swallowing the poison, and sedation may be necessary. There are no specific antidotes.

Benzene hexachloride (BHC) and lindane (gamma-BHC)

Benzene hexachloride is similar in action to DDT. Both are soluble in paraffin and other oils, and tend to accumulate in the body fats. About 20 g may be fatal.

Aldrin, chlordane, dieldrin, endrin and toxaphene, somewhat more complex hydrocarbon insecticides, differ little in their toxicity from DDT or BHC. The treatment is as for DDT.

'Glue-sniffing' and other toxic inhalants

In recent years, a new form of self-abuse and addiction has appeared, mostly amongst schoolchildren and teenagers. This is the deliberate inhalation of commonly available substances such as glues, cleaners, lighter fuels, type erasers, etc., having an organic solvent; these produce symptoms similar to alcohol intoxication very rapidly and cheaply, but may proceed to hallucinations, stupor, coma or death.

Some household and craftwork adhesives such as Evo-Stik have a toluene solvent which, if inhaled from a plastic bag, increases the danger of asphyxia. Other solvents include amyl acetate, ketones, ethers, trichlorethylene (Trilene), paint thinners and solvents. Although fatalities are relatively uncommon, they do occur, usually from cardiac arrest due to direct toxicity on the heart muscle. Long-continued abuse may also lead to cardiomyopathy and liver damage.

Another variety of 'sniffing' consists of inhaling butane or propane squirted directly into the pharynx from small cylinders of compressed gas such as those used for lighter fuel. Death can ensue with dramatic suddenness, possibly from a vagal inhibitory action from chilling of the largyneal mucosa by the expanding gas. Nothing may be found at autopsy.

27

Poisoning by plants, flora and fungi

Attention has already been drawn (p. 305) to the dangers of the black berries of deadly nightshade (*Atropa belladonna*) and henbane (*Hyoscyamus niger*), and to the lethal monkshood (*Aconitum napellus*), all parts of which are highly poisonous (p. 309), to yew and laburnum (p.310), to yellow jasmine (gelsemium), and to the classic spotted hemlock, the source of coniine (p. 311).

Children are almost invariably victims, suffering the pangs of curiosity whilst sampling the 200 or more British plants which may cause them harm. Reference to a few of the more common may be made more useful if they are grouped by their common sites of natural growth.

Waterside

Three children died in 1947 from eating the roots of water dropwort (*Oenanthe crocta*) in mistake for sweet flag which North Country anglers sometimes eat. The plant is one of the umbelliferae—like horsebane (*Oenanthe phillandrium*), spotted hemlock (*Conium maculatum*) and fool's parsley (*Aethusa cynapium*).

Another waterside umbellifer, the white flowering cowbane (*Cicuta virosa*), has a blistering yellow sap which makes the roots as poisonous as those of water dropwort. Dropworts and cowbanes flower in July and have roots looking rather like small parsnips.

Celandine, marsh marigold (*Caltha palustris*) and the large water buttercups or spearworts (*Ranunculus lingua* or *R. flammula*) have an irritant stem sap like the dropwort.

The fungi *Amanita phalloides* (deathcap toadstool) and *A. muscaria* (fly agaric) have been referred to elsewhere as sources of fatal poisoning. An excellent illustrated guide to the poisonous fungi has been published in the King Penguin series (Penguin Books).

Country

In the woods the anemone is poisonous when fresh, and the bulb and roots of the daffodil, wild hyacinth and bluebell are all poisonous; those of the autumn Crocus are rather less so.

The foxglove is dangerous in all parts, although of course not very seriously so: it is the source of medicinal digitalis (*Digitalis purpurea*). Occasionally the cuckoo-pint (wild arum) causes intestinal upsets. The berries of yew and of deadly nightshade (*Atropa belladonna*) are highly poisonous, as are those of the laburnum, cherry-laurel (*Prunus laurocerasus*), spurge-laurel (Daphne laureola), and lily of the valley (*Convallaria majalis*). The woody nightshade (*Solanum dulcamara*) berry is not significantly poisonous. Holy berries, Honey suckle, guelder rose, dwalf elder, bryony (black or white) and rowan, mezereum and bird cherry are all occasionally sources of inconvenience rather than of serious poisoning. Snowberry (planted for pheasant coverts), privets, purple berries, and the red fruits of berberis are all moderately poisonous.

Town

Among the flowers and shrubs grown in urban gardens, the monkshood (*Aconitum napellus*), sometimes called wolfsbane, is undoubtedly the most poisonous of all English plants (p. 309). Though a wild flower, it is often cultivated in gardens, and the root is sometimes mistaken for horseradish.

Laburnum, juniper and daphne (*D. mezereum*) seed are mildly poisonous, and the kernels of almonds produce hydrocyanic acid in small quantity.

American poison ivy (*Rhus toxicodendron*) causes severe dermatitis among people who are sensitive, but the condition has no more than a nuisance value, never menacing life like the allergic blistering and oedema of some acute reactions; the poison of the ivy, an oil, remains active in the dead leaf. The primula (*P. obconica*) causes much the same reaction. Waste land and rubbish heaps grow two further poisonous plants, the large white flowering thorn apple solanum (*Datura stramonium*) and hemp, often found in air raid wastes during the 1939–45 war. Either constitutes a potential danger to life, especially among children.

The *treatment* of poisoning by these plants and by fungi is largely a matter of common sense. Evacuation of the stomach, the administration of stimulants and the maintenance, if necessary by controlled respiration, of adequate oxygenation form the basic principles. The use of one of the more modern antihistamine preparations may afford rapid relief, but it is as well not to indulge in any specific remedy on the off-chance of success when the shot is a blind one. The general principles cannot miscarry and should be pressed unremittingly while further inquiries are being made about the exact nature of anything suspected to have been eaten.

Index